Power and Knowledge

THE BODY, IN THEORY **Histories of Cultural Materialism**

The Subject as Action: Transformation and Totality in Narrative Aesthetics by Alan Singer

Under the Sign: John Bargrave as Collector, Traveler, and Witness by Stephen Bann

Simulacra and Simulation by Jean Baudrillard, translated by Sheila Faria Glaser

The Deluge, the Plague: Paolo Uccello by Jean Louis Schefer, translated by Tom Conley

Philodemus in Italy: The Books from Herculaneum by Marcello Gigante, translated by Dirk Obbink

The Tremulous Private Body: Essays on Subjection by Francis Barker

Picturing Silence: Emblem, Language, Counter-Reformation Materiality by Karen Pinkus

The Gay Critic by Hubert Fichte, translated by Kevin Gavin

The Abyss of Freedom / Ages of the World by Slavoj Žižek / F. W. J. von Schelling, translated by Judith Norman

The Body and Physical Difference: Discourses of Disability edited by David T. Mitchell and Sharon L. Snyder

Constructions of the Classical Body edited by James I. Porter

An Utterly Dark Spot: Gaze and Body in Early Modern Philosophy by Miran Božovič

The Pedagogical Contract: The Economies of Teaching and Learning in the Ancient World by Yun Lee Too

Cutting the Body: Representing Woman in Baudelaire's Poetry, Truffaut's Cinema, and Freud's Psychoanalysis by Eliane DalMolin

Staging Masculinity: The Rhetoric of Performance in the Roman World by Erik Gunderson

The Culture of the Body: Genealogies of Modernity by Dalia Judovitz

Power and Knowledge

Astrology, Physiognomics, and Medicine under the Roman Empire

Tamsyn S. Barton

Ann Arbor

The University of Michigan Press

First paperback edition 2002

Published in the United States of America by
The University of Michigan Press
Manufactured in the United States of America
∞ Printed on acid-free paper

2005 2004 2003 2002 5 4 3 2

A CIP catalogue record for this book is available from the British Library.

Library of Congress Cataloging-in-Publication Data

Barton, Tamsyn, 1962–
Power and knowledge : astrology, physiognomics, and medicine under the Roman Empire / Tamsyn S. Barton.
p. cm. — (The body, in theory)
Includes bibliographical references and index.
ISBN 0-472-10425-X (alk. paper)
1. Science—Rome—History. 2. Occultism and science—Rome—History. 3. Astrology—Rome—History. 4. Physiognomy—Rome—History. 5. Medicine—Rome—History. I. Title. II. Series.
Q127.R7B37 1994
509.37—dc20 94-14241
CIP

ISBN 0-472-08852-1 (pbk : alk. paper)

This book is dedicated to my teachers.

Contents

Acknowledgments

First of all, my thanks go to Geoffrey Lloyd; the thesis from which this book came was very much the result of a dialogue between us (whatever he thinks!). He has been patient and good-humored beyond the bounds of (unremunerated) duty for the last three years. Next, I owe thanks to all the people who have read and commented on parts of earlier drafts. Before Geoffrey there were three participants in the game of "Musical Supervisors" in my first year who gave shape to my thesis: Keith Hopkins, who made me persevere with tedious astrological treatises against my will; Mary Beard, who encouraged a vague interest in physiognomics; and Richard Gordon, who put me off doing magic, as he was writing a book about it, which was obviously going to be much better than anything I wrote.

Since then I have had constructive criticism from other readers: Jaś Elsner, Onno van Nijf, Sitta von Reden, Jim Porter, Peter Singer, Nick Thomas, the anonymous readers of my fellowship dissertations and of the book itself. Valérie Huet has given me invaluable initiation into the mysteries of Roman art, while Pete Callaghan referred me to crucial artistic examples. John Crook was kind enough to spend some time discussing the possibilities of analyzing the rhetoric of Roman jurisprudence with me. I am also particularly grateful to Paul Cartledge, who read the whole draft a couple of months before I submitted it, when he had much better things to do. My examiners, Richard Gordon and John North, saved me from many errors in print. No one could have done a more thorough job than Richard, in particular. The audiences at various seminars, workshops, and conferences at which I have presented my work have contributed to its development more than they would ever imagine. (In this context I should mention Simon Goldhill's skepticism, which changed the shape of my introduction.) Particular collective thanks go to the people involved in the Cambridge "C" caucus *après*-seminar pub gatherings and to the participants in "X" seminars. Had I listened to them all more, doubtless this work would have been improved.

Thanks, too, to all the people who helped me with computers, especially in the last stages (where I have to mention Tina Lendari); without them no thesis or book would have reached the light of day.

For financial support I have to thank first Newnham College, Cambridge, which gave me a research fellowship while I was still in the third year of my graduate studies. Grants from the Henry Arthur Thomas Fund of the Faculty of Classics, University of Cambridge, and the Welsford Fund in Newnham assisted with travel for research and conferences.

Other sorts of support are at least as important, if the Ph.D. student and aspiring author is to keep going to the bitter end: my thanks for everything else to friends in Newnham, to my family, to the Ware family, to Francis Sullivan, and to Peter Singer, who probably suffered from the production of this book more than I did.

Editions and Abbreviations

Where there may be confusion over which edition is referred to in references I have given the edition used. Unless stated, all texts in Kühn (K), *Scripta Minora* (*SM*), or *Corpus Medicorum Graecorum* (*CMG*) are by Galen.

Affect. = Περὶ τῶν ἰδίων ἑκάστου ψυχῆς παθῶν. In *SM* 1.

Anat. Admin. = Περὶ ἀνατομικῶν ἐγχειρήσεων (K.2.215–731).

Anthologia Latina. Ed. D. R. Shackleton-Bailey. Leipzig, 1982.

Alexander of Tralles, De Oculis = Περὶ ὀφθαλμῶν (frr. from Philumenus and Philagrius. Ed. Puschmann. *Berliner Studien für Classische Philologie und Archäologie.* 5, 2. Berlin, 1886.

Anecdota Graeca = *Anecdota Graeca et Graecolatina, Mitteilungen aus Handschriften zur Geschichte der griechischen Wissenschaft.* Ed. H. Rose. Amsterdam, 1963. Berlin, 1864.

Anecdota Oxonensium = *Anecdota Graeca e Codd. Manuscriptis Bibliothecarum Oxonensium.* Ed. J. A. Cramer. 1963 (1836).

Anon. = Anonyme Latin: *Traité de physiognomie.* Ed. J. André. Paris, 1982.

Aphth. = *Aphthonii Progymnasmata.* Ed. H. Rabe. Leipzig, 1926.

Ars. Med. = Τέχνη ἰατρική (Spurious? K.1.305–412).

Caus. Procat. = Περὶ τῶν προκαταρκτικῶν αἰτίων. *Galeni de causis procatarcticis libellus a Nicolao Regino in sermonem Latinum translatus.* Ed. K. Bardong (Latin and Greek translation). *CMG* Supp. 2. Berlin, 1937.

Caus. Puls. = Περὶ τῶν ἐν τοῖς σφυγμοῖς αἰτίων (K.9.1–204).

CCAG = *Corpus Catalogorum Astrologorum Graecorum.* Ed. F. Cumont et al. Brussels, 1898–.

Comp. Gen. = Περὶ συνθέσεως φαρμάκων τῶν κατὰ γένη (K.13.362–1058).

Const. Art. = Περὶ συστάσεως τέχνης ἰατρικῆς, πρὸς Πατρόφιλον (K.1.224–304).

CMG = *Corpus Medicorum Graecorum.* Berlin, 1908–.

CMGSO = *Corpus Medicorum Graecorum, Supplementum Orientale.* Berlin, 1914–.

Cris. = Περὶ κρίσεων. German translation and Text. *Studia Graeca et Latina Gothoburgensia.* Ed. B. Alexanderson. Gothenburg, 1967 (K.9.550–768).

Decent. = (Hippocratic) Περὶ εὐσχημοσύνης. *De Decenti Habitu.* Ed. Heiberg. *CMG* 1.1.

Def. Med. = Ὅροι ἰατρικοί (Spurious, K.19.346–462).
Dem. = Περὶ ἀποδείξεως (Müller 1895).
Dieb. Decret. = Περὶ κρισίμων ἡμερῶν (K.9.769–941).
Diff. Puls. = Περὶ διαφορᾶς σφυγμῶν (K.8.493–765).
Diff. Morb. = Περὶ διαφορᾶς νοσημάτων (K.6.836–80).
Diff. Febr. = Περὶ διαφορᾶς πυρετῶν (K.7.273–405).
Diff. Resp. = Περὶ δυσπνοίας (K.7.753–960).
Dign. Puls. = Περὶ διαγνώσεως σφυγμῶν (K.8.766–961).
Diogenes Laertius = *Diogenis Laertii Vitae Philosophorum.* 2 vols. Ed. H. S. Long. Oxford, 1964.
Diss. = Arrian: Ἐπικτήτου Διατριβαί (Discourses of Epictetus).
Doroth. = *Dorothei Sidonii Carmen Astrologicum, interpretationem Arabicam in linguam Anglicam versam una cum Dorothei fragmentis et Graecis et Latinis.* Ed. D. Pingree. Leipzig, 1976.
Elem. Sec. Hipp. = Περὶ τῶν καθ' Ἱπποκράτην στοιχείων. Ed. G. Helmreich. Erlangen, 1878 (K.1.413–508).
F = *Scriptores Physiognomici.* 2 vols. Ed. R. Foerster. Leipzig, 1893.
FIRA. = *Fontes Iuris Romani Antejustiniani.* Ed. S. Riccobono, J. Baviera, C. Ferrini, J. Furlani, and V. Arangio-Ruiz.
Firmicus = *Firmici Materni Matheseos Libri VIII.* Ed. W. Kroll, F. Skutsch, and K. Ziegler. Leipzig, 1913 (All trans. from Rhys Bram 1975).
Germ. = Germanicus(?), *Aratea.* Ed. A. Le Boeffle. Paris, 1975.
Glauc. = Πρὸς Γλαύκωνα θεραπευτικά (K.11.1–146).
Grenfell-Hunt = *The Oxyrrhynchus Papyri.* Ed. B. P. Grenfell and A. S. Hunt. Vols. 1–17. 1898–1927.
Hephaestion of Thebes = *Hephaestio Thebanus: Apotelesmaticorum Libri III.* Ed. D. Pingree. Leipzig, 1973.
Hermog. = *Hermogenis Opera.* Ed. H. Rabe, Leipzig, 1913.
HN = Pliny, *Historia Naturalis* (Natural History).
Ideler, *Phys. med. gr.* = *Physici et medici graeci minores.* Ed. H. T. Ideler. Leipzig, 1841, 3 vols.
IGR = *Inscriptiones Graecae ad res Romanas pertinentes.* Ed. R. Cagnat, Paris, 1911–27.
In Hipp. Epid. = Εἰς τὰ βιβλία τῶν Ἐπιδημιῶν Ἱπποκράτους ὑπομνήματα, in *CMG* 5.10.2.2. Ed. E. Wenckebach and F. Pfaff. Berlin, 1934–56. (K.17A.300–17B.344).
(In Hipp.) Progn. = Εἰς τὸ προγνωστικὸν Ἱπποκράτους ὑπομνήματα. Ed. J. Heeg. *CMG* 5.9.2. Berlin, 1915: 196–378 (K.18B.1–317).
Inst. Log. = Εἰσαγωγὴ διαλεκτική. *Galeni Institutio Logica.* Ed. K. Kalbfleisch. Leipzig, 1896.
K. = C. G. Kühn: *Claudii Galeni Opera Omnia.* 22 vols. Hildesheim, 1965 (Leipzig, 1821–33).
Lib. Prop. = Περὶ τῶν ἰδίων βιβλίων. In *SM* 2 (K.14.8–48).
Loc. Aff. = Περὶ τῶν πεπονθότων τοπῶν (K.8.1–452).

Manilius = Manilius: *Astronomica*. Ed. G. P. Goold. Leipzig, 1985 (All translations by Goold, Loeb Classical Library, Cambridge, Mass., 1977).

Marcellinus: *De Pulsibus* = Περὶ σφυγμῶν: *De Pulsibus*. Ed. Schoene, Festschrift zur 49. Versammlung deutscher Philologen und Schulmänner. Basel, 1907, 448–71.

Med. Cogn. = *Galen on Examinations by Which the Best Physicians Are Recognized. CMGSO* 4. Ed. A. Z. Iskandar (Arabic and English trans.). Leipzig, 1988.

Menander Rhetor = "*Menander Rhetor.*" Ed. D. A. Russell and N. G. Wilson. Cambridge, 1981.

Meth. Med. = Περὶ μεθόδου ἰατρικῆς (K.10).

Nat. Fac. = Περὶ δυνάμεων φυσικῶν (K.2.1–214).

Nom. Med. = (Περὶ τῶν ἰατρικῶν ὀνομάτων) *Galen über die medizinischen Namen*. Ed. M. Meyerhof and J. Schacht (Arabic with German trans.). *Abh. d. Preuss. Akad. d. Wiss., phil.-hist. Klasse*. Berlin, 1931.

Opt. Med. = Ὅτι ὁ ἄριστος ἰατρὸς καὶ φιλόσοφος, in *SM* 2 (K.1.53–63).

Ord. Lib. = Περὶ τῆς τάξεως τῶν ἰδίων βιβλίων, πρὸς Εὐγενιανόν. In *SM* 2 (K.19.49–61).

Origen, *Philocalia* = Φιλοκαλία *Origène: Philocalie 21–27, Sur le libre arbitre, introduction, texte, traduction et notes*. Ed. E. Junod. Sources Chrétiennes. Paris, 1976.

Part. Med. = *De Partibus Medicinae*. Arabic and Latin versions in *CMGSO* 2.

Paul. Al. = Εἰσαγωγικά. *Pauli Alexandrini Elementa Apotelesmatica*. Ed. E. Boer. Leipzig, 1958.

Pecc. = Περὶ τῶν ἰδίων ἑκάστου ψυχῆς ἁμαρτημάτων, in *SM* 1 (K.5.58–103).

Phgn. = Φυσιογνωμομικά. In Aristotle, vol. 14, *Minor Works*. Loeb Classical Library, Cambridge, Mass.

PHP = Περὶ τῶν Ἱπποκράτους καὶ Πλάτωνος δογμάτων, in *CMG* 5.4.1.2. *De Placitis Hippocratis et Platonis*. Ed. P. de Lacy. 3 vols. Berlin, 1980 (K.5.181–805).

Pistis Sophia. Coptic with English translation. Ed. C. Schmidt. Leiden, 1978 (page refs. to the trans.).

Plenit. = Περὶ πλήθους (K.7.513–85).

Praecog. = Περὶ τοῦ προγινώσκειν, πρὸς Ἐπιγένην. *Galen on Prognosis*. Ed. V. Nutton. *CMG* 5.8.1. Berlin, 1979 (K.14.599–673).

Praesag. Puls. = Περὶ προγνώσεως σφυγμῶν (K.9.205–430).

Progn. See *In Hipp. Progn.*

Protr. = Προτρεπτικὸς λόγος ἐπὶ τὰς τέχνας, in *SM* 1 (K.1.1–39) Also ed. Kaibel. Berlin, 1894.

Puls. Ant. = Περὶ σφυγμῶν πρὸς Ἀντώνιον φιλομάθη καὶ φιλόσοφον (Spurious: K.19.629–42).

Puls. Tir. = Περὶ τῶν σφυγμῶν τοῖς εἰσαγομένοις (K.8.453–92).

Purg. Fac. = Περὶ τῆς τῶν καθαιρόντων φαρμάκων δυνάμεως (K.11.323–42).

QAM = Ὅτι ταῖς τοῦ σώματος κράσεσι αἱ τῆς ψυχῆς δυνάμεις ἕπονται. In *SM* 2 (K.4.767–822).

San. Tu. = Ὑγιεινά, in *CMG* 5.4.2. Ed. K. Koch. *De Sanitate Tuenda libri VI.* Leipzig, 1923 (K.6.1–452).

Scribonius Largus, *Compositiones.* Ed. G. Helmreich. Leipzig, 1887 (and see Deichgräber 1950 for edition of foreword).

Simp. Med. = Περὶ κράσεως καὶ δυνάμεως τῶν ἁπλῶν φαρμάκων (K.11.379–12.377).

SM = *Claudii Galeni Scripta Minora.* 3 vols. Ed. J. Marquardt, I. Müller, and G. Helmreich. Leipzig, 1884–93.

Somn. Dig. = Περὶ τῆς ἐξ ἐνυπνίων διαγνώσεως (K.6.832–35).

Spengel = *Rhetores Graeci.* 3 vols. Ed. L. Spengel. Leipzig, 1853–56.

Suetonius, Περὶ βλασφημιῶν. Ed. J. Taillardat. Paris, 1967.

Sympt. Diff. = Περὶ τῶν συμπτωμάτων διαφορᾶς (K.7.42–84).

Syn. Puls. = Σύνοψις περὶ σφυγμῶν ἰδίας πραγματείας (K.9.431–549).

Temp. = Περὶ κράσεων. *De Temperamentis libri III.* Ed. G. Helmreich. Leipzig, 1904 (K.1.509–694).

Tetrabiblos = Ἀποτελεσματικά. *Claudii Ptolemaei opera* 3.1. Ed. F. Boll and E. Boer. Leipzig, 1940.

Thrasybulus = Θρασύβουλος (πότερον ἰατρικῆς ἢ γυμναστικῆς ἐστι τὸ ὑγιεινόν). In *SM* 3 (K.5.806–98).

Ulpian, *Mosaicorum et Romanorum legum collatio.* In *FIRA,* 2:541–81.

UP = Περὶ χρείας μορίων. Ed. G. Helmreich. *De Usu Partium libri XVII.* Leipzig, 1907–9 (K.3.1–4.366).

Us. Puls. = Περὶ χρείας σφυγμῶν. In *Galen on Respiration and the Arteries.* Ed. D. J. Furley and J. S. Wilkie. Princeton, 1984, 185–228 (K.5.149–180).

VS = Philostratus: *Vitae Sophistarum* (Lives of the Sophists), Loeb Classical Library.

Ven. Eras. = Περὶ φλεβοτομίας πρὸς Ἐρασίστρατον (K.11.147–378).

Ven. Eras. Rom. = Περὶ φλεβοτομίας πρὸς Ἐρασιστρατείους τοὺς ἐν Ῥώμῃ (K.11.187–249).

Ven. Sec. = Περὶ φλεβοτομίας θεραπευτικόν (K.11.250–316).

Vict. Acut. = Ἱπποκράτους περὶ διαίτης ὀξέων νοσημάτων βιβλία καὶ Γαλήνου ὑπομνήματα. Ed. G. Helmreich. *CMG* 5.9.1. Berlin, 1914 (K.15.418–919).

Introduction

My book is entitled *Power and Knowledge.* It may be viewed as a collection of case studies in three Greco-Roman disciplines: astrology, physiognomics, and medicine. It focuses on treatises on these arts, which could loosely be described as products of the "Second Sophistic," although examples are included from the first to the fourth centuries A.D. In the introduction I have first of all to justify putting medicine on a level with the other two for the purposes of historical investigation, abandoning the usual distinction between science and pseudoscience. I also have to justify my use of the terms *power* and *knowledge* in relation to the three subjects of inquiry. In my chapter on astrology this general argument is supplemented by particular consideration of the sense in which astrology is constituted as knowledge, in the context of its history.

As well as following the traditional approach of Classical scholarship in general, and recent work on ancient science in particular, I draw on a number of ideas from different modern disciplines. Lévi-Strauss claimed three "mistresses" in Marx, Freud, and geology; perhaps the three following clusters of ideas are my paramours. At any rate they are not entirely unexpected bedfellows. First, I draw on the work of philosophers, historians, and social scientists who have worked in the sociology of knowledge, in particular those who have tended to relativize knowledge in relation to its social context. I show how this has shaped my research program, which I set against the background of the historiography of ancient science. Second, I draw on the literary-philosophical studies that come under the rubric of the New Rhetoric, which have used classical rhetorical theory to break down the model of value-free communication and thus laid the foundations for the angle I take in looking at science as rhetoric. Third, I draw on the work of Michel Foucault, taking his analyses of power as coextensive with the social to rephrase the work of the sociologists of knowledge in political terms and to reinvest the New Rhetoric with a political element. I adapt some of his notions of power to link the three parts of my book.

Finally, I arrive at the question that inevitably haunts inquiries with this theoretical background—the implications of my views of the interrelations of power and knowledge for the status of my own history. This introduction is itself, first of all, a reaction to the methodological demands exercised by my theoretical perspective. If knowledge is constructed by power, and rhetoric that aspect of communication that involves power, as I argue, what is the status of this book? A reflexive reaction to the relativism I espouse turns my analytical gaze back on myself and my own rhetoric. Hence, I present my intellectual genealogy, gesturing toward the forces exerted on the construction of this academic work. It is, after all, a matter of intellectual honesty.

Here the skeptical reader might intrude to point out that the last time you should believe a rhetorician is when she says that she is being honest. I hope that the skeptical reader will remain to overshadow what follows, not in the sense that the book will be always looking over its shoulder timidly at imagined critics but, rather, to set the certainties of academic style in their proper context, against other arguments. The following account of my research should be seen as acknowledging its character as a rhetorical exercise, which ultimately derives any solidity it has from the reaction of the audience. This "grounding" of the discourse will not be seen as exempting it from further questions about either its lack of reflexivity or its ability to persuade according to the usual criteria for judging classical scholars.

The Sociology of Knowledge

Understanding knowledge as rooted in social practice changes the way one writes the history of science.[1] It problematizes the notion of "pseudoscience," which has dogged historical investigation into phenomena like astrology and physiognomics. Science, according to this understanding, like knowledge in general, loses the transhistorical guarantee afforded it by traditional history of science; what meaning is left to counterfeit coins when the currency is no longer valid?

It goes against the grain of traditional practice to give the disciplines once designated as pseudosciences a place in the history of science or knowledge, not just because astrology relies on astronomy and mathematics and therefore had an important positive role in keeping scientific knowledge alive,[2] or even because physiognomics may have been taken seriously by Aristotle, but because their claim to be a *scientia,* or τέχνη (*technē*), was as strong (or as weak) as medicine's. That is to say, their claims to be "knowledge" in their contemporary context were as strong; they were "sciences" of the past. Indeed, one of the positive reasons for choosing the Greco-Roman world to examine these disciplines is that it is a world in which the three disciplines that I examine were competing on very much an equal footing, in which medicine had no more institutional backing than astrology and physiognomics and often actually sought to improve its persuasive arsenal by co-optation of material from the latter two disciplines, as we shall see.[3]

There are two interrelated themes here. First, I want to draw attention to the problems raised by a rationalizing history of science, a history that isolates scientific discourse from any involvement in social practice, hallowing it in some domain in which the real presents itself without credentials. Second, there is the theme of the unfathomable nature of unverbalized reality, which surfaces both in particular cases of scientific knowledge and in my more general notions of epistemology.

The theme of the relativity of knowledge runs through the book and, indeed, was the impetus for the research. Here I explain the background to that (relatively) heterodox philosophical position and how it has affected my research.

Traditional Orthodoxy: Scientific Realism

Broadly speaking, realists say that the entities, states, and processes described by science really do exist, independently of investigators,[4] and that mature scientific theories and their constituent propositions are true. Realism grounds itself in the technological success of science. Here I have no space to grapple with the subtleties of the various alternatives to realism apart from relativism, another umbrella term, which I shall explore presently. I am merely sketching out the crucial opposition from the point of view of my own historical concerns.

Philosophers tend to be concerned with specifying what should count as legitimate knowledge. Hence, a particular interest in the demarcation criteria for science resulted from the realism already outlined. Science was reliable, true knowledge, so philosophers had to find out what it was that made scientific research such a successful system for producing knowledge, as opposed to other systems. This interest in finding such criteria was based on an essentialist premise, that science existed as an object, a coherent entity or method, however difficult it might be to pin down. Demarcation criteria have never satisfactorily been formulated.[5]

A realist philosophical position sets a program for the history of science. First, knowledge tends to be seen as cumulative. Thus, whatever deviations or halts along the way there may be, the important history is of the progress toward truth. Such history will be evolutionist. Second, knowledge will be seen as individualistic and mentalistic; the context of justification will be kept separate from the context of discovery.[6] Such history will chronicle the achievements of the "great men" of science. Third, scientific knowledge will be treated as special and distinct, whatever failures in demarcation may occur. Such history will tend not to set science against a broader canvas. Finally, scientific knowledge is its own explanation: there is no need to invoke any sociological explanation, except where error is involved.[7]

Sociological Heterodoxy

Unsurprisingly, most philosophers of science have been reluctant to relinquish their role as experts on scientific knowledge in favor of sociologists, who in their ignorance are only likely to subvert cherished ideas about truth and knowledge.[8] Once, indeed, sociologists felt they had to stop their excavations at the gate of the Citadel of Science. (This was probably out of respect for science rather than philosophy.) Thus, Marx, Mannheim, and Durkheim all offered various schemes for making knowledge relative to social context, but even in worlds of class struggle and "total ideology" a clearing was allowed for science in the Hobbesian jungle; even where the sacred was demystified science remained sacralized and sociological analysis taboo.[9] Mertonian "sociology of science" contented itself with examining the way science organized and regulated itself, giving attention to relationships between scientists, while leaving the content of scientific theory in a "black box," for unexamined assumptions.[10]

The way, however, was in fact opened up for sociologists by philosophers who doubtless had no interest in what the former might make of their work.[11] While the later Wittgenstein remains enigmatic, the sociologists of knowledge could take inspiration from his insistence on the unfathomable nature of unverbalized reality, and the rootedness of accepted knowledge in social practice, and read his work as depriving scientific truth of life outside the language game.[12] Philosophers of science like David Bloor were encouraged to provide sociological accounts of mathematics.[13]

Another important contribution to the sociologists' armory was Quine's argumentation for the underdetermination of theory by evidence,[14] which problematized Popper's principle that scientific premises should be falsifiable. As the physicist-turned-philosopher John Ziman observes, arguing that Popper's criterion is strategically sound but tactically indefensible, it is rare that a definite theoretical prediction is subsequently confirmed by experiment.[15] A theory is usually validated by much less compelling evidence: if it yields results that "fit with" the experimental data. Thus, much room is left for sociological explanation.

But the "revolution" in thinking about science in society is usually traced back to a historian. Thomas Kuhn most famously turned Quine against Popper in an account that replaced a "Whiggish" evolutionary history of science as progress with a series of revolutions in thinking.[16] The incommensurability of the successive frameworks or paradigms obviously put in jeopardy the fruitfulness of any timeless criteria of what should count as good theory, what should count as explanation.[17] Kuhn further gave the impetus to ontological relativism: in his model electrons, for instance, only exist within the framework of electron theory.[18]

Kuhn thus raised the specter of relativism before science with particular urgency, and, if he was cautious about the implications of such a model, the new sociology of scientific knowledge which made an appearance in Britain in 1969, espoused the "revolution" with a vengeance.[19] Two schools have become prominent in the discipline. The Edinburgh school, based at the science studies unit at the University of Edinburgh, followed up the ideas of earlier sociologists of knowledge, Barnes and Mackenzie taking up Mannheim's line in using social interests as an explanatory resource,[20] while Bloor followed Durkheim with his use of "social imagery."[21] It was the Edinburgh school that started the philosophical debates about relativism in the sociology of knowledge.[22] Frustrated with the failure of the relativists to convince philosophers, the Bath school, based at the Science Studies Centre at the University of Bath, moved for a program of "empirical relativism," with the aim of letting the philosophical issues lie, while getting on with empirical studies, which were to stand or fall on their merits.[23]

Both schools agree, however, on the demand for "symmetry" in explanation.[24] This demand is made in accordance with the thesis that "rational norms and true beliefs in natural science are just as much explananda of the sociology of science as are non-rationality and error," as Mary Hesse puts it.[25] It was she who most elegantly supported this thesis, known as the "strong thesis," in an article that finds in its favor on "hermeneutic" and "critical" grounds. Hesse, who claims in this article to steer a course between the extremes of metaphysical realism and relativism, had done much to weaken the crude realists' grip with her work on the theory-laden nature of observation and the creative role of metaphor in science. In this article she tackled the age-old reply to relativism: the charge of "self-refutation" by pointing out that it rests on an equivocation over what concepts of knowledge and determinism are operating.[26] Thus, unable to find an argument to destroy the strong thesis, she ends by saying that, though this conclusion does not imply that there is no necessary truth, it does imply that such truth cannot provide analytic premises for explanations in the history of science. The point at which explanations must stop is in local consensus.

Thus, she accepts that cognitive terminology has to be explicitly redefined to refer to knowledge and truth-claims relative to some set or sets of cultural norms and also follows Barnes's advocation of a redescription of science in more sociological terms.[27] But after all this support of a relativist thesis she effectively shies away from any more radical consequences that her arguments might have for the writing of history, in another article, entitled "Reasons and Evaluations in the History of Science." Here she demands that we recognize the preferable nature of our own science, so that we can compare "what really happened" in, say, Priestley's experiments with phlogiston.[28] She sees no escape from the necessity of demarcating the subject matter of the history of science in accordance with the recognition of what it is in the past that exhibits causal continuity with our own science. Having attacked the rationalists' assumption that our language, rationality, and science will reveal the presuppositions of any possible language, rationality, and science, she turns round and asserts:

> A proper historical perspective neither involves uncritical accumulation of every minor writing of forgotten figures, nor is it necessarily vitiated by the imposition of our standards of rationality on an alien age. . . . So long as we take science as our subject-matter we are bound to such forward-looking history in the limited sense that we regard as important what we recognize of our rationality. (1980, 20, 21)

and she goes on to argue again that causal continuity with modern science is essential.

In my view she is not making her philosophical innovations do much historical work. How is one to reconcile stopping explanations at local consensus with using what we recognize of our rationality as the criterion of what we select to write about? Surely the kind of loosening of the boundaries of modern science for which she argues in her other article has important implications for the ways in which we may write its history. The minimum consequence of the strong thesis is that the reasons a thinker may have taken on a particular program like the Copernican universe might have been quite different from the reasons that would appeal to today's scientists and philosophers.[29] Writing this sort of forward-looking history and excluding "minor figures" might well prevent understanding of such factors. It could be argued that it is minor figures who define what is characteristic of a period. The consequences of her redefinition of knowledge as relative to cultural norms surely are that a better historical account will be given by an attempt to recover a fuller picture of what was accepted as knowledge and, indeed, the nature of the cultural norms that shaped the epistemic field. Yet it is obvious from her comments that she simply cannot see the point of a history of science that does not lead up to modern science in some way. It is my contention that a history of ancient science should include a history of astrology and physiognomics as well as medicine, if the rationales of investigations into nature in the period are to be understood. Her historical program would put these disciplines off the agenda.

I shall also be arguing that evaluation in relation to modern science distracts from this sort of historical project. But Hesse claims that the relativist drive to abstain from evaluations of past science is unsatisfactory and unhistorical: "Some elements of inductivism are bound to enter our view of past science, since what counts as such is partly determined by its historical continuity with our own" (1980, xv). While I acknowledge that discussion of past "science" is inevitably value laden, the values reflected in my discussion will reflect a different evaluative base; the continuity from past to present will lie rather in my rereading of the past on the basis of some current theory, and any inductivism will result from understanding shaped by such theory.

Barnes and Bloor give a slightly different version of the strong thesis, in a programmatic paper for the Edinburgh school. Though their interpretation poses problems that I shall be discussing, their historical program makes more sense as a consequence of their philosophical position. They abandon Hesse's dualistic terminology, which separates rational from irrational, and argue that all beliefs are on a par with one another with respect to the causes of their credibility: "It is not that all beliefs are equally true or equally false, but that regardless of truth and falsity the fact of their credibility is to be seen as equally problematic" (1982, 23).

Thus, they aim to show the contingent circumstances affecting the production and evaluation of scientific accounts, in a sociological appreciation of the processes by which statements of fact are accredited and rejected. They demand that, regardless of how the sociologist evaluates a belief, she or he must ask how it fits with local modes of cultural transmission of knowledge, local methods of socialization and social control, goals valued locally for political or technical reasons, and the general configuration of power and authority.[30] These are questions that are valuable, and, indeed, I shall be asking some of them myself.

But, before placing myself firmly in their camp, I need to deal with some of the problems raised by their thoroughgoing relativism. First, I would like to introduce some refinements to any simple view that it is merely consensus *tout court* that is at issue. There are several dialectical engagements at work in the production and evaluation of scientific accounts; more will emerge. Here I just want to mention the dialectic between existing styles of reasoning and the social context. Paul Hirst argues that rejection of "some universal and independently grounded standard of truth" in combination with an appreciation of the value of sociological contributions to explaining the rise and fall of bodies of knowledge need not entail the view that it is simply consensus that creates knowledge (1985, 100). He picks up on Ian Hacking's "muted relativist" arguments (1982) that the truth-and-falsehood (positivity) of propositions depends on the styles of reasoning appropriate to such propositions. These styles arise in historical contexts and depend for their existence on contingent events.[31] Hirst mentions the theological, legal, and "empirical-scientific" reasoning of early modern Europe as examples. Hacking himself cites the Renaissance medical, alchemical, and astrological doctrines of resemblance and similitude in specifying alternative possibilities for truth-and-falsehood as evidence for such relativism. Ancient versions of the doctrines of resemblance were operative in all three disciplines that I examine, though rarely explicitly formulated, and they specified particular possibilities of truth-and-falsehood that are foreign to modern scientific styles of reasoning. Greek philosophers, however, also elaborated certain styles of logical reasoning more acceptable to modern philosophers of science, which were sometimes brought into play by writers such as Galen, and they interacted with other elements of the social context, such as the agonistic context, and indeed with his sensory perceptions in the elaboration of his pulse theory. Certainly, it was not just a matter of simple consensus. But, to follow up my remarks on Hesse, in recognizing this limited autonomy of styles of reasoning from the context of particular social influences, we are not compelled to make value judgments concerning the styles themselves. The rationality of styles of relativism does not seem open to independent criticism since the very sense of what may be established by that style depends on the style itself, as Hacking points out.[32]

I will return to the issue of evaluation. My main disagreement with Barnes and Bloor, however, is over their desire to have it both ways in their claims for their research. Their relativistic stance sits ill with their claims to be really scientific (incorporating no evaluative attitude toward science). They actually advertise their discipline of a determinist sociology of knowledge as being *positive,* on a par with cognitive psychology (1982, 22). Bloor claims to be "more than happy to see sociology resting on the same foundations as other sciences" (1976, 144). Surely, they should take up Hesse's redefinition of knowledge in relativist terms and situate their own work in a sociopolitical context, rather than simply exploiting the traditional connotations of science in order to guarantee their project. In doing so, they only court the self-refutation charge. Here is a theme to which I shall return—designating it henceforward as "the heffalump trap." This is the trap that entices scholars who have undermined the "neutral" status of science or truth then to exploit the old connotations in their favor, thus courting the charge of self-refutation. They dig a trap, set the bait, and fall victim to it, like A. A. Milne's Pooh, because of a lack of reflexivity about their intentions: to get the honey at all costs.[33]

The Historiography of Ancient Science

In the first chapter I shall be considering debate among historians of the early modern period over the way to write the history of science, in particular the place of astrology in it. Here I want to survey the historiography of ancient science. It is a field in which little work has been done, so I am grateful to be able to draw on the recent work of P. N. Singer (unpub.) and J. T. Vallance (1990).

In the eighteenth and nineteenth centuries it was usual for scientists to include in their works a "historical introduction," in which they summarized the prehistory of the field and placed their work in that tradition. Such were the origins of the history of science in general. In the nineteenth century the historians of medicine responsible for the editions and scholarly surveys drawing together so much dispersed information on which we must still often rely were either retired or practicing doctors. For them the medical writings of the ancients still promised to furnish empirical findings that might actually be useful to the practicing doctor, even if the model of the body had changed.[34] While historians of other ancient sciences and twentieth-century historians of medicine could not claim such direct practical benefit, there were still many former scientists as well as philologists working in the field, and there remained hope that there would be some direct benefit for modern scientists.[35] It was felt that the modern scientist needed to form an appreciation of his or her predecessors. So a constructive critique, an evaluation that separated out the valuable insights of the past from the failures, themselves instructive as a negative model, was necessary.[36] The former doctor Karl Sudhoff founded his *Archiv* in 1920, in imitation of Ostwald's "Classic" series, founded twenty years earlier, in order that modern scientists should have easy access to scientific writings of the past.[37]

The historical prescriptions of scientific realism are unsurprisingly evident. Authors and editors such as Puschmann (1878, 1921), Müller (1891, 1923–), and Meyer-Steineg (1913) were keen to isolate the rational in Greek science, to celebrate its "discoveries" on the road to modern science or, at the very least, the mode of investigation that pointed in the right direction. Periods of advance and retreat on this road were set out. This was all the more daunting as a task for former scientists such as the chemist and physicist Pierre Duhem, the chemist J. R. Partington (1939), and the physicist Sambursky (1963), for whom antecedents for their sciences were less easily demarcated. It was not only the scientific backgrounds of historians that led to this modern perspective; it was also the influence of those who took in ancient science as part of historical research focused on the history of science up to the modern period, such as Duhem, Paul Tannéry, Alexandre Koyré, and Lynn Thorndike.[38]

It is also important that the chief institutional organizers and propagandists for the history of science as a whole in the first half of the twentieth century were specialists in ancient science. George Sarton, who more than any other fostered the history of science in America, and Charles Singer, who established a department of History of Methods in Science at University College, London, in 1923, were doubtless influenced by their need to gather support and respect for the discipline in their programmatic statements. Thence, presumably, the "surprisingly unhistorical focus of these utterances," which "preserve a tone surely long absent in every other field of investigation" (Kragh 1987, 18). Here are some of Sarton's recommendations, as summarized by Kragh:

a) The study of the past is of no value in itself, but is justified solely through its relevance for contemporary and future science.
b) Science is "systematized positive knowledge, or what has been taken as such at different ages and in different places." "The acquisition and systematization of positive knowledge are the only human activities which are truly cumulative and progressive." The historian ought to evaluate earlier contributions in relation to their predecessors; and when making his evaluation, he should focus on whether the development concerned constituted a step forward. The extent to which this was the case can be

judged by using modern standards of progress and rationality. On the basis of these standards, the historian will determine when the science of the past was based on true scientific principles and when it was merely pseudo-science. (Sarton himself refused to consider the physiological theories of Galen, about whom he wrote a book, because he regarded them as speculative fantasies.)

c) Socio-economic conditions have no deep influence on the life of science. The kind of history of science Sarton advocated and practised is internalistic, focussing on science as an isolated, autonomous system and on the geniuses who set it up.
d) When looked at in a historical perspective, science is an unmitigated good. It is the great benefactor of mankind, truly democratic and international. The study of the history of science will not only help prevent new wars, it will also build bridges between humanistic and technico-scientific cultures.

Charles Singer followed Sarton in Britain, emulating both his efforts to institutionalize the history of science and his prescriptive method. Launching a new scholarly series, "Studies in the History and Method of Science" (1917–21), with reference to the model of Sarton's journal *Isis,* he proclaimed that history could teach "the method by which knowledge had been gained."[39]

Meanwhile, in Britain specialist studies were appearing on particular ancient disciplines: those of T. L. Heath on mathematics (1913, 1921), T. E. Lones on *Aristotle's Researches in Natural Science* (1913), A. L. Peck on zoology (1937), W. H. S. Jones on medicine (1947), and general handbooks of ancient science were written by a classicist (Farrington 1939, 1944–49). The extent to which the ancient world was canonized in their myth of origin can be seen from the title of W. A. Heidel's *The Heroic Age of Science* (1933). The focus was on the "highlights" of Greek science and technology—Democritean atomic theory, the mechanical innovations of Hero of Alexandria, and, of course, the development of astronomy; while in medicine the focus was on the observation of the difference between veins and arteries, the suggestion of the naturalistic cause for epilepsy in the Hippocratic treatise *On the Sacred Disease,* and the Hellenistic anatomical discoveries of Erasistratus and Herophilus.

Vallance has isolated "recent dramatic shifts in focus" in the history of ancient science (1990, 716f.). First, it is now accepted that ancient science cannot be separated from its ethical and philosophical background. This is certainly the most widespread development.[40] Second, he notes, scholars of ancient science have "not remained wholly unaffected by work on science and . . . society by the likes of Popper, Kuhn, Feyerabend, Lakatos, Habermas and Foucault . . . some idea of the social and cultural context in which scientific ideas developed is now widely seen as useful to any appreciation."[41] Third, and relatedly, the revolutions in anthropology "which have exposed 'civilized' societies to the kinds of examination hitherto reserved for 'primitive' peoples, have led to comparison between the types of scientific explanation offered in ancient Greece and aetiological 'mythical' stories in Greek and other cultures." Thus, previous "enemies of scientific progress" such as Plato have been reappraised. Finally, Vallance refers to comparative research on Greece and China. If any single scholar has been instrumental in these three shifts of focus, it is surely G. E. R. Lloyd, who has used a great variety of work in social anthropology on particular issues such as zoological taxonomy, for instance. He has also taken on board philosophical problems that have arisen as a result of social anthropology, such as the relations between traditional and scientific patterns of thought and the problems of translation between cultures, and the consequent dangers of distortion in the application of our concepts to another culture. He has recently moved into comparative research on China.[42]

Lloyd has also looked to the social context of science. In *Magic, Reason and Experience* (1979) Lloyd surveyed, in the final chapter, the possible explanations of the origins of this new approach. Using comparative evidence from the Near East and elsewhere, he turned to the political and legal practice of the Greeks to explain what was exceptional in Greek thought, isolating the "possibility of radical innovation, the openness of access to the forum of debate, the habit of scrutiny, the expectation of justification, and the premium set on rational methods" as the crucial factors. He also looked at the more immediate context, remarking on the lack of anything like the modern institutional setting, and on the influence of rhetoric on natural science, thus breaking down any crude distinction between the natural scientist aiming at the truth and the deceptive rhetorician. He also pointed to the sometimes esoteric nature of natural scientific doctrines, in Pythagorean number mysticism and medical treatises only understandable to the initiate.

Finally, Lloyd has considered some of the recent developments in the history and philosophy of science already outlined, rightly pointing out that they have been ignored by commentators on ancient science (1983). Though expressing reservations about the Kuhnian model, he remarks on the salutary effects of Kuhn's work. He refers to the problems with demarcation criteria in a recent book (1987) and, in 1983 in particular, broadens the range of what may be included in the history of science. He considers physiognomics in his discussion of Aristotle's zoological taxonomy, not following those who would like to excise such "folklore" from the Aristotelian corpus. Here, with his approach, as with Pliny, these bits of folklore are interesting because they can be seen in interaction with so-called scientific modes of thought. He also mentions the fact that some astronomers were also astrologers and acknowledges that astrology gave impetus to astronomy.[43] In 1979 he notes that for the Greeks the elaboration of traditional beliefs, like divination, could constitute progress just as much as in the case of "those other disciplines we accept more readily as arts, crafts and sciences" and suggests that traditional beliefs were elaborated in imitation of the sciences.

There is much that I will develop here, but in one important respect I will be moving in a different direction from Lloyd, as a result of the difference in our philosophical stances.[44] For him it is an important question to ask, as at the end of *Science, Folklore and Ideology* (1983), whether the ancient disciplines on which he has worked are worthy of being called scientific. There are some positive responses, not only is there a new style of inquiry: "key methodological notions, including the value of empirical research, of the application of mathematics to the physical world and of an axiomatic deductive system,"[45] but also there are specific genealogies, "successful applications" of these methods, like "the discovery of the nervous system . . . exact descriptive work in anatomy, zoology and botany . . . the discovery of the diagnostic value of the pulse."[46] For my purposes, as I have explained in my discussion of Hesse, evaluation based on philosophical criteria, whether derived from a modern philosophy of science or from ancient philosophers made canonical because of subsequent developments, is not useful. Asking how good their science was has led scholars to ignore astrology and physiognomics, except insofar as they throw light on the "real" sciences of antiquity, and to stress a particular side of the medical corpus. My interest is in seeing what common rules of discourse are operating in all three disciplines and in isolating the peculiarity and specificity of ancient knowledge claims. In doing so, I lay stress on different texts from those that have previously received attention.

Two examples will serve to illustrate the difference between my project and a more traditional history of science, for which I take Lloyd as the least traditional example. For him the subsequent development of the science is important and exerts an influence on his elucidation of contemporary debates. Take the issue of quantification in ancient science. He concludes his chapter on "Measurement and Mystification" in *The Revolutions of Wisdom* with the comment: "What was needed was measurement directed and confined to determinable issues or a clear-cut awareness of the question of the directedness of measurement" (1987, 282). From my more limited perspective what is important is how quantification functioned in its local context. Quantification receives less consideration in my work than other aspects that seem more salient and more peculiar to the ancient context anyway. But, to take the case of the pulse, for instance, the ways in which measurement was attempted furnishes some interesting indications of what had persuasive cachet. Herophilus had used meters derived from music to define different pulse types, but this was not a success with his followers. What might have been persuasive to us, the use of a water clock to time pulses precisely, is also rejected by doctors after Herophilus. Galen uses ratios for rhythm and numbers to define varieties in ways that allow extremely complex permutations. The choice of numbered tables to present varieties of pulse is itself interesting as a development of divisions made according to the rules of rhetoric (see chap. 3).

Lloyd has reservations about the quantificatory excesses of the ancients' pulse theory, which come under his heading of mystification. In my explication of the more baroque complexities of pulse theory, as indeed with regard to esoteric doctrines in general in ancient science, I attempt to translate mystification into more sociological terms, as a result of the institution of the master-pupil relationship. This is an area in which religious discourse remains influential: the model of initiation is important, and the comparison of teacher to guru is not always inapposite.

The other institution that I regard as crucial for explaining the developments in ancient science on which I focus is the ἀγών (*agōn*), or public debate. Lloyd, taking the long view, isolates the ἀγών as the pivot for the "revolution of wisdom" in Greek science. It is the expression of the ideal of openness to criticism, a philosophical ideal crucial for the subsequent evolution of science. Whereas he notes cases in which this ideal was not translated into practice, the importance of the ἀγών is that it is the place where challenges may be made. Here "the rhetoric of rationality offers the material for its unmasking" (1987, 336); it is the crucible of debate, an agent of reduction to something nearer the right answer, for instance in public dissections, in which a clearer understanding of the body may be obtained.

I look at a different function of the ἀγών, as the molder of particular styles of persuasion. My rereading of it comes in the light of modern ideas about rhetoric, as does my understanding of it as an archetypal feature of ancient science. The ἀγών, however, was the site at which ancient theories about how to argue, formalized as τέχναι (*technai*) of rhetoric, were put into practice. Perhaps the roots of this institution of public debate lie in athletic and musical competitions.[47] Certainly, the ἀγών of the Second Sophistic is above all the arena for a spectator sport, the sport of rhetoric. Here is the place at which a doctor wins clients without treating a single patient but, rather, by discoursing on a pile of bones[48] or talking the audience through the dissection of an animal or even (the absurd extreme, which epitomizes the power of rhetoric for the ancients) by arguing that his opponents' patients are still ill despite their claims to health.[49] Here critical scrutiny on the part of the mass of spectators may be inhibited by awe.[50] To be sure, in some senses, the members of the audience, or at least a significant proportion of them, are connoisseurs of the game: they must be seen as worldly-wise about evaluating the claims made by performers; they expected a degree of hyperbole. It is in such a light, I think, that the mismatch between ancient theory and practice that Lloyd notes must be seen.

And it seems that (in my period at least) the ἀγών, far from narrowing down the options in any direction, encourages the proliferation of answers to questions. An impressive rhetorical tactic seems to have been to cap one's opponent by making subtle distinctions that he had missed. What evolves from the importance of this context of argument is this peculiar, local criterion of the τέχνη (*technē*): the emphasis on subtle distinctions, which seem highly unconvincing to us now. For me the ἀγών is less appropriately seen as an instrument of development in any sense of progress toward modern science than as a clue to the specificity of ancient "science": it defines a "style of reasoning" that can be seen to recur in all three of the bodies of knowledge that I consider and, I suspect, in most other bodies of knowledge formalized into τέχναι.

One of my examples of the proliferation effect is in Galen's pulse theory, which is part of a tradition much acclaimed by historians of science—the use of the pulse for prognosis and diagnosis.[51] Again, I am not concerned with the long perspective, in which the discovery of this use of the pulse is obviously important. Here my secondary theme derived from the sociology of knowledge comes into play: the "unfathomable nature of unverbalized reality." The point is made clearer by considering Chinese pulse theory. Scholars have tried to combine incommensurable systems of pulse doctrine in attempting to make sense of the Greek and the Chinese material in terms of a monolithic perceptual reality, with which modern scientific instruments are in a presumed one-to-one correspondence.[52] There is no reason why the three should be expected to match with one another, since they developed within different contexts of medical theory in response to different needs. As the historian of science Steven Shapin comments (1982), rejecting specific verbal forms of reality is not to reject the role of sensory input; it is, rather, to write a history more sensitive to the way knowledge is always tailored to doing things; it is in the course of doing things with knowledge that the knowledge is produced. I mentioned earlier that I acknowledge several dialectical engagements at work in the production and evaluation of scientific accounts that mute my relativism; here there is a dialectic between sensory input and social context. It is extremely difficult to estimate the role of sensory input here, but it seems to have minimal explanatory value in relation to the elaborate schemes of both Greek and Chinese writers on pulse diagnosis. Galen's endless subdivisions are typical of the agonistic style; they are developed in opposition to his predecessors. More important, it is difficult to see how they could be seen as being in the "pursuit of prediction and control" in any way comparable to the practitioners of modern science. Even in the case of Galen's predecessors the theories of the pulse are in no sense commensurable with those operating today. My interest is thus in the success of his pulse lore in its contemporary context, not in a retrospective evaluation based on the use of the pulse for diagnosis within a completely different, modern model of the body.[53]

Science and Pseudoscience

C. R. S. Harris (1973) lamented Galen's failure to put together his work on the pulse with his other physiological inquiries in order to discover the circulation of the blood. He was working with the evolutionary model that sees the route of progress encumbered by obstacles of traditional beliefs, or ideological constructs—the foundations of pseudoscience. From the point of view of a socializing understanding of science, of course, the lines are not so clearly drawn. To consider how this might work in a specific context I cite Steven Shapin's comments, based on his work on nineteenth-century phrenology, as an example to show how a science, or body of knowledge, developed *both* out of interests in prediction and control *and* under the impetus of expedient social interests:

> It was not assessed in terms of one interest but used the service of both. There was a series of judgements in which both were inextricably implicated. Assuming that there is a scientific component and a symbolic or ideological one is like assuming that electrical and gravitational phenomena can be accounted for in terms of chargeless masses and massless charges.[54]

In examining the past, as with any alien culture, one usually feels compelled to operate with some version of a "principle of charity." Mine, in contrast to the classical principle of charity of modern philosophers, is not to assume that the ancients must normally be thinking rationally in our terms but, rather, to find a rationale, to make sense of apparent nonsense. Hence my evaluative practice lies in the choice of focus, in redefining as most interesting what were traditionally seen as blemishes on the face of Greek rationality, whether it be the entire disciplines of astrology and physiognomics, which have been largely excluded from the history of science, or those features defined as irrational in medicine. Finding a rationale may appear to be less than charitable, however, according to our moral ideals, where it involves exposing apparently cynical political strategies on the part of ancient knowledge peddlers. The characters that people the intellectual landscape in my depiction do not measure up to our ideals of intellectual honesty or unselfish philanthropy. Nonetheless, it is not my purpose to evaluate their behavior according to such canons; I see them as playing intellectual games by rules that were tacitly accepted.

Pseudoscience is a label that implies a deliberate falsehood on the part of its practitioners. Paul Thagard's criteria of demarcation of pseudoscience allow for self-delusion as well; he focuses on intellectual rather than moral problems. Nevertheless, his criteria illustrate the inappropriateness of such concepts with regard to the ancient world:

> A theory which purports to be scientific is pseudo-scientific if and only if (1) it has been less progressive than alternative theories over a long period of

> time and faces many unsolved problems, but (2) the community of practitioners makes little attempt to develop the theory towards solutions of the problems, shows no concern for attempts to evaluate the theory in relation to others and is selective in considering confirmations and disconfirmations.[55]

This is a definition that presupposes the ideal standards and infrastructure of the modern scientific community. (Naturally, the sociologists of scientific knowledge would argue that the standards are community myths, but what is important here is that the ideals are collectively accepted.) Some related criticisms are made in rather different terms[56] by some ancients of astrology, for instance, but Ptolemy's defense of it as a conjectural body of knowledge (στοχαστικὴ τέχνη),[57] like medicine, offers a persuasive riposte in its context, several scholars have argued (Bouché-Leclercq 1899, Long 1982). Medicine, after all, could not be said to fulfill these criteria any better. Whether we consider it to be persuasive or not, Ptolemy's defense shows that the stakes of the argument were different: the qualifications for being a stochastic art were not the same as Thagard's for being a science.

Recently, this division between science and pseudoscience has come under attack. Jim Hankinson has argued that Quintus's empirical defense of divination, including astrology, in Cicero's *On Divination* is rational in its context. His pithy depiction of the conventional dichotomy, doubtless more influential than any rigorous criteria, exposes its inappropriateness neatly:

> Science . . . is tough-minded, rigorous, methodologically sound, an enterprise dedicated to the discovery and systematization of truths about the world. Pseudo-science on the other hand is its degenerate cousin, sheltering behind a facade of scientific rigour; it is nevertheless *au fond,* nothing more than a welter of superstitions, falsehood and charlatanry. No intelligent investigator, faced with a pseudo-science, will fail on deeper analysis to show up the counterfeit for the false coin that it is. (1988, 123)

Pseudoscience, he continues, is only seductive to the impressionable and the unwary, apt to be inveigled away from the straight, difficult track of genuine learning. He goes on to deconstruct the opposition with a fresh look at both Marcus's and Quintus's arguments, which make little sense within such a framework.

The political implications of the division between science and pseudoscience have also come under scrutiny. Roger Cooter argues that the deployment of the label "pseudo-science" always fulfills a conservative role,[58] in that it reinforces capitalist ideology. One does not have to be a Marxist to see that the use of the term acts to support science's position in society. More than this, it appropriates science to its side as a powerful and persuasive weapon. In the preceding pages I have set out a few of the reasons why science should not function automatically as a talisman in this way against the danger of "being tinctured with the kind of lunacy of the things one sets out to describe" in the past.[59] When I use the term *scientific* in the following work it is with the aim of drawing attention to the high status of the body of knowledge concerned in its context—akin to its root, *scientia*—rather than using it as an accolade on the basis of any modern standards. It acts as a reminder of the inappropriateness of terms like *pseudoscience.* Given the difficulty of refuting the strong thesis, it seems unhelpful to set out the subject of the inquiry in terms of science and pseudoscience. It is surely more fruitful to consider how grounds for belief in the ancient world differed from our own and the way in which their different ordering of knowledge might be related to a different sociopolitical context.

The New Rhetoric

In Greco-Roman antiquity a great deal of self-consciousness prevails about techniques of persuasion, about ways of persuading people that you are telling the truth, offering knowledge, because of the success of the discipline of rhetoric. Here I move on to my second intellectual paramour: the New Rhetoric, which derives its roots from classical theories of rhetoric. At this point I should pause to survey briefly the history of the subject in order to justify my use of the term. Rhetoric, or the art of persuasion by artifice, suffered from the beginning from an association of moral dubiousness in contrast to dialectic, most famously at the hands of Plato in the *Gorgias.* It is still commonly seen as the use of language in the interests of manipulation as opposed to some preferred "neutral" use. But from the sixteenth century, in a reform associated with Petrus Ramus (1572), logic was completely severed from even an opposite relation to rhetoric, which was now to be concerned only with matters of style or delivery. Thus, superficiality was added to immorality in the popular conception of it: as Perelman observes (1958), it is frequently associated with verbalism and an empty, unnatural mode of expression. In the eighteenth century it seems to have sunk into irrelevancy: it became a symbol of the most outdated elements in the education of the old regime, in its formality and uselessness it seemed opposed to the needs of an egalitarian, progressive democracy.[60] This century, however, rhetoric has made something of a comeback in certain circles. Kenneth Burke put rhetoric in a central position by arguing that, far from being marginal, it was ubiquitous.[61] The ideal of a completely neutral vocabulary, free of emotional weightings, was a mirage. Semantic and poetic meanings were not in opposition; semantic meaning was a partial aspect of poetic. Thus, rhetorical theory would help understanding of how language worked. Tropes were dusted off and given a central role in cognition, first metaphor (following along the lines of Rousseau and Nietzsche) but also metonymy, synecdoche, and irony. In 1958 Perelman and Olbrechts-Tyteca began to advertise a "New Rhetoric." In a reversal of the "Ramus reform" they presented rhetoric as a theory of practical reasoning. The power of this analysis was that it gave full credit to the dimension of action, focusing primarily on the relationship of speaker and audience within a social matrix. It assimilated feeling to the quality of thought itself. Rather than seeing rhetoric as opposed to philosophy, they argued that philosophy could be seen as a branch of the discipline that appealed to the universal audience.

Here was a destruction of another transformation of the science or ideology dualism. Science had been expected to develop a neutral vocabulary, while prejudice was to be left to the vocabulary of social relations. But now metaphor was allowed a creative role in science. Even the plain style of scientific academic articles could be seen as a rhetorical form in itself.[62]

In this new vision of a world of communication permeated with rhetoric, in which the audience became all-important, objectivity came into question. Explanation had to be seen as not only being about something but also for someone. Reading writing as arguments between people undermines the usual distinctions between objectivity and value ladenness. As Edmondson argues, "values do not just enter at the level of the choice of the subject-matter or in terms of specific concepts, claims or judgements but they operate in a much more systematic and indeterminable way; evaluative positions are properties of communicative processes as a whole."[63] She points out that this view is in opposition to long-held assumptions about language. Locke thought that linguistic conventions were there to aid smooth transference of ideas from mind to mind by diminishing the influence of language on thought.[64] Hence, the ideal of plainness for optimal communication. Such assumptions may be overtly discredited, but they remain covertly influential. Bringing human feeling back into the picture of communication is thus another sociological heterodoxy that has failed to overthrow orthodoxy. Again, it alters the moral perspective. Rhetoric is neither necessarily a servile flattery, as in the Platonic model, nor must it be an arbitrary and reprehensible means of bringing the audience under the speaker's power. Edmondson argues for a more positive view of rhetoric as "argumentative procedures which are used in and responsive to specific communication situations in order to make contentions suasive for readers and hearers" (1984, 5). It can be seen as discovering in a subject aspects that aid one's interlocutor's grasp of it.

This presentation of rhetoric (as in the case of Perelman) derives from a reading of the classical authors—Aristotle, Cicero, and Quintilian, in particular. She regards Aristotle as leading a tradition in which rhetoric is not a technology of manipulation but, rather, an exploration of reasonable intersubjective communication in society (1984, 6). (For Aristotle rhetoric is the counterpart of dialectic but involves reasoning from premises that are merely probable rather than true.)[65] In the Roman world, in which rhetoric becomes a branch of politics, it is a method of educating the ideal citizen. She takes up Aristotle's threefold division of the means of persuasion into ἦθος (ēthos), πάθος (pathos), and λόγος (logos) and reinterprets them in the light of current theory. The ancient stress on the ἦθος, or personal character, of the speaker is important in view of the "modern sociolinguistic fact that any argument is perceived and understood in some relation with the propounder." As Oswald Ducrot puts it in *Dire et ne pas dire,* "Information is an illocution that can be completed only if the receiver recognizes the speaker's competence and honesty beforehand."[66] Edmondson redescribes πάθος as sensitization (1984, 17); putting the audience in a certain frame of mind is the usual translation. Avoiding the traditional view of this as potentially exploitative, she stresses the way in which the psychological mode can affect understanding, taking her cue from Aristotle.[67] Thus, she uses sensitization to illustrate the cognitive and noncognitive components in argument. λόγος (proof) is the abstract structure of argument itself, the tenor or burden of what is said expressed in purely cognitive terms, which is not equivalent to the argument itself. And the enthymeme, or rhetorical syllogism, encapsulates the way the three are blended in everyday deductions. Armed with this theoretical basis and the classical tropes, she proceeds to give an exegesis of some canonical sociological texts.

Edmondson's moral rehabilitation of rhetoric is certainly important. It needs to be seen as a normal aspect of communication rather than as a deformation of it. Yet in her eagerness to show her colleagues that she is not criticizing them for their rhetorical devices but only appreciating the way they work, she does tend to cast a veil over the presence of power in rhetoric. Here is the heffalump trap again: in her careful rephrasing of the operations of rhetoric so that it sounds neutral, she is heading straight for it. Once you bring *ideology* into *science,* as in the case of Barnes and Bloor, or *emotion* into *information,* as here, you cannot then exploit the latter term for its connotations of the neutrality that you have just impugned without a certain self-consciousness. You have to acknowledge your role as rhetorician. It is because the rhetoric of sociology is one of objectivity that Edmondson is forced to neglect the worrying potential of rhetoric, which was there from the beginning. The ancients' attitude to rhetoric was far from sanguine: because of its power, it needed to be harnessed to an ethical program.

There is a further point to be made here. Edmondson is not concerned with the reconstruction of the historically specific nature of classical rhetorical theory but, rather, in using her reading of it to reread modern sociological texts. Similarly, in using her ideas and those of the other New Rhetorical theorists in order to understand ancient texts, I am indulging in a species of presentism akin to that of the Whiggish historian of science and thus drawing out those aspects of the texts I think I can recognize as rhetorical in the modern sense. Nevertheless, there are cases in which the ancient rhetorical treatises themselves presuppose readings of technical texts, as will be particularly apparent in the case of physiognomical material; here I fall more squarely in the tradition of classical scholarship.

Michel Foucault: Power and Knowledge

I would argue that power cannot be divorced from any communication that presents itself as the truth and that rhetoric is the best heading under which to discuss this aspect of communication. Where political aims include accreditation from others, observes the anthropologist Marilyn Strathern in a volume entitled *Power and Knowledge,* coercion rests in devices used to compel them to yield certain perceptions of events.[68] Conceptual domaining is a political tool. This is a point at which I should acknowledge a debt, while again differentiating myself from the source of inspiration. My third paramour has obviously been lurking in the background all along. It is from the later work of Michel Foucault that I take many aspects of my model of power, which I have waited till now to explain. Ultimately, it is with the aid of his depictions of the coextensiveness of power relations with the social that I rephrase the contingent social interests considered by the aforementioned philosophers of science in political terms.

First, I take up his vision of power as essentially unstable, the model he develops in opposition to the traditional juridical characterizations of it as a commodity. Second, I find enormously suggestive his challenge to the old image of power as repression, by construing its role as positive. He asks rhetorically whether power would be so successful if all it did was work negatively, by repression. What gives it its hold, he answers, is that it produces effects at the level of desire; it produces pleasure: "knowledge involves the discovery of secrets . . . which gives the individual joyful power," it produces "reality, domains of objects and rituals of truth,"[69] it is a productive network that runs through the whole social body. In Foucault's work truth is linked in a circular relation to systems of power, which produce and sustain it, and to effects of power, which it induces and which redirect it. This is where he abandons ideology on the grounds that there is no pure form of knowledge and that it presupposes a subject and some kind of base for which it is the superstructure. The political question, according to Foucault, is not about error, illusion, alienated consciousness; it is about truth itself. I quote the passage from his interview with Alessandro Fontano and Pasquale Pasquino, to allow his rhetoric full play:

> Truth isn't outside power, or deprived of power . . . it isn't the reward of free spirits, the child of prolonged solitudes, or the privilege of those who have been able to liberate themselves. Truth is of this world; it is produced there by virtue of multiple constraints. And it induces there the regulated effects of

> power. Each society has its regime of truth, its general politics of truth: that is, the types of discourse it harbours and causes to function as true; the mechanisms and instances which enable one to distinguish true from false statements, the way in which each is sanctioned; the techniques and procedures which are valorised for obtaining truth; the status of those who are charged with saying what counts as true. (Trans. Morris and Patton 1979, 45–46)

As a general high-level formula, this mutual generation of power and knowledge can be brought to bear on the relations between the state and astrology, as I argue in the first chapter. But it is his concentration on the fluctuating situation at the micro level that has furnished me with the focus for more of my work:

> Power becomes effective or not, that is, power is always a definite form of momentary and constantly reproduced encounters among a definite number of individuals. Power is thus not possessed, it is in play because it risks itself. Power is won like a battle and lost in the same way. . . . At every moment power is in play in small individual parts. ("Power and the Norm," trans. Morris and Patton 1979, 59–60)

This is not merely a matter of seeing the small skirmishes as significant; it is also a way of linking them with the great war. This is significant for my enterprise in the following chapters, which is to show the interlocking of different levels of the politics of knowledge.

> Between each part of the social body, between a man and a woman in a family, between a teacher and a pupil, between the one who knows and the one who doesn't, there pass relations of power which are not the pure and simple projects of great sovereign power over individuals. Rather they are the mobile and concrete ground on which that power came to be anchored, they are the conditions for its functioning. ("Interview with Lucette Finas," trans. Morris and Patton 1979, 70)

I find the image of power and knowledge as never crystallized into finality but only permanently in a field of flux, as a battlefield upon which one can only capture and freeze moments in which one view of it triumphs, a peculiarly appropriate construction for the ancient world, where institutionalization of knowledge production was at such a low level. Second, there are also advantages in following his dramatic enlargement of the sphere of the political in that, on his model, it becomes possible to see how even the smallest theaters of conflict relate to the grand stage of traditional political history. There is both a capillary relationship, a metonymical one that links the different levels, and an analogical or metaphorical one—the same operations are visible in both arenas. I should immediately cover myself on one count here: this is not a retreat into idealism. It is not a neglect of the very real presence of physical force or violence in power relationships, on which Foucault has also focused in connection with his concept of "biopower," for I do not mean to grant to verbal rhetoric some ultimate sovereignty. Violence, however, or the threat of violence, is by no means sufficient to explain the ascendancy of the powerful.

Yet there are also serious difficulties in Foucault's ideas. He admits that the conceptions with which he is operating are nominalistic, which he justifies on the grounds that he is using a grid of intelligibility: power is neither an institution, nor is it a structure, nor a certain innate strength, it is the name given to "a complex strategical relationship in a particular society."[70] But there remains a tension between this nominalism and a claim to give power an explanatory role, as Dreyfus and Rabinow observe.[71] How can it be simultaneously both a productive principle in the practices themselves and a merely heuristic principle used for giving the practices retroactive intelligibility? This relates to two relevant problems in Foucault's work. First, there is the problem of agency. Perhaps because of his concern with our own age, in which the impersonal operation of power is all too obvious, power in his version becomes a metaphysical force that takes on all the transcendental qualities that he denies the Subject, in his revolt against humanism. In choosing rhetoric as the lens through which to view the political action with which I am concerned, I am distancing myself from these grander philosophical problems, to focus on an intentional but nonetheless socialized subject.

Second, we are back with the old self-refutation threat. Foucault typically leaves it unclear how he has solved the problems incumbent on this kind of relativism:

> I am fully aware that I have never written anything but fictions. For all that I would not want to say that they are outside truth. It seems possible to me to make fiction work within truth, to induce truth-effects within a fictional discourse, and in some way to make the discourse of truth "fabricate" something which doesn't as yet exist, thus "fiction" something. One fictions history starting from a political reality that renders it true, one fictions a politics that doesn't as yet exist starting from a historical truth. ("Interview with Lucette Finas," trans. Morris and Patton 1979, 4–5)

Is he just inheriting the tension present in the work of Nietzsche, clearly indicated as one major source of inspiration? Nietzsche's combination of a denunciation of truth as the "mobile army of metaphors, metonymies, anthropomorphisms"[72] with his use of the term to characterize unargued assertions such as the doctrine of recurrence, which he simply feels to be true, is a fine example of this tension. But what is one to make of the phrase "political reality" here, let alone "historical truth"? The context seems to undermine any transcendent quality for either. Must we substitute Hesse's social understanding of truth here to avoid seeing these statements as self-refuting?

In *Discipline and Punish* Foucault disclaims an attempt to write a history of the past in terms of the present but admits to a "history of the present."[73] This Dreyfus and Rabinow explain as an approach that "explicitly and self-reflectively begins with a diagnosis of the current situation."[74] The problem arises because Foucault takes so much care to avoid erecting a theoretical system, or to elaborate a discourse that purports to represent the truth. But this is difficult to square with the rhetorical role he wants to give his "genealogy." He needs, if not Truth, modest truths, and so it is that his history must be "grey, meticulous and patiently documentary." It is, anyway, unclear how much he succeeds since he writes history in such a manner as to infuriate historians. Mark Poster (1984) remarks on the silences that scream at the reader, the topics annoyingly placed out of the normal order, disrupting one's sense of logical sequence, the levels of analysis placed together in irritating confusion, the violation of the difference between ideas and behavior, the ignoring or reversal of simple questions of causality, the confusion of the narrative line, the failure to clarify the object of investigation, and the odd, incomplete nature of the evidential basis.

Foucault thus revels in the heffalump trap. I have said that, for a relativizing strategy to work without falling into the trap, the relativist must acknowledge his or her role as rhetorician. This, of course, does not solve all the problems. You can get out of the crude-form heffalump trap by pointing to your activity as rhetorician, but it is impossible to do so continually, while operating as one. There remains the kind of tension that led de Man to see rhetoric as fated to a condition of deceit and mystification from which it is ceaselessly trying to escape.[75] The only answer is that of the reflexive writers, such as Ashmore (1989) and Woolgar (1988), who urge us to stop seeing reflexivity as a problem and to enjoy the creative possibilities it offers. There is no doubt, however, that this kind of reflexive style can alienate many readers and thus fail as rhetoric. In this introduction I have been concerned only to leave my rhetoric in an ironic frame, leaving the next move to the audience.

In choosing not to follow Foucault's refusal to allow closure on his work, I am accepting my own role as rhetorician. One of the most important contributions of rhetorical theory to an analytics of power comes with its sensitivity to audience. The audience sets the initial terms of consensus; the rhetorician can only work from there. This points up the fact that power can never be seen exclusively as a one-way relation, with passive acceptance responding to active force; both sides must have a role in constructing it. One of the problems with Foucault's work has been its neglect in historical analysis, if not in theory, of the role of resistance to power. So it is that I am writing with no assumption of passive acceptance on the part of my readers but, rather, with some acceptance of how they have set the terms in advance. In that awareness I am making the kind of closure Foucault would not in setting out my theoretical basis. To most readers the historical style in operation will seem less alienating than in theory. It is in an engagement with such readers that some of my axiomatic beginnings here will appear to be lost in a rhetoric of truth; the ironic frame will fade into the background. This arises more from a desire to engage with the classical scholar and the historian in general according to the rules than from real disengagement from a commitment to a kind of relativist history. In fact, the tradition of classical scholarship offers great opportunities to reassess larger questions about the status of science such as I have been addressing, since in its preoccupation with the classical world, and as a result of the relative dearth of evidence, it has always brought a great variety of sources together, using many different scholarly techniques, in order to throw light on particular texts. There was always implicit insistence on linguistic and cultural specificity.[76] The thrust of such a style of inquiry thus naturally tends to work against the Whiggish impulse.

Finally, after this sketch of my intellectual genealogy I should say something more on the implications of my relativism for the status of this history. One of the ideas that seems to be behind Foucault's contorted observations on truth and fiction seems to be that of the mutual implication of past and present. I trust that the muted form of relativism I have adopted allows the possibility of a degree of translation; it would be hard to justify this study if I regarded past and present here as incommensurable in the strong sense. What I want to undercut, however, is any apparent insistence that my approach offers the real truth about the ancient world or even that it is an objective one; it is clear enough from a glance at the historiography of this century that, as the text unfolds in time, the meaning changes. The ephemerality of the concerns of this introduction will be all too obvious in a few years' time. My argument so far has tended to suggest that a rationalizing approach is anachronistic, but, obviously, the goal of regaining a past perspective is marked by historicity as well. The theories of the sociology of knowledge, of the New Rhetoric and of Foucault on power and knowledge, can themselves be examined as part of the sociology and politics of Western society. Furthermore, I could be myself subject to sociopolitical investigation; my views could be seen to derive from biographical contingencies: Cambridge is, after all, a site of power struggles over knowledge. All such possibilities would not undermine the project, for the reasons Hesse outlined in dealing with the strong thesis: a different concept of knowledge is operating, which does not need to be guaranteed free of social influence. I would not claim that my approach is intrinsically better than that of the rationalizing historian in its "program of truth"; its merits and demerits will have to be weighed up according to the extrinsically agreed criteria (the appropriate "styles of reasoning").

To stretch the concept a little further this work could be seen as being produced for the modern equivalent of an ἀγών (*agōn*). As discussed, ἀγῶνες are recognizably rhetorical and, thus, inevitably raise a degree of skepticism; on the other hand, they are persuasive to the extent that they are intrinsically relative to audience. The word ἀγών can be translated as "battle." We as scholars are involved in a battle of knowledge. The ground over which the battle rages is irretrievable as a whole. There is a plurality of truths, and, crucially, our knowledge of the ground can only be mediated. I can only hope to be persuasive in constructing my image of the intellectual life of the period; even if I admit that the "grid of intelligibility" is one imposed by present concerns, I would still argue that the mesh is not so coarse as to provide a perverse reading and that it is a grid that will reveal a picture not previously apparent. Whether I have succeeded or not can only, of course, emerge from dialogue with my audience.

Chapter 1

Star Wars in the Greco-Roman World

Magic, that most fraudulent of the arts, has held complete sway throughout the world for many ages. Nobody should be surprised at the greatness of its influence, since of all the others it has embraced three more that hold supreme dominion over the human mind; medicine . . . religion . . . and astrology, because there is no one who is not eager to learn his destiny or who does not believe that the truest account of it is to be gained from watching the skies.

—Pliny, *Natural History*

And finally, I must thank the Royal Society for supporting the publication financially. [I] . . . hope that its subject-matter will not be too great an embarrassment to that august body . . .

—J. D. North: *Horoscopes and History*

Part 1. The Rise and Fall of Astrology

Introduction

Historians are still suffering from embarrassment about taking a serious interest in astrology. The apologetic tone[1] of North's preface suggests that even in 1986 there is a fear among scholars who might otherwise have worked on the topic of being "tinctured with the kind of lunacy they set out to describe."[2] There is extraordinarily rich material available—the twelve volumes of the *Catalogus Codicorum Astrologorum Graecorum* are some testimony to the voluminous outpourings on the subject in classical antiquity—yet it has excited little serious historical study. Nor have comments like Pliny's (at *HN* 30.1.1–2) invited a reassessment of the importance of astrology. Despite the efforts of classical philologists such as Usener, Boll, and Cumont and of historians of religion and culture such as Warburg, Saxl, and Cassirer since the end of the nineteenth century to publish the long-neglected texts and emphasize their autonomous conceptual value,[3] the texts have been largely ignored by mainstream historians. There is a great discrepancy exemplified in the different attitudes evident in this chapter's two epigraphs that is revealing about the politics of intellectual life today.

In challenging the social and political historian's neglect of astrology,[4] I am putting into question the rationalizing program, the strategy of ignoring those domains of the past that can in no way be annexed to the intellectual empire of the present. Such a program risks rationalizing away the very aspects that reveal ancient life in its specificity. S. J. Tester, the author of a history of Western astrology (1987), aptly refers to a "McCarthyism" among classical scholars studying ancient science, concerned that there are too many Greeks engaged in un-Greek activities. Despite the traditional classical procedure of sifting through a great variety of evidence that may throw light on particular texts, in this case perhaps there has been an emotional investment in tracing a particular legacy of Greece in modern science, which excludes consideration of less welcome inheritances such as astrology.

As discussed in the introduction, I am also putting into question ideas at the core of a rationalizing history of science, a history that isolates scientific discourse from any involvement in social practice, hallowing it in some domain in which the real presents itself without credentials. But social context is all-important in the explanation of the attitude toward astrology that has prevailed. The image of the superstitious anachronism of contemporary popular astrology lurks in the back of scholars' minds. George Sarton, one of the important figures in the history of science referred to in the introduction, is certainly an extreme case, with his vitriolic condemnations of "the astrologic nonsense that has done so much harm in the Western world and still poisons weak-minded people today." The incongruousness of his moral tone is now slightly ludicrous: he refers to the great astronomer Hipparchus' interest in astrology as a "betrayal" and demands "all honour to the relatively few men like Cicero, who had the insight and courage to resist the astrological avalanche."[5]

If the shifts in the ideological landscape of modern scholarship examined in the introduction have left Sarton marooned, the descendants of his viewpoint are still with us. The historiography of seventeenth- and eighteenth-century science furnishes an interesting parallel. Patrick Curry (1985) sums up the state of the scholarly field. He describes historians as divided into two camps espousing opposite tendencies. First, there are those, of whom Frances Yates is probably the most famous,[6] who claim to attempt "to understand the past in its own terms." This approach grew out of a reaction against a Whiggish history of science and proclaimed the importance of Hermetic magic, Neoplatonism, alchemy, and astrology in contributing even to those developments in seventeenth-century science regarded now as ancestors of present-day science. On the other hand, there are those who present themselves as taking a more matter-of-fact approach, in the footsteps of Sarton: what was science then is science now, and the same goes for the occult.[7] This latter group are anxious to emphasize the more narrowly "internal" development of science and its relative autonomy from metaphysical and especially from social context—"at least to weed out the less desirable kinds of influence." As Curry observes, this crude polarity of science and nonscience that they set up serves only to obscure genuine historical questions and to generate countless pseudoproblems of "radical incoherence." Thus, Vickers asks questions such as: "Why do the most vehement attackers of magic retain occult beliefs and habits?" or "How can Bacon's speculative philosophy coexist with his rigorous logical method based on observation and experiment?"[8] Obviously, what seems incompatible to Vickers now need not have been perceived as such by the historical actors.

Curry is less critical of the former group, though he is cautious, since reassessments of Yates and company have not always gone in their favor. He accuses them of eliding differentiations of magic and science that are in play in the historical periods they discuss. Clearly, too, claiming to study the past in its own terms is too optimistic: history, as discussed in the introduction, must always be a history of the present. Curry reserves the truly scathing remarks, however, for the second group's presuppositions.

More recent and subtle exponents of the sociological/metaphysical approach can be found in Curry's edition of a collection of articles on astrology (1987). Particularly interesting is Keith Hutchinson's "Towards a Political Iconology of the Copernican Revolution." The shift toward a heliostatic conception of the universe has long been considered a standard testing ground for philosophical accounts of rational criteria for evaluating competing scientific theories, as he remarks. But he situates the shift in the context of the centralization of political power and of Baroque aesthetics. Noting that there had been a strong commitment to a heliostatic universe before persuasive evidence was available, and considering the political messages that Renaissance observers drew from the heavens, he argues that there are strong grounds for thinking that changing conceptions of the way in which society should be ordered were instrumental in effecting the reordering of cosmology. But he refines the meaning of *instrumental:* "changes in society appear to operate to generate an aesthetic sense as to what is an appropriate portion of the physical universe in which to seat the solar power." This is no crude depiction of the functioning of political ideology but, rather, an empathetic exploration of the social background to the changing tastes of the seventeenth century.

There has been no account of the rise of ancient astrology in terms of a revolution of wisdom. From the perspective of the twentieth century it is, at first blush, hard to understand how the rise of astrology could be seen as in any sense comparable to a scientific revolution. But as Richard Lemay, another contributor to Curry's volume, reminds us:

> Conceptually, the effect of the Scientific Revolution was to render it nearly impossible for historians henceforward to grasp the different scope of ancient science, of its epistemology and orientation. . . . Inevitably, these [concepts, tools] greatly differ from our modern apparatus in lexical, semantical and structural fashion all at once. (1987, 60)

Perhaps the model of a revolution of wisdom will not appear so inappropriate after all, once something of the context of "ancient science" is reconstructed.

Yet all this flurry of reexamination of fundamental presuppositions about the subject among historians and philosophers of science seems to have had only limited impact on studies of ancient science, of which astrology remains on the margins, rather than being considered in relation to other ancient "scientific" disciplines. Historians of science are the only scholars who have looked at astrological practice, but they have normally been concerned only with what they could learn of contemporary mathematics or astronomy, not with astrology itself, let alone with setting it in its social or even intellectual context.[9] Social historians, on the other hand, have not known what to do with the rich material at their disposal. They have used the circumstantial detail of astrological treatises to indicate something of the potential of contemporary human life. Because of the nature of the texts, this tends to produce either numerous nuggets of incidental information such as those in Thorndike (1913) or Macmullen (1971) on ancient occupations, which make for turgid reading en masse,[10] or conclusions of such generality that they seem too bold for their provenance, such as the following: "In a more sinister way, a proliferation of manuals of astrology, of dream-books and sorcery-books show with how much anxiety a new public of half-educated men needed to remain in control of a life whose pace had quickened."[11]

One can see that the astrological sources might be mined for both sorts of information, the more specific and the more general. I cannot see, however, that the trajectories of historians so far have looked promising as strategies for dealing with the rich evidence available. Frederick Cramer is one of few historians who has taken astrology seriously and written about it within its social context (1956). He has amassed much valuable evidence and produced a very readable work. Yet he seems almost completely unaware of the problems with taking ancient evidence at face value, and he has an inclination toward elaborating wildly speculative hypothetical accounts when no evidence is available.

My strategy is both to bring together consideration of astrology's political role with some exegesis of astrological practice and to bring together this exegesis of its practice with examination of other disciplines, avoiding the genealogical type of inquiry that obscures the question of contemporary interrelations. Ancient astrology offers a contrasting case to our organization of knowledge, illustrating the artificial, historically specific nature of boundaries between knowledge and pseudoknowledge, intellectual discipline and technical craft, science and mysticism. Astrology sprawls across these boundaries in such a way that the anachronism of applying them to the ancient world becomes clear. It is time for the stigmas attached to the "margins of science" to be seen for what they are, part of the present-day operations of power in legitimating different discourses.

In abandoning our perceptions of astrology as intrinsically marginal and dubious, we are led to undertake a new sort of inquiry, an inquiry into the connections between its knowledge status and political change. We are driven to ask questions about the context in which it is constructed as a plausible discipline, to look at how powerful people adopted it, created the consensus on its truth to which Pliny referred (see epigraph), confirmed the reason (*ratio*) it claimed.[12] At this crude level of analysis truth appears as a function of power.

Yet there is, secondly, a reciprocal relation: once constructed as truth or knowledge, it becomes a source of legitimating power. If we see astrology in this light, we can then examine its legitimating function in fields as diverse as medical practice, Mithraic cult,[13] and the usurpation of imperial power. It is this last aspect that forms part of my concern in my account of the authorities' relations with astrology, in which I attempt to suggest what made it suitable for such an important political role. It here becomes clear that these two directions of influence I have outlined are only analytically separable and cannot be treated in isolation from each other because of the complexity of the relationship between power and knowledge. These two interrelated points, then, form my theme in part 1.

The third point is that, looking positively at astrology's rationale and the way it was practiced, rather than taking its irrationality as given or enumerating its logical breakdowns with a scornful pity, we can solve the problems of the apparent absurdities. It becomes evident that these aberrations have function and coherence. Indeed, they fit with contemporary intellectual style and religious thinking, laying claim to the kinds of truth implicit in both discourses. The strategies of astrologers, which aim at appropriating the power of knowledge by restriction, make a parallel at a lower level to the strategies of the political authorities. And they are more successful in their attempts to control it. I shall be concerned with this level, that of intellectual politics, in part 2.

Astrology as Knowledge?

The sense in which astrology became knowledge is not simple precisely because of the enormous gulf between the ancient intellectual domain and our own described by Lemay, as will become clear in my account. But Pliny's remark cited in the epigraph to this chapter is a significant marker of the difficulties of reconstruction. This acknowledgment of widespread certainty about the truth of astrology is set within a context of doubt about its practitioners, expressed frequently in other parts of that great rambling work, the *Natural History* (especially bk. 7). The ambivalence that seems evident here is a part of a recurrent syndrome, where divination is concerned, a syndrome that I will be discussing in this chapter and the next. But what is also crucial is that, as the quotation from Pliny suggests, and as I shall be illustrating in chapter 3, similarly ambivalent views are held about medical science, which has not suffered from the same kind of skeptical modern scrutiny as ancient astrology.

And in the case of astrology the question of its status is further complicated because of the very different sets of beliefs that could be seen as falling under this category. Skepticism might be directed only at one branch of the discipline. It is genethlialogy, or horoscopic astrology, concerning itself with individual nativities, that is the focus of my investigation, since it is this part of the discipline that becomes the locus of conflict. The term is normally associated, however, with other branches, such as astrological ethnography, concerned with the effect of the stars on the people of different regions, or astrological meteorology, which will sometimes also be included in my discussion of views on astrology. Geminus, for instance, the writer of an astronomical work in about 50 B.C., seems to endorse aspects of genethlialogy, while being skeptical about astrological meteorology.[14] I am not generally concerned with astrolatry, or star worship, though elements of it are usually submerged in notions of astrological influence. Further difficulties arise in establishing astrology's status because the classical terms (ἀστρολογία/ἀστρονομία) were usually used by the ancients to cover both what we call astronomy and astrology.

It is important, too, in consideration of ancient skepticism about astrology, that the context and direction of the polemic are grasped. Sextus Empiricus' blistering attack on astrology in his *Against the Professors* must be seen in the context of his attacks on grammar, rhetoric, geometry, arithmetic, music, and philosophy, in short the ancient curriculum.[15] In effect, he furnishes better testimony to the extent of astrology's inclusion in the curriculum than to widespread second-century skepticism about it.

There are also questions about the precise context of its standing as knowledge. My account of the relations between the authorities and astrology concentrates on the official attitude to astrology, an attitude that certainly presupposes acceptance of its status as knowledge for hundreds of years. The official attitude certainly reveals an expectation that this acceptance is shared by the mass of the people in the empire, whether this could realistically be seen as the case or not. One could certainly argue that the official attitude shows acceptance only on the part of the sociopolitical elite, rather than acceptance on the part of the intellectual elite. Of course, such boundaries are difficult to draw, but genuine questions about who accepted astrology and in what sense can still be asked. Consideration of all the evidence available is beyond the scope of this work, and in the end such questions admit of no definite answer. The evidence marshaled in this account furnishes at least grounds for believing in the existence of extremely widespread acceptance of the truth of astrology in some form and in the operation of very different guidelines about what constituted knowledge.

Astrology, then, as we shall see, occupied a far more central position in any plausible map of ancient bodies of knowledge than one could anticipate from a modern perspective. It had not always occupied this position but, rather, moved in from the social fringes and out to them again. My theme here is power and knowledge at the highest political level, and to substantiate my thesis about their mutual implication I have to follow the history of astrology's changing place in the world of antiquity beyond the period with which I am mainly concerned, looking back to the third century B.C. and forward to the seventh A.D.

Astrology, Divination, and the Fall of the Republic

It is striking that astrology in any form was marginal to Roman elite politics until the Late Republic. There are a mere two testimonies to its existence that can be taken seriously as evidence for the second century B.C. In these examples the new form of divination appears only as appealing to the masses, with the elite attempting to prevent this.[16] To set astrology's later rise to prominence in context it is necessary to examine the place of state divination in general in the Roman republic, recently considered by J. A. North.[17] Of private divination, as he observes, we hear little. The main source is Livy, who accords divination a conspicuous role in his narrative (which survives for the years 219–167 B.C.). He records the prodigies, omens, and divine signs of all sorts and the priestly consultations and rituals that followed year by year. The archival material he used very probably bears some relationship to the senatorial records, the *Annales Maximi.*[18]

There are three groups of diviners who emerge from the reports.[19] First, there was the college of augurs, who were originally concerned with interpreting the movements and cries of birds, though by the first century B.C. and probably for some time before that the auspices were generally taken by feeding the sacred fowl. (Refusal to eat was seen as a sign of disfavor.) Auspices had to be taken before public action of any sort, but augurs had particular responsibility for the religious aspects of popular assemblies, including the interpretation of signs such as thunder and lightning that occurred before or during these. Second, there were the *XVviri sacris faciundis* (literally, the Fifteen Men for Doing Sacred Things),[20] the keepers of the Sibylline Books, a set of poems in Greek supposedly bought from a prophetess by the last king of Rome. They were consulted more rarely, perhaps as a last resort, about prodigies (anomalies seen as signs from the gods), and about the introduction of new cults. When the keepers' advice was sought they would consult the books and make recommendations for the necessary ritual accordingly. The third group is more confusing. The name *haruspices,* traditionally associated with Etruria, is used to describe interpreters of both prodigies and the entrails of sacrificial animals. We cannot be sure whether the two groups are one or whether North's suggestion should be accepted that the group consulted by the senate about prodigies is of higher status than the group of entrail interpreters. These entrail interpreters may have been originally distinct from the officials responsible for deciding whether a sacrifice was accepted by the gods in Roman divination, but in our evidence the two techniques are intermingled. This may have been a gradual process that took place throughout the Republic, as Schilling argues (1979).

The keynote of Roman divination remains clear, however: it was a matter of establishing and maintaining the *pax deorum* (peace of the gods) in relation to the city. Divination, like other religious activity, is closely implicated in political activity; indeed, it is an integral part of it. The auspices were taken by a magistrate at prescribed times in the exercise of his office, such as before assemblies or battle. The power of *auspicium* (taking the auspices) was a concomitant of *imperium* (political authority); the magistrate had to carry out the ritual properly in order to guarantee his magisterial action. The significant feature of Livy's accounts of divinatory action is that expiation seems to take precedence over interpretation. It is more important to prevent the impending disaster than to be precise about its nature. Roman extispicy (entrail reading) seems to have been originally a matter of insuring divine favor rather than of divination of the future as in Etruscan tradition. It functioned to provide semisolicited divine communication, since sacrifices had to be performed anyway. Normally, if there arose any problem with the entrails (such as enlarged or diminished organs), this would be taken to mean that the victim was rejected by the gods, and new victims had to be selected until accepted (*perlitatio*). Obviously, a run of problematic entrails was a bad omen. Schilling, however, argues that Roman extispicy took on some of the Etruscan techniques: the kind of disaster threatened was indicated more specifically. The case of Decius and Manlius, described in Livy (8.9.1), in which death for the commander but victory for the army was the interpretation, is set in the earliest period (340 B.C.), but prediction of this sort remains rare till the second century B.C. And the examples of prediction by haruspices, which do occur for the years from 140 to 44 B.C., hardly do more than narrow down the nature of the disaster portended for the community—to bloodshed, fire, defeat, civil discord, and so on.[21]

In contrast to Livy, Cicero, in his work *On Divination* of 45 B.C., does focus on divination of the future in the stronger sense of prophecy, or prediction. It is important to remember, however, that, as a philosophical treatise, this work is strongly influenced by the Greek model. Indeed, as North observed, he has seemingly coined the word *divinatio* as a translation of the Greek μαντική (*mantikē*). This text must therefore be treated with caution as evidence of changes that had taken place in Roman religion. Yet it is clear that the precise nature of what is portended is now at issue. For instance, the portents of the Catilinarian conspiracy mentioned in Cicero's poem on his consulship were interpreted in detail by *haruspices:* when Natta's statue and the bronze tablets of laws were struck by lightning, because the Nattas were of noble birth, either a threat from among the nobility or danger to the nobility was threatened as well as the overthrow of the laws.[22] In Cicero's *On the Responses of the* Haruspices, he quotes the *haruspices* as predicting danger for the Senate and statesmen as a result of dissension among the nobility and the rule of one man, if their recommendations are not followed (19.40). There are other pieces of evidence relating to the first century B.C. A rare instance of a prediction that is strongly positive and a personal omen for the presiding magistrate is that reported as being afforded to Sulla in the early first century, in which an image of a gold crown appears on the liver, which Sulla is commanded to eat.[23] Again there are elements of prophecy in the use of the Sibylline Books in the first century, as is clear from Cicero.[24] Some of the prophecies reported may incite skepticism, but even these, as North remarks, speak at least of contemporary expectations.

While North is wary of extrapolating from first-century evidence to the earlier Republic, Raymond Bloch argued that the ancient Roman conception of the prodigy as an inevitably dire sign of the rupture of the *pax deorum* began to change as a result of Greek influences, under the pressures of the Second Punic War (218–201 B.C.), into a conception of a prodigy as a presage of the future.[25] He also points out that that it was the haruspices who introduced the idea that a prodigy may portend something favorable.[26] His idea of development would seem to be supported by Weinstock's finding (1951) that the Etruscan haruspices, more inclined to a degree of interpretation anyway, were influenced by Greek horoscopic astrology in their interpretation of lightning in the Hellenistic period, though it would clearly be risky to be precise about the timing of the shift. For North this "adjustment" to more explicit prophecy is not a significant change but, rather, a minor issue. Yet, if Bloch is right, at least to note a process of development, this links interestingly with the gradual disappearance of the reporting of prodigies, documented by MacBain (1982), which begins with the Social War (91–87 B.C.). This disappearance at least is a dramatic shift; whether it is a change in the perception of what is worth reporting in the sources or a change on the ground is unimportant. MacBain focuses on the end of the need for a symbolic unification of Italy, with Rome's grant of citizenship to the defeated Italians, as an isolable factor contributing to the shift. He notes Livy's famous comment from the perspective of the Augustan period: "I am not unaware that, because of the same heedlessness that leads people generally to believe that the gods foretell nothing, no prodigies at all are announced in public or reported in histories" (43.13.1), and, most interestingly, observes that the public prodigy gives way increasingly to the private omen relating to the personal fortunes of the great military figures of the Late Republic and to the emperors after them. He cites the last twenty books of Julius Obsequens's *Book of Prodigies,* which cover 86–12 B.C., together with Suetonius' *Lives of the Caesars.*

We may expect political shifts to be mirrored in religious shifts in Rome, since religious activity is so much a part of the political process. Here is surely the crux of the matter: there is a process of mutual reflection between religious and political institutions because they are aspects of the same power relations. North, who takes his cue from this perspective, focuses on the lack of a single identifiable authority in charge of all this religious activity and links this with the diffusion of political power characteristic of "middle" Republican institutions. None of the people in the three groups mentioned above functioned exclusively as diviners or, indeed, as religious officials, nor were they the only people responsible for divination. Both the taking of auspices and the public sacrifices necessary for extispicy to take place were mainly the province of magistrates. North also points to the further involvement of "lower-class" specialists, experts in the techniques of sacrificing (*victimarii, popae*) or of the reading of the auspices (*pullarii*). Possibly the *haruspices* who read the *exta* (in contrast to the Etruscan *haruspices*) were of this social level.[27] Thus, we have, in its hierarchical organization, almost a mirror of society. Further, the Senate maintained ultimate control over religious matters and does not seem to have been generally compelled either to request or to act on priestly advice.[28]

North brings out the particular style of middle republican divinatory activity by contrasting it with that of the Greek μάντις (prophet): it "a) lacks emphasis on specifically prophetic utterance, b) lacks identifiable prophets or holy men, c) produces anonymous teams of diviners who display an oblique, or reticent relationship to their divinatory techniques." The μάντις, on the other hand, might typically be commemorated by name, with the emphasis on his heroic achievement and ancestral tradition. North also tentatively contrasts this with the Etruscan tradition, in which *haruspices* are individually commemorated in at least one monument,[29] and with the individual diviners celebrated in the myths of the regal period.

In Rome, at least, the celebrated individual diviner is to be associated with the powerful individual. This shift from groups of diviners who remain unnamed to celebrated individuals can be related to the shift from expiation to more complex interpretation. The celebration of individuals is related to their possession of specialized, complex skills, of which the most highly valued is specific prophetic utterance. Cicero's *On Divination* reveals that by the first century B.C. the simple yes-or-no response of the sacred fowl to questions of a ritual nature attracted a good deal of scorn from some quarters.[30] Something more sophisticated, more in tune with the new Greek learning, was required. Further, the records of divinatory activity in the republic do not seem to suggest that its role in decision making was an important one. Something that promised more precise guidance was likely to appeal to the powerful individuals now emerging. Even if these functionalist explanations are too crude, what clearly is important is that the keeping of a personal diviner serves as a sign of the appropriation of power.

Indeed, it is with the return of the individual diviner and his specialist skills from the monarchical past that the political stage is set for the entrance of the astrologer. The collapse of the balanced distribution of power that constituted the Republic was signaled by the reappearance of such figures in tandem with the new political giants: Gaius Gracchus and his loyal friend Herennius Siculus (father or grandfather of a consul), who acted as his personal *haruspex,*[31] Sulla and his Gaius Postumus,[32] and Caesar's Spurinna,[33] (though Caesar is associated with a contemptuous attitude, being above divinatory advice when it suited him). Verres, the provincial governor accused of extortion who was prosecuted by Cicero, is also given his *haruspex,* Volusius; perhaps Cicero is here offering a parody of greatness.[34] These diviners are *haruspices,* but they are not the anonymous members of an official group established for consultation by the Senate.[35] There had always been *haruspices* for private divination, but they do not show up significantly in the records we have. The effect of their reappearance in this semipublic capacity is to make it seem as if they have come loose from their political moorings in the same way as their patrons. It was these diviners, above all, who were to find themselves facing astrologers, from outside the official religion altogether, as rivals.

Since astrology has not attracted much serious attention from historians, there has been little attempt to give any historical explanation of its relatively sudden rise to prominence. Much has been attributed to the influence of the Stoic Posidonius on elite Romans in the generation before Cicero and Caesar in making astrology intellectually respectable. But, as A. A. Long (1982) observes, the older authorities who formed this consensus, such as Cumont, were writing at a time when it was fashionable to see Posidonius' trademark everywhere.[36] Long rightly casts a skeptical eye over the evidence for Stoic enthusiasm for astrology in the early period. It is true that in Stoicism the existence of the gods requires divination[37] and that astrology would suit the Stoic search for natural signs revealing the order of the universe, but the evidence is scanty.[38] Long also has doubts about Posidonius' interest in astrology, although he admits that the evidence in favor of Posidonius' interest is more impressive than that for the early Stoics.[39] This is the period in which horoscopic astrology takes off in the Hellenistic world, and it could be seen as a natural move from other sorts of divination. He concludes, however, that astrology was at most a subordinate feature of Stoic interest in divination.

Long is surely right to recognize that the Stoics cannot be convincingly isolated as the determining factor in the rise to prominence of astrology in Rome, though he overstates the case against their interest, in this period. It seems clear that Stoic ideas, as generally diffused among the ruling elite, did lend themselves to the support of astrology, and that their concept of cosmic συμπάθεια (harmony) binding together the heavens and the earth became the first axiom of philosophical astrology. It was already prominent in the work of the Augustan Manilius. But surely equally important in preparing the ground was the place in an aristocratic education of a basic knowledge of the stars, their myths, and meteorological associations, thanks perhaps largely to the concerns of Alexandrian poetry.[40] Varro illustrates the extent to which the stars have become part of the curriculum: he devotes the entire ninth book of his *Disciplines* to *astronomia.*

As I have been arguing, however, it is to changes in the political arena in the first instance that one must look in order to make sense of the change in status of the discipline. It is hardly an accident that the rise of astrology coincides with the fall of the Republic. The first Roman aristocrat we find associated with a belief in astrology was the consul Octavius, killed when Cinna and Marius took Rome in 86 B.C. According to Plutarch, the astrological diagram that lured him to his death was found with his dead body.[41] Less dramatically, Plutarch also records that Sulla, apparently not content with the advice of his *haruspex,* was advised by Chaldeans too.[42] By the time of Pompey, Crassus, and Julius Caesar, contemporary evidence shows astrology preparing to play a major political role.[43] In Lucan, Nigidius Figulus, the polymathic friend of Cicero, who was the first Roman astrologer of eminence, is portrayed as employing astrology as Caesar crosses the Rubicon to prophesy the end of the astral cycle and the beginning of a new era.[44] Suetonius, another later source, attributes predictions of imperial power for Octavian in 63 and 45/44 B.C. and for Tiberius in 42.[45] What is significant is the nature of the stereotypical role of astrology, whether the cases are well founded or not. Crucially, horoscopic astrology is associated with the struggle for *individual* power.

We have already seen that the political changes that prepared the way for astrologers also threw the individual *haruspex* into prominence. There was now a certain rivalry between the two arts. While the *haruspices* had tradition and the state religion on their side, the astrologers had their novelty, and, where the *haruspices* specialized in prodigies, the astrologers could provide both answers to immediate questions (catarchic astrology) and information about the whole of life. But there was also a certain crossover. If the references to one Sudines as both an astrologer and a *haruspex* do not simply reflect later confusion, this goes back to the third century.[46] Both Nigidius Figulus and Varro seem to have tried to compare and perhaps combine the two disciplines, and Tarutius of Firmum, the learned astrologer and friend of Varro and Cicero, who calculated the horoscope of Rome,[47] was, argues Bouché-Leclercq (1896), a *haruspex* who extended his interests beyond his original art. Furthermore, Weinstock (1950) argues persuasively that Gaius Fonteius Capito, interpreter of the Etruscan Books of Tages and the author of the work on thunder (*Tonitruale*), which combines astrological elements with the traditional haruspical brontoscopy, of which fragments survive, was also a contemporary of Varro.[48] Apart from the interpretation of lightning and other celestial phenomena, there were common domains of interest in the finding of divine or astral influence on the viscera.

The evidence cited in Bouché-Leclercq (1896) and Weinstock (1951) suggests that it was the *haruspices* who were modernizing their art with astrological additions. But *haruspices* did not entirely give way to astrologers. Sulla, seemingly undecided about whose merits were greater, seems to have lent an ear to both a *haruspex* and an astrologer.[49] And *haruspices* do continue to figure in such tales for a long time: Tiberius reinforced the Augustan edict of A.D. 11 with particular reference to *haruspices;* it was by haruspical techniques that his father gave a prophecy of imperial power for Vespasian;[50] Larginus Proculus, described by Suetonius as a *haruspex,* was said to have predicted Domitian's death by the haruspical technique of brontoscopy, though another source describes him as an astrologer;[51] and several *haruspices* were reported by the third-century historian Dio Cassius to have warned Caracalla to beware of 8 April (79.7.2). Severus Alexander was supposedly well versed in haruspicy and augury as well as astrology; *haruspices* predicted his rule and an astrologer predicted his death.[52] Torelli (1975) finds epigraphic evidence of *haruspices* up to the third century at least. In A.D. 319 Constantine forbade private consultation, only traditional public haruspicy being allowed.[53] As late as Aurelian, there is a prohibition on soldiers' consulting them. But the signs in the Republic were that *haruspices* were losing their grip on political life.

A crucial occasion for the rivalry of these two divinatory styles was, of course, the *Iulium sidus,* the comet that appeared shortly after the death of Julius Caesar and shone for seven days during some games Octavian was celebrating.[54] The *haruspices,* with their expertise in interpreting thunder, could attach the appearance of comets to a ready-made theory. Comets were for them a species of lightning, inflamed torches hurled by thundering deities. Their official interpretation was that the comet presaged a new order. One Baebius Macer reports that the *haruspex* Vulcanius went before a popular assembly proclaiming that the comet was a sign of the end of the ninth (penultimate) *saeculum,* an ominous prediction,[55] though a favorable version could suggest that a glorious new era would be inaugurated under a savior. Also according to his prediction, he collapsed and died in the assembly. It was hardly a hopeful inauguration of a new era.

There was clearly some disagreement about the meaning of the portent. Dio Cassius (45.7.1) says that, while some called it a comet and associated it with the usual (negative) consequences, the majority ascribed it to Caesar, interpreting it to mean that he had become immortal, a version accepted gladly, if not actively supported by Octavian. He was reported by Suetonius as having a star put on the head of Caesar's statue.[56] This notion of catasterism, or translation to the stars, had more in common with astrological beliefs in their most popular form. Astrologers did concern themselves with comets and doubtless had their say on this one.[57] Interestingly, Pliny, having quoted the official version from Augustus' memoirs, suggests that Octavian secretly saw the comet as the star of his new birth as the adopted son of Caesar, an interpretation Cramer ascribes to Theogenes, who had, according to Suetonius, already functioned as his astrological advisor.[58] This must, of course, remain speculation. At any rate, the *haruspices'* traditional authority was clearly being eroded.

Astrology offered a particularly appropriate style of legitimation, in its more sophisticated development of the familiar beliefs in the signifying power of the heavens, a new designer version of the old omen lore for the individuals who had ousted the chorus as protagonists on the political stage. It, like traditional divination, was a learning dependent on books, but it promised to answer better the new demands made of traditional divination, demands for subtlety and precise information.

Astrology Established: The Role of Capricorn

Astrology was firmly constructed as a legitimator with Augustus's establishment of the principate.[59] The *Iulium sidus* belonged to the realm of traditional omens, but the *princeps*'s publication of his birth sign on coins to be seen all over the empire accorded astrology a new, superior status. Suetonius says that Augustus made his horoscope (*thema*) public and issued a silver coin with Capricorn, his birth sign, on it. He attributes Octavian's confidence to a consultation with the astrologer Theogenes in 44 B.C. and sets the publication of the horoscope some unspecified time soon afterward.[60] As Libra was Augustus' Sun sign, there has long been some debate about the role of Capricorn: both signs are given prominence by the poets.[61] Bouché-Leclerq and others argue that it was the "chronocrator" of the month of conception (the sign designated as presiding over that month), despite Suetonius' specification that it was his birth sign. Meanwhile, Riess (1896) and others argue that, as the sign in which the Moon was at the hour of the birth, it was the determining "birth sign." Gundel (1926) argues that it was the sign in which Augustus's "Lot of Fortune" was to be found as well as where the Moon was, which would help explain the cases in which Capricorn is to be found portrayed with the attributes of Fortune and Manilius' use of *felix* of Capricorn.[62]

Whatever Capricorn's precise relation to Augustus's birth, it is probably significant that it was seen as the birth sign of the Sun, in that the winter solstice takes place in Capricorn. According to Suetonius, he was born just before the sun rose. As Dwyer (1976) points out, a clever astrologer could have suggested to the young Octavian that Capricorn was an auspicious sign for this reason. Given the associations the *princeps* cultivated with the sun and Apollo in the early years, it fits well.[63] Dwyer himself suggests that, on the basis of Nigidius Figulus' commentary on the sign of Capricorn, it is to be associated with Pan and his role in restoring the rule of the gods, saving the world from the tyranny of the Titans. He goes further and suggests that, before Actium, the theme of the righteous revenge of the son is implied by the myth narrated by Nigidius. Thus, Capricorn may have first of all symbolized Octavian's just revenge on the killers of his adoptive father, Julius Caesar, and, only after Actium, liberation from tyranny. Capricorn is also associated with rule over the West in the poets.[64] Dwyer connects Capricorn's rule over the West with Aeneas' westward journey. In addition to all this speculation, it is worth noting that Augustus's principate was inaugurated under Capricorn.[65]

Kraft (1967), who provides photographs of several examples, argues that the appearance of Capricorn on coins from at least 41/40 B.C. onward is to be linked in another way with Octavian's careful self-presentation. He claims that the sign was used first of all against Mark Antony. The first surviving coin with the sign of Capricorn may have been minted by Q. Oppius, the *praefectus classis* (prefect of the fleet) based at Cyrene in 41/40, a partisan of Octavian, who set Capricorn by the head of the Venus of the Julian family, sometimes with the half-moon.[66] Glass pastes and cameos with Capricorn on them, mainly Italian, were also produced before Actium. Examples show Capricorn with a bearded Octavian; or a young Octavian's head over a ring (Caesar's signet ring, pointing to his heirship), with Capricorn, corn ears and a poppy; or with a child riding on its back over the waves, identified as Octavian and dated to the 40s.[67] Hölscher even identifies one depiction of Capricorn on a glass paste as dating from the period of reconciliation with Antony, as Octavian's head is placed above the intertwined signs of Capricorn and Leo, Antony's conception sign.[68] But the sign only played a small role in the public presentation of Octavian before Actium. The first appearance of Capricorn on Augustus's own coins in 28 B.C. was on the obverse of a *denarius* (silver coin) from the Eastern mint, together with Augustus's head, with the crocodile of Egypt and the legend *Aegypto capta* (Egypt taken), referring to the victory over Antony. *Aurei* (gold coins) and *denarii* of the same type followed, while from 27–20 B.C. *tetradrachms* (coins worth three *denarii*) from Asia showed Capricorn with a cornucopia on its back.

How were these representations of Capricorn connected with the "propaganda war" against Antony, in Kraft's view? One of the later coins (19–16/5 B.C.) may depict a figure identified as Eileithyia, goddess of birth, with Capricorn.[69] Two years before, the Senate had declared the birthday of Octavian a lucky day, to be celebrated annually, while that of Antony was to become an unlucky day (Dio Cassius 51.19.2–3). The gist of the message of the coins Kraft translates as follows. Octavian "was born" (under Capricorn), in a frequently used phrase going back to Cicero, "to save the Roman State" (*natus ad reipublicae salutem*), born to be the *vindex libertatis populi Romani* (defender of the freedom of the Roman people).[70] *Libertatis vindex* was the legend on the Asian coin (*cistophorus*) of 28 B.C., which was followed in 27 by two series of *cistophori* with Capricorn as one of three reverses, a series traced to Chios.[71] In both the *Libertatis vindex* coin and the Capricorn coins the reverse is always surrounded with an Apolline laurel wreath, which seems to have been specifically designed in opposition to Mark Antony's Dionysiac ivy wreath.[72] The birth sign was found in conjunction with the *clipeus* (shield) and the *corona civica* (civic crown), referring to the honors given Augustus by the Senate in 27 B.C., in Spanish coin issues, both of Augustus and of Tiberius, in his memory. It was also found on coins from the Eastern mint with the legend *Signis (Parthicis) receptis,* referring to his diplomatic victory over the Parthians of 20 B.C., an achievement meant to wipe out the shame of three defeats,[73] the last two of which were associated with Antony. While Augustus was born to save the state, then, Antony was born to destroy it.

Coins also show Capricorn together with a rudder, globe, and cornucopia, the marine and terrestrial attributes of the goddess *Bona Fortuna,* which fits with Gundel's association of Capricorn with Augustus's Lot of Fortune. The globe surely also refers to Augustus's *potestas* (power) over land and sea. They first appeared in the East and from 20 B.C. in the West. One coin with a cornucopia, from the Lugdunum Mint, is found with the legend *IMP. XI* (referring to the number of triumphs celebrated by Augustus), which suggests a date after Tiberius' Pannonian War in 12 B.C. For Hölscher, above all, taking all these particular associations into account, the Capricorn is guarantor of the *aurea aetas* (golden age). The variety of ingenious interpretations possible illustrates the flexibility of astrology as a tool of legitimation and the condensation of meaning possible in one symbol.

Capricorn is also found in apparently private contexts, on a vast number of antefixes (the terracotta fixtures on gables), some as late as the second century A.D. On these the goddess of Victory holds two Capricorns by their tails or is simply depicted between them. On the most common type Victory stands on a globe from which the Capricorns project. The antefixes seem to have originally represented a trophy that must be associated with Actium, perhaps the statue that Augustus erected in the newly dedicated Senate House after his Actium triumph in 29 B.C., as Hölscher suggests.[74] He also comments that the antefixes' wide dissemination in Rome and central Italy indicates the extent to which the people could show in their private as well as their public possessions their identification with Augustus's new era of peace after the end of the civil war. It is significant that a theme such as *Victoria,* made so public by its dissemination on coins, usually with a different set of elements, is also found in these less-public contexts. The Capricorns on the pediment of the *lararium* (shrine of the household deities) of the House of Menander are another example, probably related to the imperial cult.[75]

But in most cases in which the Capricorn is displayed we can tell that it is not there in a purely personal capacity but, instead, as a statement of a link to the imperial house. The heraldic style of the double, opposed Capricorns holding a *clipeus* is found, for instance, on a fresco in Stabiae, in the "Room of the Planisphere" off a portico whose roof tiles link it explicitly with Narcissus, *Augusti libertus* (former slave of the emperor).[76] Many instances are fragments of temples of the imperial cult, as with altar reliefs from Bologna and Rome, and the capital from the temple of Augustus in Puteoli.[77] Another marble bas-relief from Carthage, of Augustus's head with Capricorn in the same position as on the Vienna cameo (see below), may have been linked with the imperial cult.[78] Several of the bas-reliefs from Gaul showing Capricorns are related to the legion XXII *Primigenia* (founded in 39 by Caligula), though not all can be traced. In fact there were five legions with the sign of Capricorn in the area anyway.[79] From Pannonia Inferior there is a gravestone of the latter half of the first century A.D. with Capricorns, globe, and lunar crescent from the legionary camp of Ulcisia (north of Budapest), which presumably relates to one of these legions. A sarcophagus from the same province now in Budapest (Capricorn with globe) may be similarly explained, as may a tombstone from Piedmont with Capricorn and lunar crescent, though Cumont suggests that the frequent appearance of Capricorn on tombstones may be connected with its role as the gate through which souls ascended to the sky.[80] It is clear, anyway, that the sign was extremely widely disseminated throughout the empire from Augustus onward.

While cheap glass pastes, such as those made before Actium, may have been used for gifts to political clients, even mass-produced for recruitment, gems are one group of artifacts designed for restricted circulation. Some of the motifs on the coins recur, while those such as the portrayal of Augustus as Neptune after Actium tend to be restricted to the gems. In one gem Capricorn seems to stand for Augustus: a carnelian shows Capricorn with globe and trident. Here, as in the Stabiae fresco, is something like a coat of arms.[81] The "Actium victory cameo,"[82] a costly sardonyx piece, is another example. It shows on the obverse a togate Augustus in a *quadriga* (four-horse chariot) drawn by tritons over the sea, triumphantly holding up a branch and a scepter. However, familiar motifs from the coins recur. The front of the chariot is decorated by a *corona civica,* and the two outermost tritons hold globes in their upraised right hands. A victory bearing a crown surmounts the globe of the triton on the left, while two Capricorns bearing the *clipeus virtutis* surrounded by a laurel crown top the globe held by the triton on the right. A less costly sardonyx cameo shows Augustus with the laurel crown of victory, held up by two Capricorns.[83] This, dated to A.D 10–14, is one of a frequent type, popular from Augustus onward, showing a pair of Capricorns, tails outward, supporting Augustus's head on the *clipeus virtutis* or on a portrait medallion, itself surrounded by a laurel crown.[84]

The famous *gemma augustea* of Vienna,[85] or Vienna cameo, shows the potential of gems to present a complex variety of themes; indeed, this gem verges on the category of a historical relief, as Hölscher (1988) comments. This precious article certainly belonged to a rich owner, perhaps even to a member of the imperial household.[86] Here the sign of Capricorn is linked with a variety of features typical of Augustan self-presentation. Augustus is portrayed as the *cosmocrator* (ruler of the universe) in heroic seminakedness on a double throne under which Jupiter's eagle has alighted, holding a scepter in his left hand and in his right a *lituus,* the augur's crook, which shows that wars are fought under his auspices. On the left throne is *Dea Roma. Oecumene* (the inhabited world) is crowning Augustus with the *corona civica, Oceanus/Chronos/*Saturn is in front, while *Tellus* (the earth), or *Italia,* with a cornucopia in her lap, together with two children, leans against the throne. All faces are turned toward Augustus. The sign of Capricorn, on a disk with rays on it (the Julian star, or the sun), is between the heads of *Roma* and Augustus, whose feet rest on the weapons of conquered enemies. Center-left is a figure who seems to be dressed as the *princeps iuventutis* (leader of the youth), presumably Germanicus. The gem can be dated from the depiction of the figure descending from a triumphal chariot on the left. According to Pollini, this is the occasion of Tiberius' solemn entry to Rome, a triumph over the Illyrians having been postponed after the Varian disaster.[87] The barbarians on the right then refer to the future: it seems that Tiberius is on his way to Germany in A.D. 10. The Scorpion on the trophy being erected by a Roman legionary may refer to Tiberius' birth sign. Hölscher (1988) supports this view by suggesting that this is an important link between the upper and lower parts of the gem, as the standard is directly below Tiberius, and part of its subtle symmetry in reflecting Augustus' sign. Here, then, astral backing for the whole dynasty, from Julius Caesar to Germanicus, may be implied.

The birth sign of Augustus was an important feature of the public presentation of Augustus all over the empire, showing him as destined for his historic role. It was taken up again, first by Tiberius, in his twentieth year, who issued Augustan coin types,[88] and then by later emperors sporadically, often in cases in which their legitimacy was in question.[89] Hölscher notes that Capricorn might have special meaning for the Flavians, as the sign under which Vespasian took power and

Domitian began his reign. It was also very often used by Titus, whose Sun sign it was: he could with justification claim faith in his destiny.[90] It was a feature that recurred in imperial art up till the third century A.D., presumably in an attempt to appropriate Augustus's success and claim legitimate succession to that ideal. In this later usage, Hölscher argues, the theme is above all of peace and security. What is striking is that Augustus seems to have been the first to bring the sign to such prominence. The only Hellenistic forerunners to these themes were the Capricorns used on the coins of Ptolemy, king of Mauretania, and on autonomous pieces of Sabrata and other African towns.[91]

And no other star sign achieved comparable status. I have been able to discover only one coin from the early empire in which the same idea was followed with another sign. This was a silver minting of Queen Pythodoris Philometor of Pontus, with Tiberius' head on the obverse and the sign of Libra, with a star between the scales, on the reverse. This is clearly paired with an issue of three years later showing Augustus with Capricorn.[92] It is true that there are the different zodiac signs on legionary standards, which Domaszewski (1892) tried to associate with the birth signs of different founders, arguing that Caesar's legions had Taurus, Augustus' Capricorn, and Tiberius' Scorpio. In fact, as Ritterling (1925) argues, this is clearly not the only reason for the choice of legionary badges. Domaszewski was right, however, to draw attention to the preeminence of zodiacal, or star, names for the standards, and the case remains strong for a link between Julius Caesar and Taurus (implying a link with the House of Venus?) and between Augustus and Capricorn.[93] But the problem of Tiberius' birth sign is not yet solved. He was born on 16 November,[94] which would suggest that the sun was in the last degree of Scorpio. Yet the place of Libra in the last book of Manilius (4.558)[95] and the coin of Queen Pythodoris made Voigt (1899) suggest that Libra was Tiberius' sign. Perhaps both Scorpio and Libra played their roles in his horoscope: Housman (1913) points out that the Moon on his birthday was in Libra.

It is also worth mentioning, in the context of Augustan ideological use of astrology, an important element of Augustus' monumental complex on the northern side of the Campus Martius (the Field of Mars). The obelisk that stands in Piazza Montecitorio, in front of the Italian Parliament in Rome, was the Gnomon, or shadow caster of a giant instrument (the *Horologium Augusti*), as it says on the inscription of the pope who moved it in the eighteenth century. The instrument was described by Pliny as a marvel in his *Natural History* (36.72). Augustus had the ship that carried the obelisk laid up in dry dock in Puteoli for all to see (36.70). Buchner (1988), in his excavations, uncovered part of the north-south bronze meridian line, with the remains of names of the signs of the zodiac and reference to the seasons (in Greek) along it. It was, however, at a higher level than the Augustan instrument and had probably been resited higher up, perhaps by

Domitian in his restoration of the area in A.D. 80, in order to compensate for the rising of the Tiber. Buchner's dramatic discovery seemed to substantiate his claims for the shape of the whole structure on the ground, yet a recent article has cast doubt on the reconstruction.[96]

Buchner claimed that the instrument was a sundial, telling the time of day, as well as a meridian instrument, recording the extent of the sun's shadow at noon each day and, therefore, the progress of the days of the year, marked by day lines. Schutz shows that there is no justification for regarding the instrument as more than a meridian line, recording the progress of the sun through the zodiac. There was no intricate network of lines. Buchner used his reconstruction of the line network to show that there was a complex and precise relationship between the instrument and other monuments on the Campus Martius. Schutz's arguments not only destroy the line network but also show that Buchner's choice of the exact site of the obelisk was made arbitrarily, in order to establish the connections with the other monuments.

Buchner's argument was that the obelisk was turned to face the Mausoleum of Augustus, which had been erected fifteen years before, and that it was also orientated in relation to the Ara Pacis (the Altar of Peace, dedicated to Augustus by the Senate in 9 B.C.). Indeed, his theory was that on Augustus's birthday, the shadow moved about a hundred meters along the equinoctial line, to point directly toward the altar in the evening. Buchner followed Kraft's line in seeing this as a visual representation of the idea that Augustus is *natus ad pacem* (born for peace). He also saw the globe on the top of the obelisk, mentioned by Pliny, as the image of Augustus's domination of the world.[97]

Unfortunately, it seems that any relationship between the instrument and the monuments concerning Augustus's death and achievement in bringing peace is a general one resulting from their being sited near each other, rather than a precise geometrical one. Furthermore, Augustus's birthday is no longer especially significant in this.

Some elements of this ideological complex remain, however. The obelisk was from Heliopolis, the City of the Sun, in Egypt. It was undoubtedly connected with Augustus's association of himself with the Sun, by means of Apollo. It was the first of Rome's many obelisks and also represented the peace that came after victory over "Egypt" (over Mark Antony). Furthermore, we know from Pliny that the instrument was designed so that the edge of the paving coincided with the day of the winter solstice, the day when the sun's shadow at noon was at its longest. Thereafter, the shadow moved back down the line until the summer solstice. Thus, the role of Capricorn was made visible, at least to those who could read Greek. With Augustus began a new day and a new era.

The obelisk in Schutz's reconstruction was in fact even larger than in Buchner's, thirty-one meters rather than twenty-two, and, even if the paved area was much less wide, the instrument must have dominated this part of the Campus Martius. It is striking that on the base of the Antonine column recording the resting place of Antoninus and Faustina, there is a depiction of the obelisk held by the genius of the Campus Martius opposite *Roma.*[98] Together with the other monuments in the area, in particular the Mausoleum, this was a project that was far more appropriate to a monarch than to a great man of the Republic, and it was perhaps more acceptable in an area under Agrippa's control, which was technically outside the city.[99]

In an even grander gesture of public faith in his stars, according to Dio Cassius, Augustus actually published his horoscope "in a decree."[100] Gundel argues that this publication of his horoscope may have been a move to quell rumors of his impending death, which were caused by a comet.[101] Though this is difficult to prove, it would nicely symbolize the shift from the older style of omen lore to the new. We have seen how Augustan artists were quick to pick up on the new style of legitimation; we shall see that the poets did not neglect it.

Astrology Established: Poets, Philosophers, and Other Intellectuals

Augustus's publication of his astral backing (in whatever form) is a dramatic indication of the political construction of astrology as knowledge, which leads me to stop the chronological narrative and take stock of the status of the discipline in general. I referred in the introduction to an embarrassment among scholars when it came to astrology and to the existence of descendants of the Sartonian view that the honorable course for people of any era was to be skeptical of the validity of the discipline. This may be seen in the way in which students of the period often undervalue the contemporary intellectual status of astrology. This tendency is perhaps more evident in the case of historians of philosophy, who are often concerned to defend philosophers of whom they approve from contamination by astrological beliefs.[102] There were certainly philosophers who did take astrology seriously, most notably Stoics, but it is important to remember that philosophers were not the only authenticators of knowledge in the ancient world. I shall be returning to the question of the sense in which astrology becomes knowledge throughout this chapter, but there are one or two points to be made here in order to clarify the situation.

First, there was a relatively sudden move to general acceptance and wide use of astrology among the elite. Perhaps the most obvious sign of astrology's new popularity was the adoption of planets' names for days of the week. This relied on the astrological concept of planets as "rulers of time." Augustan literature also furnishes ample evidence of the way in which astral lore suddenly became fashionable in court circles. Bouché-Leclercq refers to it as "*une manie littéraire.*"[103]

Augustan poets could build on traditional Alexandrian literary themes but give them a new emphasis. Catasterism, or translation to the stars, following the eponymously titled work attributed to Eratosthenes, is a favorite theme. It becomes the ordinary form of compliment to a great man. A place for Augustus in heaven is offered between Scorpio and Virgo by Virgil,[104] Germanicus in his Latin version of Aratus refers to Capricorn's taking Augustus up to heaven.[105] Ovid follows suit, and it is in his *Metamorphoses* and *Fasti* most of all that catasterism becomes the natural end to many a legend.[106] In Horace not only is there reference to the Julian star but also to his pondering a poem on Augustus's translation to the stars.[107] Dicks (1963) finds a further ten references to catasterism in Horace, including a tongue-in-cheek proposal to catasterize the usual butt of his insults, Canidia, in an epode in which he proposes to recant to avoid her spells (17.41).

Aratus of Soli, who in about 280 B.C. composed the *Phaenomena,* a versification of Eudoxus' astronomical treatises, was, of course, the ultimate Alexandrian model for writing about the stars. Montanari Caldini (1973) has shown the way in which Germanicus (if he was the author) has altered his model in his "translation" of the Greek poet's famous poem on celestial phenomena and the weather to take account of contemporary astrological ideas. This shows particularly in the fragments of his *Prognostica,* in which, departing from Aratus, he considers the meteorological effects of each of the zodiac signs, the movement of the planets through the signs, their phases, and their "stations." Admittedly, he only delineates the effects generically and restricts himself to astrometeorology, in order not to depart too much from his model. Virgil, likewise restricted by his models, in the *Georgics* only discusses the stars as signs of the seasons, though he refers twice to the stars as knowing destiny in the *Aeneid* (4.519, 9.429).[108] Some felt constrained to offer *excusationes* (excuses) for failing to deal with this type of subject.[109] On the other hand, Manilius, the author of the *Astronomica,* who is clearly an astrologer only at second hand, is actually attempting to be a modern Aratus, writing a new kind of didactic poem for the new order.

This is the only work of this period fully occupied with astrology that has survived; for the most part it is the extra ingredient that is de rigueur. Compliments, for instance, gain a touch of class with an astrological allusion, as in Horace's *Odes* 2.17.17–25. Here he congratulates Maecenas on having escaped with the help of Jupiter the baleful influence of Saturn on an occasion in the theater and talks of the harmony of the stars controlling their destinies, in a passage in which the use of technical astrological terms is evident. Horace has himself, he says, been saved from a falling tree by Faunus (who has associations with Mercury). Insults similarly look more impressive with astrological allusions. Ovid, in his *Ibis,* attacks his addressee:

> You were born unlucky . . . no star was favourable or propitious at your birth, Venus didn't shine, nor did Jupiter in that hour, neither sun nor moon were in an auspicious place, and he whom shining Maia bore of great Jupiter didn't direct his rays in any way profitable for you. On you weighed the star of Mars, who only presages savagery, nothing ever peaceable and the star of the aged wielder of the scythe. (209–16)

Equally, consolations are felt to gain force from reference to celestial events: the author of a *Consolation to Livia,* on the death of Drusus, assures her that at his passing:

> Sidera quin etiam caelo fugisse feruntur,
> Lucifer et solitas destituisse vias:
> Luciferin toto nulli comparuit orbe.
> Et venit stella non praeunte dies:
> Sideris hoc obitum terris instare monebat
> et mergi Stygia nobile lumen aqua. (405–8)

> Indeed they say also that constellations fled the sky and Lucifer left his usual path: Lucifer was seen by no one in the whole world. And day came without the star appearing first. This warned that a star's destruction threatened the earth and that a noble light would be submerged in Stygian water.[110]

In other passages Horace warns Leuconoe not to inquire by means of the stars into the length of their lives and refers in passing to his *Genius,* as the *natale comes qui temperat astrum.*[111] Propertius allows astrology more than a passing mention, actually allowing half a poem to an astrologer called Horus, a son of Babylonian Horops, who proceeds to produce the proofs of his knowledge of the art at tedious length, before advising the poet to write elegy and to beware of the Crab, perhaps referring to the "decan" belonging to Venus.[112]

One of the more amusing aspects of the fashion for astrology is the way in which traditional seers are suddenly presented as knowledgeable about the stars from Augustan poetry onward. Anyone with claims to knowledge of the future cannot ignore astrology and maintain credibility, as Bouché-Leclercq has commented. Virgil makes Aeneas add astrology to Helenus' oracular and augural skills and gives the Etruscan Asilas the ability to read the stars as well as entrails, auspices, and thunder. Calchas, according to Propertius' astrologer, neglected astrology to his cost, while in Statius' *Thebaid,* the poet, commenting on the folly of divination in connection with Amphiaraus and Melampus, includes astrology in the divinatory arts.[113] A sign of the extent to which astral matters have pervaded poetry is given by Quintilian's recommendation, in his *Oratorical Instruction* (1.4.4), to his pupils that they should learn *astronomia* to understand the poets.

Poets were traditionally the fount of wisdom in antiquity, and in this case they do furnish some index of the general attitude to astrology. The assertion of F. E. Robbins in the introduction to the Loeb edition of Ptolemy's *Tetrabiblos* that "with few exceptions everyone from emperor to lowest slave believed in it" may seem a little sweeping in the face of the problems of evidence that are always with us in the study of the ancient world. If, however, we substitute *took seriously* for *believed,* it is on balance easier to support than to contradict this opinion.[114] Historians who have considered the question have broadly concurred with Robbins's view, which is itself derived from the authorities specifically concerned with the history of astrology.[115] In consideration of this question it is important not to assimilate ancient criticisms of astrology to modern rationalist objections.

There are three important points to be considered under the heading of ancient criticisms of astrology. First, philosophical objectors to astrology were mainly embroiled in arguments with other philosophical schools, and thus they fail to engage with astrology itself much of the time.[116] The arguments about free will and determinism, which I examine later in the context of the church, are a prime example. The philosophical objectors certainly fail to engage with scientific astrology, as represented by Ptolemy. Second, many criticisms of astrology can be understood in the context of the double image of people such as diviners and doctors, people who potentially wield the power of essential knowledge but are found in individual cases to be either pretenders to the art or abusers of it.[117] The argument that the disciplines are frequently let down by their practitioners is extremely common and the stereotypes of the Good and Bad experts omnipresent.[118] In the latter case condemnations of astrology are often moral objections that testify all the more to its power. Excessive commitment to it, such as is exhibited by bad emperors or women who ought not to be meddling with men's affairs anyway, as in Juvenal's sixth satire, is worthy of disapproval, but the art is rarely dismissed completely.

Some indications of how seriously it was in fact taken by a variety of intellectuals may be gained from close examination of their remarks. Skepticism may be mistakenly inferred by selective consideration of remarks without attention to context. Seneca, in the *Pumpkinification of Claudius,* makes cynical comments about the astrologers who were wrong about Claudius' death (3.2).[119] But in philosophical works he follows the Stoic line on astrology. In the *Consolation to Marcia* he writes of the Sun, Moon, stars, and five planets:

> . . . pursuing their different courses and striving to stem the headlong whirl of heaven. On even the slightest motion of these hang the fortunes of nations,

> and the greatest and smallest happenings are shaped to accord with the progress of a beneficent or maleficent star. (18.1–3)

The context attaches this view firmly to the Stoic universe bound by rigid laws and a fixed chain of causes. In the *Natural Questions* Seneca explains astrologers' mistakes:

> Since everything in nature moves according to the same laws of fate, all things may be signs for him who can read them. . . . Now the observations of the Chaldaeans take into account the powers of the five stars, but surely all those thousands of stars do not shine for nothing. What else is it that introduces such great errors into the work of those skilled in casting natal charts except that they allot so few stars to us? One star influences one person, another influences another. They carry on their work in duties that have been distributed among them. However it is more difficult to know what power they have than to doubt that they have power. (2.32.7–8)[120]

Here is the "double image" syndrome, in which respect for the art coexists with scorn for practitioners.

There is also ambivalence in Stoic attitudes to divination in general. Marcus Aurelius follows Epictetus in criticizing those who resort to divination when they have the resources within themselves to live well.[121] But Epictetus' remarks, though not addressed specifically to astrology, make it clear that it is the attitude toward divination that must be correct, not that one should not resort to it. There should be neither fear nor greed. Rather: "We should come without previous desire or aversion, as the traveller enquires the road of the person he meets without any desire for that which turns to the right rather than to the left" (*Discourses* 2.7.10).

The astrologer Firmicus Maternus enjoins a similar attitude in the first book of his *Mathesis*. As for Marcus, who used an astrologer himself,[122] he clearly sets the astrologer beside the doctor as a professional who has had many successes but, like every mortal, has limitations: "Hippocrates, after healing many a sick man, fell sick himself and died. Many a death have Chaldaeans foretold, and then their fate has overtaken them also" (*Meditations* 3.3, cf. 4.48.1).

A passage in which Tacitus comments on astrology has been taken for evidence about Stoic views.[123] The historian is discussing the question whether it is fate or chance that governs the revolutions of human affairs, in a rare personal digression brought on by the appearance in his narrative of the famous astrologer Thrasyllus, who appears as the man who taught Tiberius the art that enabled him to predict the future rule of Galba. Tacitus refers to the debates on this subject between the "wisest of the ancients and their disciples" and mentions a group of people who hold the conviction that heaven does not concern itself with the beginning or end of human life, or with people at all, and that therefore the good suffer while the evil prosper. These would most easily be seen as the Epicureans. He contrasts them with another group of people who believe that, though there is a harmony between Fate and events, it is not dependent on the wandering stars but, instead, on primary elements and on a combination of natural causes. This group leaves humans the capacity of choosing their lives, maintaining that, once the choice is made, there is a fixed sequence of events. Certainly, this would be the view of some Stoics, though not all.[124] It is not clear how much we may trust Tacitus as a source on philosophy. But aside from this question the view as it is somewhat confusedly expressed here is not necessarily at odds with astrology. It was never a Stoic view that everything ultimately depended on the stars, but only that the stars were a part of the chain of causes that went back finally to God/Nature.[125]

This passage is interesting for Tacitus' own views and for those that he attributes to most people. After his own statement of suspension of judgment on the question of free will and his cautious review of two streams of philosophical thought on the subject, he continues:

> Most men, however, cannot part with the belief that each person's future is fixed from his very birth, but that some things happen differently from what has been foretold through the impostures of those who describe what they do not know, and that this destroys the credit of a science, clear testimonies to which have been given both by past ages and by our own. (trans. M. Grant)

Significantly, he then seems to align himself with "most men" (*plurimis mortalium*) by promising immediately after this passage that he will relate Thrasyllus' son's correct prediction of Nero's death when the time comes.[126] These remarks of Tacitus, framed by two correct astrological predictions, are particularly important, because the generally positive attitude toward the validity of astrology must be set against the sardonic remarks he makes about astrologers elsewhere. These are presumably examples of those who destroy the credit of astrology by their impostures; Tacitus then is yet another illustration of the double image syndrome.

A couple of other cases may suffice here to indicate the pervasiveness of astrology in circles normally held up as examples of "rationalism" and "practicality." First, there is Vitruvius the engineer and author of *On Architecture,* probably written between 31 and 26 B.C. In relation to the subject of sundials he launches into an astronomical survey describing the movements of the Sun, Moon, and planets through the zodiac. He concludes, before moving on to the dials, with some remarks on astrology:

> For the rest, as to *astrologia,* the effects produced on the human course of life by the twelve signs, the five planets, the sun and moon, we must give way to the calculations [*ratiocinationes*] of the Chaldaean [astrologers], because the casting of nativities [*genethlialogiae ratio*] is special to them so that they can explain the past and the future from astronomical calculations. Those who have sprung from the Chaldaean nation have handed on their discoveries about matters in which they have approved themselves with great skill and subtlety. (9.6.2, trans. F. Granger)

He seems to have considered the discipline as a perfectly legitimate branch of astronomy.

Second, there is the very interesting case of Galen, which illustrates the danger of misinterpretation of skeptical remarks because of an urge to distance an ancestor of modern medicine from disreputable associations. Galen certainly ridicules Pamphilus' use of the "sacred herbs of the demons and decans" from a Hermetic text, as has often been pointed out.[127] Yet the polemic takes him in another direction in *On the Natural Faculties,* in which he sharply objects to the Methodist school of medicine whose members hold in contempt omens, dreams, portents, and any kind of astrology (πάσης ἀστρολογίας), and he says that he has dealt with these matters more fully in another book about Asclepiades.[128] In the Arabic version of his commentary on Hippocrates' *Airs, Waters, Places,* translated by Toomer (1985), he refers specifically to the *genethliakoi,* or natal astrologers. The passage is unfortunately fragmentary. Most are charlatans, he says (probably he is objecting to their lack of knowledge of astronomy and geometry, but he may be making this charge against doctors, as often), and then there is a lacuna, which the translator says logically demands some qualification along the lines of "but some are genuine scientists."[129] This would seem to be supported by his list of approved astronomers, which includes the astrologer Apollinarius.[130] And in the *On Prognosis* he sets ἀστρονομία, clearly in the context meaning astrology as well as astronomy, alongside other liberal arts abused by the rich and powerful in Rome:

> They do not see the particular beauty of each study and they cannot stand intellectuals. Geometry and arithmetic they need only in evaluating expenses and improving their mansions, ἀστρονομία [*astronomia*] and divination only in forecasting whose money they are going to inherit. (trans. Nutton, 72, 29–74, 2 = K.14.604–5)

Presumably, to judge from his *On the Critical Days,* the honorable use of astrology is in medicine (K.9.901ff.). Here, while refuting the application of number symbolism for judgment of the course of a disease, he advocates consideration of Moon phases, in particular throughout book 3,[131] but also of Moon phases in relation to the zodiac. He mentions the importance of the position of the Moon in the zodiac at conception and birth, or the beginning of anything, and further speaks of "benefic" and "malefic" planets and their effects in relation to the influential planets at birth, following "Egyptian astrologers," whose remarks on the effects of the moon he has found true (Egypt was the home of iatromathematics, or astrological medicine).[132] He is not prepared to discuss the causes of the effects of the aspects (K.9.913, 1ff.). No scholar has challenged the genuineness of this treatise, but it certainly poses a problem for those who would like to excise as spurious those parts of the Galenic corpus that take on board astrology.[133] Vivian Nutton is anxious to save Galen here; he says that Galen

> certainly did not accept without demur the teachings of the astrologers, far from it. . . . Whereas some of his contemporaries, like Pamphilus and Xenocrates, were less scrupulous about what they accepted, Galen's reliance upon astronomy and dreams is conditioned by the rational uses to which they are set and by the logical demonstration by which they are tested. (1979, 172)

Nutton seems to accept one of Galen's most common representations of himself here,[134] without considering how rational uses might differ in the contemporary context. In *On the Critical Days* Galen claims to have tested Egyptian astrologers against his experience; the interesting point is surely that astrology can be seen as a rational adjunct to medicine.

Astrology in Imperial Politics

As later Constantine was to make the Christian God his ally, so Augustus took the macrocosm as his, in a very public way. But it was not such a neat solution to legitimating his rule as it might first appear. Such an ally was by definition outside his control, for, if controllable, it would forfeit belief, since it had no tradition to sustain it. To put it another way, the *pax astrologica* was more difficult to maintain than the *pax deorum,* since astral legitimation was no imperial monopoly. While the Republican system of government always retained the possibility of being vulnerable to disturbance, it was hardly as pregnant with the seeds of dissension as the new astrological dispensation of imperial power. Augustus had to try to restrict access to this reservoir of power. It was in A.D. 11 that he issued an edict proscribing consultations either about death or without witnesses, an edict that was to see frequent use and revival under his successors.[135]

Perhaps because of the nature of our sources, it is in the reign of the next *princeps* that we first find the anecdotes illustrating the dangers of this new alliance. Tiberius is one of the emperors most strongly associated with astrology in our later sources, particularly where he is portrayed as the archetype of the "bad" emperor. At any rate, he elevated Thrasyllus, the man known as his teacher of astrology,[136] whom he met while in exile in Rhodes. Thrasyllus, an Alexandrian grammarian, was a versatile scholar, who remained long famous as an authority on astrology.[137] His elevation was such that he was able to found an illustrious dynasty, his great-grandson becoming a consul in 109.

Tiberius is portrayed as employing an occult cabinet: the satirist Juvenal represents the old emperor as shut up in Capri *cum grege Chaldaeo* (with a herd of astrologers).[138] Their job was to locate those marked out for great destinies, so that they could be destroyed (Dio Cassius 57.19.3–4). Similar stories are told of Domitian, another bad emperor par excellence:

> Domitian, of course, had not failed to take careful note of the days and hours when the foremost men had been born, and in consequence was destroying in advance not a few of these who were not even hoping for the attainment of power. (Dio Cassius 67.15.6, trans. E. Cary)

He is certainly reported to have had Mettius Pompusianus, whose "imperial" horoscope was public knowledge, exiled to Attica and executed on this account and only to have spared Nerva because an astrologer said that he would die soon anyway.[139] An alternative rationale could lead to the same result: Balbillus, probably Thrasyllus' son, is supposed, presumably retaining an element of haruspical interpretation, to have advised Nero that only the execution of several senators would avert the consequences threatened by a comet.[140] Suetonius reports this in connection with the executions that took place as a result of the Pisonian and Vinician conspiracies (*Nero* 36). The theme of power exercised from behind closed doors recurs in the accounts of the reigns of the bad emperors. Nero's wife, Poppaea, apparently a precursor of Nancy Reagan in this respect, kept her own retinue of Chaldeans for her secret councils. It was their nefarious activities that secured her marriage to the emperor, in Tacitus' account (*Histories* 1.22). Caracalla, of course, followed in this line but took it to extremes. Herodian relates how, suspecting traitors everywhere around him, he scoured the country for *magi,* astrologers, and soothsayers and, finally despairing even of the staff he had found, ordered his righthand man to find a *magus* to tell him the time and manner of his death and whether anyone was plotting to seize the government (4.12.3–4).

"Good" emperors, like Vespasian, who made Mettius Pompusianus a consul,[141] and Titus, did not fail to investigate the genitures of senators when rumors went around, but they pardoned them ostentatiously. Titus actually is said to have warned two that they were in great danger from someone else: Domitian, as it proved, of course (Suetonius, *Titus* 9.2). Naturally, we are not bound to believe these tales; what is significant is that they were common currency. As Hopkins notes, commenting on one such tale:

> Political power and legitimacy rest not only in taxes and in armies, but also in the minds of men. The myths made up and told about emperors were part of the mystification which elevated the political sphere above everyday life. The stories circulated and were told whether they were true or not. (1978, 235–6)

They also cannot have failed to reinforce astrology's status as knowledge.

Emperors also consulted astrologers about the succession. Such uses of the art are reflected in the strange account of Hadrian's choice of L. Ceionius Commodus (Aelius Verus) as his successor. The author is attempting to explain away this apparent error on the part of such an expert in astrological matters:

> The emperor was acquainted with the horoscope of Verus . . . and adopted a man whom he did not really think suitable to govern the empire merely for the purpose of gratifying his own desires. . . . For Marius Maximus represents Hadrian as so expert in astrology, as even to assert that he knew all about his own future. (*SHA, Aelius Verus* 3.8–9)[142]

Caligula, according to Suetonius' grandfather, did his best to save Thrasyllus from error about his own succession. Since the astrologer was supposed to have said to Tiberius, when consulted, that Caligula had no more chance of becoming emperor than of crossing the bay of Baiae on horseback, Caligula insisted on constructing a bridge across the bay so that he could perform this feat (Suetonius, *Gaius* 19.3).

Unsurprisingly, there are stories of correct astrological predictions of future greatness for almost every emperor.[143] Augustus himself was supposed to have been predicted to be the ruler of the world on the day he was born by no less an astrologer than Nigidius Figulus, once he found out the hour of his birth.[144] The verdict was apparently confirmed in 44 B.C. in Apollonia by Theogenes, who threw himself at his feet on seeing the birth chart (Suetonius, *Augustus* 94.12). In fact, according to Suetonius, Augustus' destiny was literally marked on his body: he had marks on his chest and abdomen in the shape of the constellation of *Ursa Major* (the Plough), which was, of course, the constellation around which all the others revolved.[145] Tiberius, himself promised the purple when a child by Scribonius (Suetonius, *Tiberius* 14.2), was credited with seeing in Galba a man "who would one day taste of imperial power" by means of the astrological skills he had learned from Thrasyllus,[146] while Agrippina, inquiring on Nero's destiny, was told that the stars indicated that he would indeed become emperor but would kill his mother, which allowed her the chance of an immortal response: "*Occidat, dum imperet!*" (Let him kill me, so long as he becomes emperor!)[147] Vitellius' parents were reputed to have opposed any advancement for him on the grounds of his frightening horoscope. He, of course, scoffed at such promises and thus escaped Nero.[148] In Otho we have a clear case of what frightened the emperors most: he was encouraged to revolt by Ptolemy Seleucus,[149] and four days after the adoption of Piso, in January, 69, "the astrologers also urged him to action, predicting from their observation of the heavens revolution and a year of glory for Otho" (Tacitus, *Histories* 1.22, trans. M. Grant).

Astrologers are frequently to be seen catalyzing rebellion, and others did not fail to use their advice. Tacitus paints a portrait of events in July, 69: "after this speech from Mucianus, the other officers crowded round Vespasian with fresh confidence, reminding him of the responses of the heavenly bodies" (Tacitus, *Histories* 2.78, trans. M. Grant). As Tacitus goes on to comment, Vespasian actually retained Ptolemy Seleucus himself when he gained the throne. Nerva too was persuaded by astrologers, primarily because he was in peril of his life, since astrologers had denounced his imperial horoscope (Dio Cassius 67.15.5–6).

What perhaps worried emperors even more than the danger of astrologers working for others was astrologers working out when they would die. Fear of magic was of course lurking behind such worries, but from any point of view an emperor whose death date was known was a dead emperor. Predicting an emperor's death was highest treason, but there are references to such predictions in our sources. When Tiberius left Rome in 26 the astrologers predicted that he would not come back. In the event this was seen to refer to his retreat from Rome rather than his demise. Caligula was supposedly informed by the astrologer Sulla that his death was very definitely imminent. For Nero they predicted that a day would come when he would be deposed.[150] Domitian lived in fear of various astrologers' predictions of his death, though he attempted to confute one and declared the day before his death that the next day the Moon would be stained with blood in Aquarius (where the maleficent planet Saturn had been at his birth).[151] Septimius Severus knew himself, from his horoscope, that he would not come back from his campaign in Britain. But, according to Dio, he was careful to place the Ascendant in different places in the two depictions of that horoscope, which he had done on the ceilings of the rooms in the palace in which he heard lawsuits (Dio Cassius 77 [76] 11.1). In this way no one else could work out his death date. Severus Alexander was supposedly an adept in astrology, but it helped him little. He was told by Thrasybulus that he would die by the sword of a barbarian, but, according to the irony demanded of divination by narrative, it transpired that this was no honorable death in war but, rather, at the hand of a barbarian guard of his own army (*SHA, Severus Alexander* 27.5, 62.2–5).

The emperor was often portrayed as scoffing at predictions, to give the narrative more power. When the elder Gordian laughed at the imperial future predicted for him, his son, and grandson it was said

> that the astrologer showed him the agency of the stars and cited the passages from old books to prove that he told the truth. He even predicted . . . the day and manner of their death, and the places they would die, with a firm belief in his correctness. (*SHA, Gordian* 20.1)

The astrologer had the last laugh, because of the shortness of their rule.[152] Domitian tried to prevent an astrologer called Ascletarion from being right about the manner of the astrologer's own death: the man had said that he would be torn apart by dogs. The emperor gave orders that he should be executed and buried carefully. But a sudden shower put out the fire of the funeral pyre and made the men in charge take shelter. Immediately, a pack of dogs fell on the corpse and ripped it to pieces![153] Dio Cassius, who does not say the man was an astrologer, has the shower happen as the man is being burnt at the stake (67.16.3). Thus, the prophecy seems even more accurate. All this tended only to reinforce high opinions of astrology. In the case of Vitellius we can see a more exaggerated form of this poetic license. In Suetonius' version the astrologers responded to his edict ordering them to leave before a certain day with a prediction that he would die before the edict took effect, but in fact they were several months out. But Dio's later account presents the astrologers as correct in their prophecy.[154] Many of these anecdotes are thus obviously apocryphal, but it is the fact that they were told and retold that is really significant. They reveal the dangerous potential of an art believed infallible if only practiced properly.

It was a potential that both emperors and their rivals took extremely seriously. Dio tells us that, when the conflict between Antony and Octavian was building up, Agrippa expelled astrologers and magicians (49.43.5). And Augustus himself, perhaps in the same year as the comet that some saw as threatening his end, was said by Dio to have proscribed consultations either about death or without witnesses.[155] It was the case of Drusus Libo that drove Tiberius to take action, in A.D. 16. The young man's ambition was exploited by astrologers, dream interpreters, and magicians. When the story came out he committed suicide. Two *senatus consulta* (senatorial decrees) were then passed against astrologers and magicians, exiling them from Rome and Italy, the second more severe.[156] One of those involved in the Libo conspiracy, L. Pituanius, was thrown off a rock; as for another, L. Marcius, the consuls conducted him outside the Esquiline Gate, and there, after sounding the trumpets, they inflicted punishment *more prisco* (in traditional fashion), which involved beating to death with rods (Tacitus, *Annals* 2.32).

There are no fewer than eleven cases involving the indictment of high-ranking Romans, charges of *maiestas* (lèse-majesté) and the use of astrology recorded in the first century; seven cases in all are reported up to 371 of astrologers or other diviners indicted on *maiestas* charges under the edict of A.D. 11, despite their slighter interest for ancient historians, while there were probably no less than ten *SCs,* or edicts, between 33 B.C. and A.D. 93.[157] There was Lepida, said to have consulted by means of Chaldeans about the family of Caesar; Lollia, rival of Agrippina for Claudius' hand, who was accused at the behest of Agrippina of having sought to know from Chaldeans and others about the *princeps'* marriage, who was exiled and who committed suicide; and Scribonianus, son of the rebel against Claudius, who was exiled for inquiring about the end of the emperor's life and died soon afterward. Antistius Sosianus in A.D. 66, while in exile, rifled the files of the exiled astrologer Pammenes in the hope of securing a pardon from Nero and found the horoscope of M. Ostorius Scapula and data implicating P. Anteius Rufus. Both committed suicide to forestall execution.[158]

The repressive laws obviously had no permanent effect (cf. Tacitus *Annals* 12.52). It was not in every circumstance that the law was applied in all its rigor. It was thought in the first place that the science itself should not be punishable but only the profession.[159] But positions hardened under pressure. Diocletian's edict of 296 was conserved in Justinian's *Codex* (9.18.2): "It is in the public interest that people learn and exercise the art of geometry. But the mathematical art [astrology] is punishable, it is absolutely forbidden."

Denise Grodzynski (1974) has made a particular study of the laws of the fourth century preserved in the Theodosian Code condemning divination and magic. The two were totally assimilated, she argues, for the first time, and from 358 became one of the five major crimes.[160] In principle any private magical or divinatory act could be punished by death, as a crime agaist the state, except from 319 to 357, when the constitutions of Constantine only laid pain of death on haruspices themselves and not on their clients.[161] Constantius II condemned all diviners, even *vates* (prophets) and dream interpreters, and their clients. Between 358 and 371 possibly even the public practice of haruspicy or augury as part of religion was outlawed. Succeeding emperors made more precise the cases in which the death penalty was to be applied.[162] In fact, in cases in which the consultation clearly was about private affairs, the guilty might escape with property confiscation or torture.[163]

Grodzynski argues that political circumstances such as the instability of the empire are not sufficient to explain the general increase in severity of punishments in the Late Empire and that the explanation of this change as being part of the struggle against paganism is incomplete. The target is more specific than paganism. The laws of the Theodosian Code, above all after Constantine, put the accent on the reprehensible character of the *curiositas divinandi* (the desire to know in divination, 9.16.5). This desire to know what is forbidden is more subject to penalty than divination per se. Such audacity could only be of diabolical origin, and thus deserved the strictest punishment.

Before examining the peculiar features of the Christian battle with astrology, however, it should be said that there are also some continuities between pagan and Christian emperors as regards their attitude to astrology. We hear of an attempted coup involving the astrologer Heliodorus under a Christian emperor in 371. Valens, following the example of Vespasian with Ptolemy Seleucus, seems to have made the offender his court astrologer. Valens also had tortured and butchered a man found with a horoscope labeled "Valens," though he claimed it was his brother's birth chart.[164]

There is some evidence of recurrence of the old pattern in palace revolutions, despite the sorry state of our evidence between Theodosius and Justinian. Pingree (1976a) has reedited a fascinating set of three "coronation-horoscopes" from the fifth century preserved in a later Arabic source (al-Qasrani) as well as three others from Greek sources. All three coronation-horoscopes share a pessimistic attitude to the prospects of the rulers, though in the case of two of the subjects it is made clear that the horoscopes were cast optimistically before the coronation. The implication is that an astrological advisor is relieving his patron, apparently the emperor Zeno, of worry about rivals' chances of imperial power, by showing astrologically how they are bound to fail.

Pingree reconstructs the picture as follows: in the first two cases "our" astrologer has gotten hold of copies of the horoscopes cast by the rivals' astrologers for the coronations, while in the third case our astrologer has cast a horoscope himself for the known date of the rival's assumption of power. The first horoscope was cast at 9 A.M. on January 12, 475, for the coronation of Basiliscus as emperor of the East, after Zeno had fled Constantinople with his wife, mother, and household gods on the ninth day of his consulship.[165] Horoscopes may originally have been cast for both Basiliscus by the astrologer of one Illus, who was supporting Basiliscus. At any rate, Zeno's astrologer was proved right, if he analyzed the horoscope to reassure Zeno, for Basiliscus was overthrown after two years.

The second, cast on July 18, 484, tells us that the usurper Leontius had chosen his moment to be crowned at Antioch after consulting two astrologers (Neugebauer and Van Hoesen, L484). Here again the astrologer of Illus, who supported Leontius too, may have been involved. How did the astrologers get it wrong? Our astrologer's answers follow what I shall be calling the agonistic model: they ignored such and such variables, which would have revealed that Leontius was doomed to fail. Leontius had rebelled against Zeno; our astrologer may well be the Maurianus who was consulted by Zeno about the succession in 486, according to the sixth-century historian John Malalas.[166] Pingree argues that the same astrologer was responsible for another horoscope (Neugebauer and Van Hoesen, L440), which analyzes the career of a grammarian, Pamprepius of Panopolis. Pamprepius was associated with the revolt of Leontius, and his horoscope records that he went from Athens to Byzantium and there became associated with a great man and, pretending to be a wizard, or one initiated, became quaestor, consul, and patrician before being put to death as a traitor, presumably in 488 with Leontius.

The third of the three coronation-horoscopes was probably cast when Zeno conferred presents and titles on Theodoric Valamer, a potential rival, in order to persuade him to withdraw to his capital at Novae.[167] Pingree also connects with Zeno's astrologer a horoscope cast in 463, which was interpreted as presaging that the son of the emperor Leo would die at 5-1/6 months (Neugebauer and Van Hoesen L463). Zeno (Tarasicodissa at this time) had been offered the hand of Leo's daughter Ariadne, and the astrologer may have persuaded him that he need not fear for his succession. The precision of the date of death may imply retrospective interference; certainly as regards another horoscope, which was cast on the entry of Theodorus (the *praefectus Augustalis*) to Alexandria in 486, Pingree suggests that the astrologer had been forced after Theodorus' fall to correct his original predictions of great things, made when Theodorus was appointed to the prefecture. All these horoscopes, and possibly eight others, were used as illustrations in a treatise, perhaps originally one that Zeno's astrologer produced in order to advertise his successes.

We hear of nothing similar afterward. Cumont (1918) says that, after Justinian closed the schools, astrology fell from prominence till the eighth century. There must be some implication of its declining role at court in the claim of one "Stephanus the Philosopher" to be reintroducing astrology to "Rome" (Byzantium) in the eighth century.[168] Only from the ninth century is there evidence that the Byzantine emperors were again surrounded by astrologers.[169]

Firmicus Maternus, writing under a Christian emperor around A.D. 334, is actually following a trend that began with the Augustan Manilius,[170] when he sets the emperor above the influence of the stars, in an attempt to eliminate the subversive potential of astrology, though he takes it a stage further by advising that it is quite useless to cast his horoscope.[171] In his case, as well as in Manilius', there is ambivalence because of a simultaneous desire to present the emperor's rule as fated.[172] It was clearly not a compromise that elicited much imperial trust. In fact, no Latin treatises are found after his.

Astrologers saw the movements of the stars as reflecting relations between earthly potentates. The terms they used for certain configurations, such as ἐπιδεκατεία, καθυπερτέρησις (tithe), and δορυφορία (bodyguard)[173]—not only illustrate an anthropomorphizing tendency but also the desire to set the temporal order within the eternal and thus authorize it. The successive attempts of emperors and their supporters to bind the former intimately to the serene, unchanging world beyond the moon often appear rather wistful in retrospect. The emperors' relation to astrology was one of dependence as much as one of exploitation; this was why they were led, as much by belief in its power as by their realization of the political implications, to crush those who found in the stars backing similar to their own.[174]

Astrology, despite the risks for those who claimed it for their side, was very suitable as a reservoir of power, with its familiar, condensed symbols and its ability to assume the guise of religious, mythical, scientific, or political discourse. These factors may have been necessary, though obviously they were not sufficient in themselves, for its potential to be confirmed. The foregoing crude delineation of the way this potential was confirmed is meant to set the success of the discipline in a social context, since it is still necessary to stress that we should not consider its rise, or indeed its fall, in purely intellectual terms but also as sustained or undermined by particular configurations of power.

Astrology and the Christian Church

The church, once its own power was established, attempted to undermine the science of astrology. The attacks of the church Fathers are notable for their frank presentation of the power struggle between the stars and God, astrologers and the church. As long as Christianity remained a *religio illicita* (illegal religion), as Laistner (1941) remarked, longer disquisitions against astrology are rare.[175] Indeed, there were Christian writers prepared to accommodate it within their faith, for which there was ample encouragement, not only in the tale of the Magi, who followed the star that they interpreted as announcing the birth of a great king, but also in the account of the creation of the stars as signs in Genesis (1.14) and various celestial prodigies associated with Christ in the Gospels.[176] Firmicus Maternus himself was the author of a Christian attack on the mystery religions, though it is usually assumed that he wrote the *Mathesis* before he was converted. The bishop Sidonius Apollinaris, writing in the late fifth century, furnishes some indication of the extent to which astrological learning was accommodated in a Christian milieu. He refers to astrology with respect, as a mysterious and lofty matter, while remembering to condemn it as contrary to the faith on occasion. He is a rare case of a Christian writing in pagan mode, in imitation of pagan literary models, which allows a less rigorously hostile attitude to pagan learning.[177]

But the attacks of the church Fathers, when they come, show clearly why astrology was a threat. It was a subversive challenge to God's authority, which was of course vested in the church on earth. It is notable that the argument centers around the doctrine of astral fatalism. Astrology is normally discussed in the context of full-dress discourses on fatalism or in commentary on scriptural verses, in which the writers pause to eliminate any interpretation that favors the stars' direct influence on human life. As Riedinger (1956) notes, the tendency to find references to astrology, when the texts in question seem originally to have meant nothing of the sort, is indicative of the degree to which astrological ideas were current.

A further indication of the subversive potential that led to the repression of astrology is the fact that the Fathers also discuss it in connection with heretical doctrines. Indeed, it is the Gnostics who seem to spark off the first direct attacks on astrology. In the second century, when the church is far from established and united, so that heresy was not a serious threat, we find only passing broadsides from Tatian, Tertullian, and Clement of Alexandria among Christian apologists; only the brief remarks of Tertullian are directly connected with discussion of heretical sects.[178] But Hippolytus of Rome (martyred 235) attacked the Gnostics with particular emphasis on their astrology in his *Refutation of All Heresies,* taking his detailed argumentation from Sextus Empiricus.[179] He justifies this excursus, having carefully disclaimed any knowledge of the art:

> But since, estimating the astrological art as a powerful one, and availing themselves of the testimonies adduced by its patrons, they wish to gain reliance for their own attempted conclusions, we shall at present, as it has seemed expedient, prove the astrological art to be untenable, as our intention is to invalidate also the Peratic[180] system, as a branch growing out of an unstable root.[181]

Though the Gnostics are a fashionable subject of research, little work has been done on their astrological notions. Despite new papyrological evidence, there remains a problem with the source: the ideas of many Gnostic sects must be reconstructed from their Christian opponents.

It seems clear, however, that the use they make of astrological influence in their cosmologies derives from the Hermetic strand of astrological literature. In almost all of the Gnostics the stars are seen as evil powers hostile to men, degraded versions of the astral potentates and gods of Hellenism, and the devotees have the task of liberating themselves from their influence by true gnosis. The soul had to reach beyond the visible cosmos of the planets and fixed stars to the worlds from which it came. Within this framework each sect had its own esoteric teaching about the roles of astrological entities within its cosmology.[182] Gundel and Gundel observe (1966, 324) that other testimonies show that the Gnostics knew horoscopic astrology and its birth charts and not only the basic doctrines.

Origen (185/86–254/55), who remained immensely influential despite his later condemnation, illustrates the nature of the struggle between the astrologers and the church in his *Commentary on Genesis.*[183] In his uneasy compromises he shows that astrology was a serious rival. Origen summarizes his arguments as follows: "1) How our freedom is safeguarded when God knows in advance for all eternity the acts that each man is judged to have accomplished. 2) How the stars are not agents, but signs. 3) That humans cannot have accurate knowledge of these signs, but that they are revealed for the sake of powers greater than humans. 4) The reason for which God has created these signs is in order to obtain knowledge for the powers will be examined" (23.6.20–30). He elaborates a Christian version of astral fatalism with his notion of the divine writing. This moving writing, formed of letters and characters traced by God's hand in the sky so that the δυνάμεις θεῖαι (divine powers) can read them, prefigures all cosmic events from creation to consummation. This is done to instruct the celestial powers and make them happy, in uncovering for them all divine mysteries and all kind of knowledge and in some cases to intimate to them their precise orders for the missions entrusted to them (20.29–39). Interestingly, he also allows evil powers access to this knowledge, remarking explicitly that, if demons execute actions prefigured by the stars, they do not do so because they read the "writing" to discover the will of God but only because they act maliciously of their own volition, as the good powers act freely when they follow orders (21.1–12). He also seems to admit that the stars are not inert objects manipulated by the divine but, rather, animated, intelligent entities. Saint Pamphilus, in his work *In Defence of Origen* (9), affirms that this doctrine was not yet heretical.

He sets the course of the debate on free will, astral fatalism, and Divine Providence, dangerous shallows from which the only escape lay in the uncompromising authoritarianism of Augustine. The obvious parallels between good Divine Providence and bad Astral Determinism led the church Fathers to betray the arbitrary nature of their predilections from the point of view of secular reasoning. The influence of the stars was unacceptable, because humans had to have free choice about whether to sin or not, but what kind of free choice was it if God was in control instead? Origen also illustrates the tendency of the Patristic writers to use the arguments of pre-Christian philosophers against astrology without giving them a central role, since the really important arguments are about whether astrology offers a threat to Christian doctrine.[184]

Though Origen stands at the head of a tradition of argumentation against astrology that repeats commonplaces from the pagan philosophers and rejections of astrological fatalism as morally dangerous ad nauseam, he also represents a turning point. Following arguments were less subtle and less compromising.[185] Most Christian apologists felt obliged to enter into detailed philosophical and scriptural discussion. Thus, in Greek, Diodorus of Tarsus (?–394), Gregory of Nyssa (ca. 335–94), Nemesius, bishop of Emesa on the Orontes (4th/5th c.), and Gregory of Nazianzus, and, in Latin, Ambrosiaster's *Inquiries* (115) and Augustine's *City of God* (5.1–11), all address themselves to the refutation of astrology in general discourses on fatalism.[186] There are also discussions of the subject in the commentaries of Basil the Great (bishop of Caesarea, 329–79) in the *Sixth Sermon of the Hexaemeron,* of Procopius of Gaza (d. 538), and of Ambrose on Genesis, and of the anonymous Arian on Job (4th/5th c.).[187] Riedinger (1956) adds many others in his list of thirty Christian apologists in the East alone, from Origen to the eighth century.

The main arguments against astrology, as mentioned, are stereotyped by the late imperial age and do not need examination in detail here. Boll (1894) has pointed out that there are two basic lines of argument from the second century B.C. to the Byzantine period. First, it is asked how it can be asserted that the physical or mental characteristics of a person depend on the configuration of the stars at birth or conception, when in fact the same bodily or mental traits are to a large extent found in all the members of one people, and, alternatively, the instances in which large numbers of people die at the same time, though they were born at different times, are brought up. The case of the destinies of twins serves frequently to illustrate the converse: How can two people under the same astral influence turn out so differently? Second, there are attacks on what the writers represent as the principles of astrogeography, insofar as it is concerned with astral influence on the inhabitants of particular regions. As Amand (1941) points out, even some of the arguments about free will derive from pagan philosophical antecedents. The apologists engage even less than their predecessors with the theory and practice of "scientific" or savant astrology, though with the better excuse that such research was seen as highly compromising.[188]

There are some individual attempts to cope with difficult contradictions that throw into relief the essentially political nature of these attacks. The tale of the Magi[189] is a case in point. At all costs these Patristic writers want to deny that this is evidence for the truth of astrology, since this would put Christ in thrall to the stars, the situation Origen attempted to avoid. The situation parallels from one point of view the situation of the emperors. As in their case, early doctrine presented Christ as legitimated by astral phenomena, while later both Christ and the emperors had to be emancipated from the influence of the heavens.[190]

The first move was to present God as "trumping" astrologers with the Star of Bethlehem. The astrologers had true knowledge of the future after all, but only till the birth of Christ.[191] Alternatively, taking their cue from Gnostics and Neoplatonists, the apologists argued that Christians, once baptized, are freed from astral fatalism, from this time. This did, however, leave astrology for pagans.[192] In the third century Christians tried other ways of getting round the difficulty. They argued that the Star was in fact no ordinary star—neither a fixed star nor a planet nor a comet—that it had moved differently from all known stars, since it had led the Magi to Bethlehem, and that it was thus not assimilable in any sense to the sorts of star that were within the province of astrologers. In short, the Star of the

Magi was a miraculous luminary, perhaps an angel or a holy spirit, and thus did not belong to the astrological repertory.[193] There remained, of course, the problem that God had chosen to reveal the birth of his son to astrologers, who knew the movements of other stars with such certainty that they could interpret the meaning of this one.[194] Gregory of Nazianzus felt obliged to add to the traditional tale in his hexameters *On Foreknowledge* that the Magi were converted, abandoned their craft, and adored Christ.[195]

It is with Saint Augustine, though, that the iron fist seems most obviously brought in to settle the argument on the difficulties of reconciling the doctrines of God's Providence, and indeed of Original Sin, with free will. Augustine developed his views on the creative religious function of power after his experience with the Donatist heresy (*Letters* 93). Not for him the cautious formulations and the moral qualms about lack of free will, which he bulldozes with his doctrine of grace and predestination. He dismisses Cicero's argument that divine foreknowledge would undermine free will, while asserting that human wills are in the order of causes that is "*certus Deo,*" determined by God (*City of God* 5.9). But he supports Cicero's arguments against astrology and brings out the old arguments that had been used in support of free will to attack the art. He admits the possibility of revelation of the future (for what of Christian prophecy otherwise?), but pagan prophecy, he says, is the work of demons who occasionally pick up the odd tip from signs of divine thought to mingle with their usual lies (5.7). What could be a clearer revelation of the nature of the struggle going on between the church and astrology?

Augustine had in his youth been a keen consulter of astrologers and enjoyed discussions with them on matters of theory (*Confessions* 4.3). Astrology was associated with the Manichaeans,[196] of whom Augustine had been one. Though later historians might look on Manichaeism as a new religion, it was regarded by the orthodox church as heretical,[197] and it influenced later heretical groups, such as the Priscillianists, followers of Priscillian, bishop of Avila, A.D. 381–85. Thus, there was particular reason, from Augustine's point of view, to crush astrology: he knew the dangers. He adds vehemence, but little else from his personal experience of astrology, in his reuse of the old arguments against it and undermines the effect of these arguments with his characterization of the art as demonic revelation, whence it gains at least an intermittent certificate of reliability. Christians such as the heretic Priscillianists could simply replace the demons by respectable scriptural figures like the Patriarchs and argue that they had eliminated the pagan superstition from the science.

But the time for such compromises was past. The church Fathers' attacks show that any Christian interest in astrology was a threat and had to be stamped out. Whatever arguments might be put forward on behalf of the art, it is the church that must decide the rules of debate. God is allowed to combine predestination with free will, while the astral divinities are not; God can insure that astrology is only veracious until Christ, or for pagans, or only occasionally as a result of angelic or demonic decipherment of God's plans. Crucially, the only such insight into the future is through prophecy authorized by the church.

And the church moved to crush its rival. In the fourth-century *Constitutions of the Apostles* (8.32.11) astrologers are put on a par with debauchers, magicians, and the philosophical rabble (philosophers being regarded even more negatively by church than by state, as heretics)[198] and refused baptism or damned.[199] The first record of council canons forbidding clergy to be astrologers or magicians comes in those of the Council of Laodicea in 365 (*Canons of the Apostles* 1.77.29), but it may be a later interpolation. The pronunciation of the anathema on those who think that astrology is worthy of belief, or that human souls and bodies are subject to the stars, in reaction to the heretic Priscillianists, recorded for the Council of 400 at Toledo, is from the first half of the fifth century.[200] This had to be repeated at the Council of Braga in 561 (*Canons of the Apostles* 2.31.9, 10), where more precise details of their astrological doctrine are preserved. The sect is also the subject of Leo I's fulminations in a letter concerning astrology:

> Merito patres nostri, sub quorum temporibus haeresis haec nefanda prorupit, per totum mundum instanter egere ut impius furor ab universa ecclesia pelleretur.
>
> Our fathers, in whose time this evil heresy broke out, rightly hunted it with great energy throughout the world so that this impious madness should be driven out of the whole body of the church. (*PL* 54.679 A–B)

But in 572 the Priscillianists were still in the sights of those who condemned astrology. At the Second Council of Braga there was even more virulent condemnation, pronouncing the anathema against Christians using astrology before they built houses, planted trees, or married (*Canons of the Apostles* 2.56.72). As for the East, the Council at Constantinople, the *Quinisextum,* which took place in the presence of Justinian in 553, vigorously attacked astrology in general.[201] Procopius, in his pamphlet attacking Justinian, records that astrologers were publicly humiliated by being flogged and driven on camels through the city. At the fourth Council of Toledo of 633, the Twenty-ninth Canon threatens clergy consulting astrologers with imprisonment in the monasteries and harsh penitential discipline.[202] We hear of figures like Eusebius, bishop of Emesa, whom his people expelled from his see on the grounds of his interest in astrology.[203]

Gundel and Gundel suggest that the church was more successful than the emperors in removing astrology from its privileged position, remarking on the effect of the *Quinisextum* on the Eastern empire (1966, 339). They are only surprised that it did not succeed completely. It is not clear how much of a setback it suffered in the East: at court it seems to have lost its high profile, as we have seen, if only for a couple of hundred years. As far as the production of the literature is concerned, even though there are problems with the dating of the material in *CCAG,* it is obvious that there is continuity. We do find evidence of its having flourished at the local level from saints' lives of the fifth to the seventh centuries, as collected by Gilbert Dagron (1984). His article admirably reveals the microcosmic version of the church's struggle with astrologers in the competition between the local holy man and the local astrologer, for the custom of the villagers or townspeople.

The vignette that illustrates most neatly the context of the sorts of astrological texts I shall be discussing occurs in the *Life of St. Symeon the Younger.* When the earthquakes of 551–57 strike, the inhabitants of Antioch go to consult both the astrologer and the Stylite saint and, in order to decide who can help them best, actually organize an ἀγών, or public debate, between them.[204]

But what also emerges from Dagron's account of this competition is a certain accommodation of astrology in the East. The situation in the West is rather different. In the time of Sidonius Apollinaris, in the late fifth century, astrology still attracts learned adherents and evinces a certain respect from him as an example of pagan learning. As a bishop, however, he feels constrained to point out that it is contrary to the faith and even to assert that his friend, the professor of rhetoric at Bordeaux, deserved his death at the hands of his slaves, for inquiring about his future.[205] Yet, it seems, from the evidence of Isidore of Seville, as if the learned discipline had declined by the sixth century.[206] Cumont (1903) believed that this showed that the Latin church succeeded where the Eastern church failed, in destroying this "superstition savante," until the twelfth century.[207] He was only contradicted by M. L. W. Laistner in 1941, who argued on the basis of library lists that "not persecution or prosecution, but the lack of manuals caused the disappearance of 'scientific' astrology in the West for four or five centuries after Firmicus composed his astrologers' handbook." This is to counterpose rather different sorts of causal factors. One might well ask why the production of manuals stopped while other writing went on. Presumably, Laistner would have to argue for lack of interest. It seems hard to dissociate this from the attitude of church and state.

All this must remain matter for speculation. I would put no great weight on the following suggestion, but perhaps Arthur Darby Nock provides an answer to the difference between the two halves of the empire. In an article on Roman religion in general (1972) he remarks that, while Greeks and Romans alike regarded prodigies as indications that all was not well with the gods' relations with the city and took some action to propitiate the supernatural, only the Romans had this formalized as *procuratio prodigiorum* (lit. "dealing with prodigies"), a regular proceeding, initiated by the Senate, and that there is nothing in Greece corresponding to *auspicia* as the concomitant of *imperium.* He goes on to argue that the control of religion was centralized in Rome to a degree unknown in Greece[208] and that those who controlled it claimed that their decisions were valid in heaven and on earth. On the consul's speech about the Bacchanalian rites in 189 he observes that this control "is legal in form, it accepts and defines the situation, and its definition is explicit, not implicit."[209] He proceeds to connect this with the Christian era, where he claims to detect a specific inheritance of the precise tendency to define not only de facto but also de jure what is permissible. It was the Roman church that early claimed the right to determine whether an offense was a mortal sin and to give absolution. In short, one can see that a plausible explanation of the different fates of astrology in East and West might be given by relating the different churches' inheritance of different pagan religious attitudes. If so, the Latin church inherited a concern for precise legalistic definition of good and evil and the desire and political means to take for itself the power to impose that knowledge.

Fatalism and Control

Ironically, considering the arguments of the church I have just been discussing, the alliance of fatalism, in our usual sense of the word, with astrology is something of a red herring, as Peter Brown perceived with regard to Late Antiquity.[210] Yet he omits mention of the reason why it is that, in his own words, "the modern scholar expects ancient men to sigh under the weight of a determinism implied in the astrological beliefs of the age."[211] It is hardly surprising that the "modern scholar"[212] sees determinism in terms of some monolithic, rigid, and oppressive force. This figure takes at face value the ubiquitous rhetoric, not only in the astrologers themselves (*fata regunt orbem, certa stant omnia lege* [Fate rules the world, everything stands under fixed law])[213] but also that in their opponents, from Carneades to Augustine.

Astrologers certainly exploited the common perception of Stoic εἱμαρμένη (Fate), as a physically and theologically justified sequence of causes, which left no room for alternative outcomes,[214] in search of certainty as the basis of their art. They aligned themselves in effect, however, with the traditional dialectical concept of Fate. Certain salient features of one's life are laid down from the start, worldly sucess or failure, children, health, and of course the date of death. Yet there is always room for partial negotiation, as it were. Thus, the Delphic Oracle told Croesus that they had been unable to divert destiny so that the fall of Sardis occurred in his sons' lifetime but that they had been able to postpone it for three years (Herodotus, *Histories* 1.91). The validity of catarchic astrology, taking astrological readings for particular enterprises, depended on this dialectic, after all. Vernant has commented on the paradoxical nature of the divinatory enterprise:

if the practitioners were really omniscient, their practical activity would be pointless. Though Ptolemy might argue that knowledge of the future enabled one to face it with a calm mind and Vettius Valens might refer to the inutility of prayer,[215] it is hard to imagine clients bothering to find out about the inevitable. Rather, they wanted more manipulable answers:

> So divinatory systems are established on the basis of more or less stable equilibria between opposite poles, in a sort of constant tension between on the one hand the formal framework, the logical structures, the grammar they put into play for a complete and rigorous codification of the event, the singular fact, and on the other the multiplicity of concrete situations, always diverse and shifting, on which people come to interrogate the oracle and to which its response must allow modification in the direction wanted by the consultant. (Vernant 1974, 18)

From the point of view of astrological theory a complete codification involved an almost infinite number of permutations of determining factors. Ptolemy, who argued for physical causation in terms of the four elements as an explanation of astrological influence, was careful to spell out the complexity:

> Why can he [the astrologer] not also perceive the general quality of his temperament from the ambient at the time of his birth, such as, for example that he is such and such and such and such in soul, and predict occasional events by the use of the fact that such and such an ambient is attuned to such and such a temperament and is favourable to prosperity, while another is not so attuned and conduces to injury. (*Tetrabiblos* 1.2.10–11, p. 7, 1–11, trans. F. E. Robbins)

In the case of astrological ethnology customs are allowed their own influence as well as all the other mixture of factors, though "the ambient" is the overdetermining cause (*Tetrabiblos* 1.2.18–19, pp. 8, 23–29, 23).

The astrologer's alliance with the stars, like the emperor's, is also fraught with attempts to control the ally. At the extreme this involved magic. Tertullian remarks on the connection between magic and astrology, an attitude increasingly espoused by the legal writers, as we have seen.[216] The legendary priest Petosiris, whose name, with Nechepso's, is given as a standard source in astrological treatises, is portrayed as a model for Hermetic astrology in being able to control the workings of destiny.[217] In Porphyry's account Plotinus' rival attempts to wither him with star spells: ὃς καὶ οὕτως ἐπέθετο, ὥστε καὶ ἀστροβολῆσαι αὐτὸν μαγεύσας.[218] (The attempt failed, as Plotinus only turned the spell back on the sender.) In the magical papyri astrological entities appear frequently, and it is clear that the Fate determined by the stars is manipulable. In one spell the procedure is given for calling up a god:

> Now when the god comes in do not stare at his face, but look at his feet. . . . You, then, ask, "Master, what is fated for me?" And he will tell you about his star, and what kind of daimōn you have, and your horoscope and where you may live and where you may die. And if you hear something bad, do not cry out or weep, but ask that he may wash it off or circumvent it, for this god can do everything. (*Papyri Graecae Magicae* [Preisendanz] 13.708–15, trans. Morton Smith)

As Gundel notes, sometimes even 'Ανάγκη and the Fates are summoned to help the magic.[219]

There is a tension between the need to show knowledge of singular events and the aspiration to total knowledge, total power, as Vernant comments. Diviners, because they have to deal with the essentially aleatory, attempt to exclude the aleatory from their perfect and complete systems of knowledge. Astrologers, if they could not achieve omniscience, or indeed the total power to control afforded by magic, attempted to mediate between the two poles of Fate and free will in such a manner as afforded them maximum power. This becomes evident with consideration of astrological practice as it appears from the texts.

Part II. Astrology in Practice

An Ancient Horoscope as Example

Historians have understandably balked at the technical complexity of astrology. As a way into this mass of data, I am going to take a finished ancient horoscope and look at the sort of raw predictions derivable from the treatises most amenable to such a project. It would have been more in keeping with the chronological focus of the other two chapters if I could have used only second-century astrologers[220] for this particular exercise. Yet the two texts I have decided to use, in particular the first, are by far the most suitable—first, because they present themselves as being simple handbooks and, second, because they match up each configuration with a precise prediction. The results of this "experiment" are therefore particularly clear when these texts are used. The way that they work is, however, typical.

The first treatise I consider is that of Firmicus Maternus, a fourth-century senator from Sicily, whose work I have had cause to mention already. The *Mathesis* (Learning) was begun in 334 and is dedicated to a patron high up in the imperial bureaucracy, for whom we have literary and epigraphic evidence.[221] It is the richest of all treatises in terms of precise predictions. The second is that of

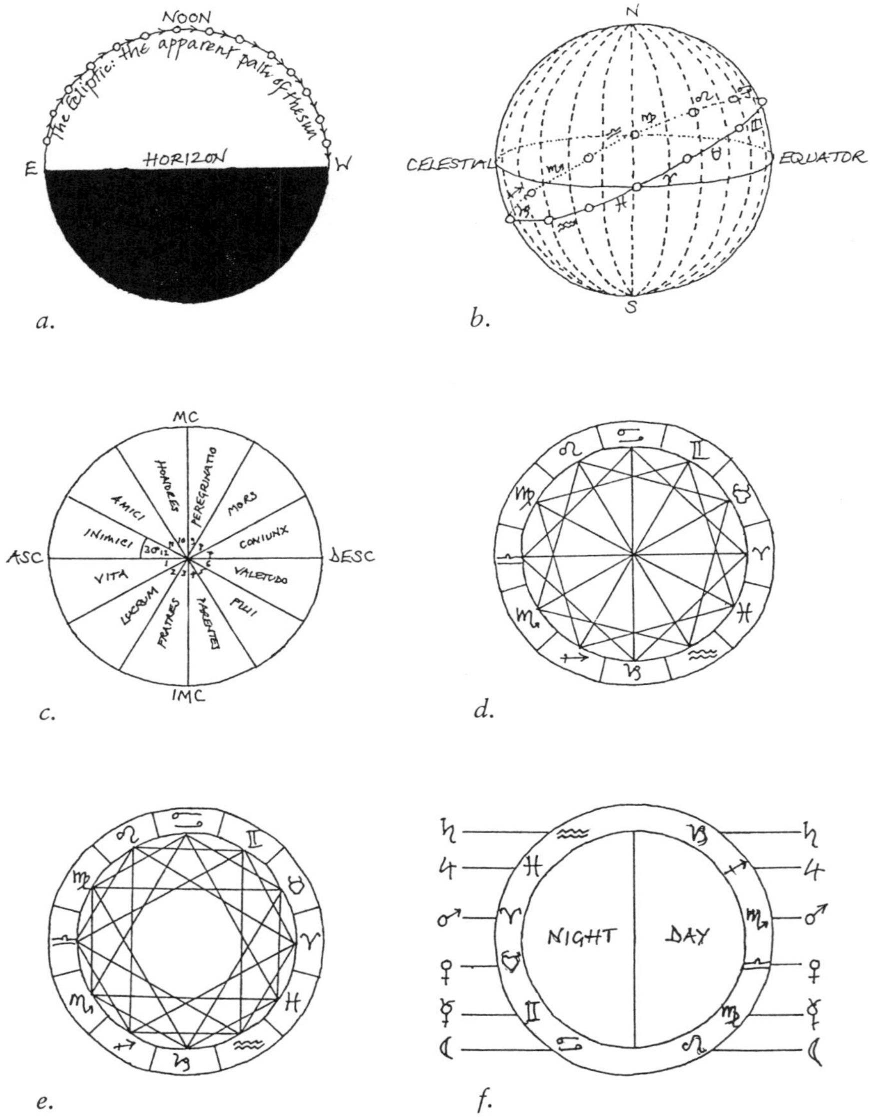

Fig. 1. *a,* Direction of the signs' movement; *b,* deviation of ecliptic from Celestial Equator; *c,* places: fixed; *d,* signs' aspects: opposition and square; *e,* signs' aspects: trine and sextile; *f,* zodiacal houses of the planets

Dorotheus of Sidon, or "the Egyptian," who flourished in the mid-first century A.D. and was one of Firmicus' sources. He wrote an astrological treatise in verse of which only fragments were available in the fourth-century astrologer Hephaestion until David Pingree (1976) published an Arabic text, based on a third-century Pahlavi source, with an English translation. This has had some obvious interpolations; there are two horoscopes from the third and fourth centuries A.D. as well as a couple of additions from Vettius Valens and from Indian astrology. Comparison with the fragments in Hephaestion suggests, however, that the main difference from the original was that the translation is an abridged version.[222]

The horoscope I have chosen also survived in Hephaestion, who excerpted it from a collection of historical horoscopes compiled by the second-century Antigonus of Nicaea, with two others that have not been certainly identified. It is interesting because it is a case (albeit retrospective) of one of the most notorious uses of astrology in our sources.[223] Though the name itself is withheld, astronomical data for 6 A.M., January 24, A.D. 76, agree very closely with the data in the text: thus, the subject, or "native," is the emperor Hadrian.[224]

When attempting to interpret a particular configuration of stars in the manner of these two ancient astrologers, one immediately runs into problems. But they are significant problems, so the best way to give an insight into astrological practice is to go through a few questions from the point of view of a naive observer. When I conceived the idea I accepted the treatises' presentation of themselves as handbooks, as the scholars in the field seem to have done,[225] and was initially as irritated as they by any failure to explain or any deviation from a standard method. But, as I shall illustrate, it soon becomes clear that the last motivation of these writers was to teach how to "cast" a horoscope.

Astrology for Beginners

Before considering how the data might have been used, some very basic information is necessary.[226] (Some of this information is illustrated in fig. 1.) You have to imagine the Earth as a globe lying in the center of a great hollow sphere, with the stars apparently fixed on the inside surface. Between the fixed stars and the Earth run the Sun, Moon, and planets on their courses. Only the five planets easily visible to the naked eye—Saturn, Jupiter, Mars, Venus, and Mercury—were known to ancient astrologers. Making the assumption that the longer it takes for them to go round the sphere, the further away they are, the furthest from the earth is Saturn, followed by Jupiter, Mars, Sun, Venus, Mercury, and the Moon.

If you draw a circle to represent the vast sphere of the fixed stars, putting the north and south poles at the top and bottom of the sphere, and halfway between them draw in the great circle, you will have drawn the Celestial Equator, an imaginary line on the inner surface of the sphere, which is a projection of the

Earth's equator. The whole sphere and everything in it except the Earth, which remains stationary, revolve on the axis between the poles in an east-west direction, taking twenty-three hours and fifty-six minutes for each revolution. The Pole Star is now virtually at the celestial North Pole,[227] and constellations can be seen to revolve round it during the night.

If you watch the western horizon at and just after sunset, and note which constellation sets with or just after the Sun, for a year, you will have made a list of the constellations lying on a great circle on the celestial sphere. The Sun has moved right round the heavens and is back where it started. This circle, lying at an angle of 23-1/2 degrees to the equator, defines the "ecliptic" (fig. 1b). (This inclination to the equator is why the Sun appears, from the center of the Earth, to move north, crossing the equator in spring, turning back at the summer solstice, when it reaches the Tropic of Cancer, and then south, crossing the equator in autumn and turning back at the winter solstice.) The Sun takes a year to travel round the ecliptic, in the opposite direction to that of its daily rotation round the Earth, as part of the spinning sphere of the heavens. As it is moving slowly in the opposite direction to that spin, it takes a short time longer than the stars to go round the Earth from east to west: twenty-four hours, as opposed to twenty-three hours and fifty-six minutes. The Sun takes around 365-1/4 days to get back to where it started on the ecliptic, but in that year the stars have been round the Earth 366-1/4 times. So the stars' day is shorter than the Sun's, which is why the constellations are not in the same place every night of the year.

Such are the apparent motions, regardless of the fact that it is the Earth that spins on its axis every day and travels round the Sun in a year. The Moon's apparent movement is very complicated, but, though it seems to wander, its plane to the ecliptic is 5°9′. The time between one Moon and the next is around 29-1/2 days, but the time it takes to go round the ecliptic is just over 27 days. When it arrives back at its starting point, the Earth and Moon have to move on for a little more than two days before the Moon is back in line with the Sun, to give another New Moon. This is because the position of the Sun against the stars is changing. The five planets also move irregularly, seeming to stand still ("in their stations"), or even move backward (to "retrograde"). All travel within a band 8-1/2 degrees either side of the ecliptic, at different rates, Mercury taking only eighty-eight days to go round but Saturn nearly thirty years. This band round the ecliptic is called the zodiac.

Here begins the elaboration of the astrologers, which was possible once they had a scheme for representing the sky. The connection with the heavens, however, becomes more and more tenuous as the elaboration goes on. The zodiac is divided into twelve "signs" of equal size (30°), an arbitrary division that has little to do with the constellations that give the signs their names and characters. (Anyway, the points at which the ecliptic crosses the Celestial Equator are not fixed: the beginning of the sign Aries [the vernal equinox] is now in the constellation of Pisces, having appeared to move backwards because of the wobble in the Earth's axis. This is the phenomenon known as the precession of the equinoxes.) If you visualize the signs in the appended birth chart (fig. 2) as a wheel that circles clockwise through the sky, following the path of the Sun as it rises in the East, climbs to midheaven at noon, and sets in the West, you can understand the schematic presentation of the appended birth chart.[228] This is a particular moment, set by the Ascendant, the point emerging in the East as the child is born. The bottom part of the chart is seen as "under the Earth," or below the horizon. The 360° of the zodiac are computed anticlockwise.

There is also nothing to indicate the "places" in the sky (those labeled *Vita, Lucrum,* etc., in fig. 2); they are simply worked out by counting sections of 30° from the Ascendant. They are visualized as stationary; the wheel of zodiac signs moves through them. In this chart the Ascendant happens to be at 1° Aquarius, so they roughly coincide with the signs. From the Ascendant are also found the cardinal points: the Descendant in the West, the *Medium Caelum,* or midheaven (MC), at the top, and the *Imum Caelum* (IMC) opposite it. These are most simply calculated by counting 90° from the Ascendant, though observation provides different answers because of regional variation, as the ecliptic lies at an angle to the equator. The MC was in fact, according to Antigonus, at 24° Scorpio.[229] It is never clear in the treatises which method should be used,[230] nor whether individual degrees or whole signs are significant,[231] omissions typical of a syndrome I shall be examining.

The seven "planets" (the term includes the Sun and the Moon) are beneficent, maleficent, or mixed in character. Saturn and Mars, and sometimes the Sun, are generally maleficent; Jupiter, Venus, and on the whole the Moon are beneficent, and Mercury is mixed. Their influence is thought to vary according to their positions. When they are in signs they are designated as "ruling," or in their "terms," the parts of the signs they are allocated (see the outer circle in fig. 2), or in their "exaltations" or "depressions," the planets have a greater influence. Further, they are said to "aspect"[232] one another efficaciously in certain angular relationships: planets 180° apart are said to be in opposition, planets 90° apart in square aspect, both unfavorable, while those 120° and 60° apart are both favorable. There is also the "conjunction," when two planets seem to coincide and thus influence each other.

A further complication, not visible in the chart, is the extra system of Lots, which offers another set of options like the places: there are Lots of Fortune (the most important, mentioned above in connection with Augustus's horoscope), of Brothers, of Travel, etc. These are calculated by counting the distances between various astrological entities and transferring the distance counted to another place on the chart.

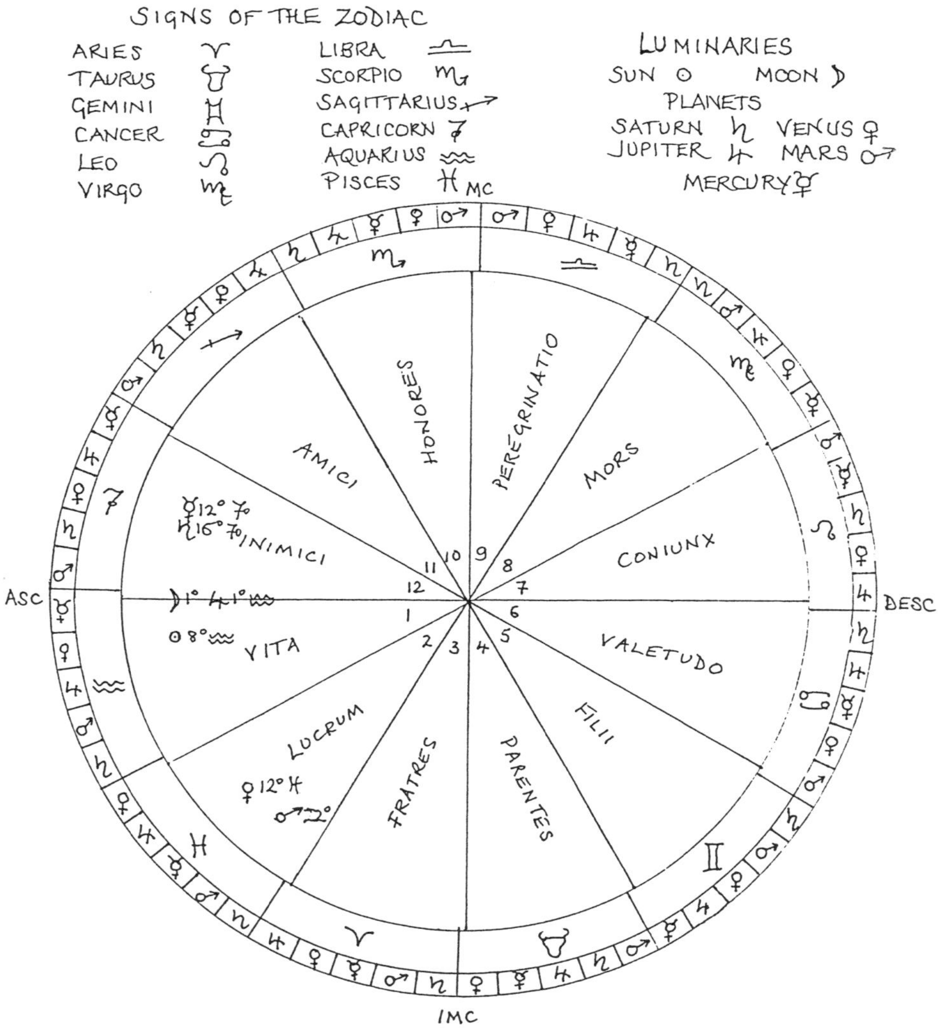

Fig. 2. Hadrian's birth chart. "Such a person was adopted by the Emperor, akin to him, and having lived with him two years, became emperor about his 42nd year, and was wise and educated, so that he was honoured by shrines and temples, and he was married to one wife from maidenhood and was childless, and he had one sister. And he was at discord and conflict with his own relatives. When he had reached about his 63rd year he died a victim to dropsy and breathlessness." (Antigonus of Nicaea)

The Horoscope Cast

> There was . . . a person having the Sun in the 8(20)th degree of Aquarius, the Moon, Jupiter and the Ascendant all three together at the first degree of the same sign, namely Aquarius, Saturn in the 16(5)th[233] degree of Capricorn, Mercury with it in the 12th degree, Venus in Pisces in the 12th degree, and Mars with it at the 22nd degree. (*CCAG* 6, pp. 67.8–68.3)

One of the first noticeable features of Antigonus' following explanation of how this explains Hadrian's biography, as given on the birth chart, is that the procedure for determining the length of life is most complicated:

> In this configuration the house ruler of the Moon (in Aquarius), Saturn (one of whose houses is Aquarius), being in his own house (Capricorn), allots its maximum number of years of life: 56; and since Venus (in Pisces) is in aspect (sextile) to it, it allots an additional 8 years, so that the total number of years is 64. After 61 years, 10 months the degrees of the Ascendant and the Moon (in 1° Aquarius) come into quartile[234] with Saturn, which however is not destructive because Venus is in aspect to it (Saturn) the second time (Venus is then at the beginning of Sagittarius, thus again in sextile to Saturn in Aquarius).[235]

These calculations were the "grande oeuvre" of astrology, as Bouché-Leclercq observes, judged most difficult by adepts, most dangerous and illegal by enemies of the art.[236] Antigonus uses postnatal configurations to add greater precision to the figures obtained from the natal chart. We know that this horoscope is abridged, but the lack of explanation of the way in which these influences yield the figure of "the 63rd year" is immediately striking.[237]

Firmicus' method, simpler in that it does not consider postnatal complications, proves instructive to compare. Taking Saturn as the "Giver of Life," we are offered innumerable variables to take into account[238] but only three answers to choose from (2.25.3): fifty-seven years if favorable, if evil thirty years or thirty months and twelve hours! The puzzled student is then given another barrage of variables just in case any conclusion has been reached:

> If the Ruler of Life or the Giver of Life, that is the Ruler of the Nativity, is in his own House, or Exaltation or terms, and if the planets in his own condition exert a favourable influence on him, that is are favourably aspected to his position, and these stars themselves that influence him are well-placed, then a larger number of years is portended. But they indicate an average age if the Giver of Life is in his own terms or in his sign or in his rising while the Ascendant is in Libra.

One more problem: here in 2.25 Firmicus equates the Giver of Life with the Ruler of the Chart, but in 3.2.23 and in 4.1.8 they seem to be different. Even if they are to be found by the same method, he offers four methods of choosing the ruler. He does express a preference for one method—which here yields Saturn but by a different route from Antigonus.

If this seems churlish in the author of a handbook, consider Dorotheus. In his third book he offers many different and idiosyncratic ways of determining the "governor and indicator of the time of the years of life." As usual, not all terms are explained, but it is clear that, while appearing to eliminate options, he is in fact piling them up so that numerous candidates emerge as possibilities. As becomes apparent with his examples, this entire procedure is irrelevant anyway, since the calculation begins from the degree of the Ascendant instead, and not the "governor of life's years" at all! The length of time it takes to conjoin with the rays of the malefics and the situation of the planets vis-à-vis one another each time this happens are the key factors. The methods of Vettius Valens, Ptolemy, and Paul of Alexandria are similarly complicated. If the spherical trigonometry involved were not complicated enough, the authors seem to go out of their way to offer incompatible systems.[239] Even Bouché-Leclercq had problems in understanding what Ptolemy was doing. The *Tetrabiblos* offers five different ways of finding the Aphetic House and the ἀφέτης (*aphetes* [sender forth]) for the beginning of life. Then the end of life must be found and the interferences en route calculated. The intervals in degrees of the zodiac must be converted to degrees of right ascension (along the equator), which are translated into years. For this kind of trigonometry the tables of the *Almagest* would be needed.

A few initial points can be made. We can isolate no straightforward chronological development in astrological theory. The astrologers are not gradually refining or even elaborating a method but, rather, indulging in free improvisation on certain themes. A reader of these texts who wished to calculate the length of life would be immensely frustrated, though doubtless impressed by the learning of the author. Certainly, the book would only serve as an aid to study in an apprenticeship of some kind. What Cramer (1956, 169) saw as the daring revelation of forbidden secrets begins to take on a different aspect with the revelation of this extreme obscurity. On Ptolemy, Bouché-Leclercq (1899, 422) makes an observation that would have been equally apt for our astrologers: "You could imagine that he felt on him the eyes of the imperial jurisconsults, who were very touchy about predictions about death."

Also notable is that Antigonus does not even mention that Hadrian died in a climacteric year par excellence (Firmicus 4.20.3). The dangers of a year that was a multiple of both 7 and 9 were well known to Augustus, who confesses his relief on his sixty-fourth birthday to his elder grandson, in a letter preserved in Aulus Gellius (15.7.3).[240] Calculations of climacteric periods often formed part of astrological theory, but this was a very basic, even vulgar example. Was this common-or-garden, straightforward numerology too unimpressive?

If one can find an obvious motive for making the procedure for determining the time of death as intricate as possible, it is more difficult in cases such as Dorotheus' extreme contortions regarding the number of children.[241] In another horoscope that I calculated using his methods I found the numbers generated ranged from two to twenty. As regards this horoscope, however, he could arrive at Antigonus' conclusion (p. 71, 2f.) that Hadrian would be childless (or have few children or else trouble from them). What is remarkable is that at least five procedures achieve a consensus on his childlessness, but after all this he destroys this consensus with his final comments. "Now I'll make all clear. . . . If one benefic aspects the place, then you should not at all despair for his children, but he will have some" (2.12.18). Firmicus is unwilling to be pinned down. In one passage he would suggest Hadrian will have children by two wives and lose them (6.32.37–38). Mostly, indications are imprecise: "The natives will be adopted by strangers or find themselves fathers of alien children, or tutors, or governors of minors. Some are forced to find their exposed children after a period of time" (4.10.10). A general idea of the intrusion of disorder into ties of blood is operative (cf. 4.19.5, 5.1.30), which makes it broad enough to coincide with another of Antigonus' retrospective "predictions" (p. 68, 10; p. 71, 6–7): that Hadrian will be adopted.

What is clear here is that answers can be flexible and that once again there is no attempt to present a standard procedure; in fact, there is rather an overriding attempt to prevent the possibility of a simple choice.

An Imperial Horoscope?

Hadrian's great-uncle (and an astrologer from Lower Moesia) apparently predicted his imperial future.[242] Does this frequent literary motif have any practical correlate in our treatises' theories, as Cramer assumes?[243] First, it should be said that the planets' positions, as described in the horoscope, are in very good agreement with the positions Neugebauer and Van Hoesen estimate for the day of Hadrian's birth.[244] Only the Moon would have been significantly different, if he was in fact born at a time other than 6 A.M. (as would the Ascendant, of course). Furthermore, it is an immediately striking horoscope to someone a little acquainted with the fundamentals of astrology, with the most important benefic (Jupiter) with one of the luminaries in her own sect (by night) together exactly with the Ascendant in conjunction with the Sun by 8° with the other planets clustered round in δορυφορία, or "attendance." Antigonus uses all these data to support his case. He exploits the metaphor of δορυφορία explicitly, claiming that it foreshadows his προσκύνησις among all; all would prostrate themselves before him.[245]

Yet even in an abridged horoscope this is not enough for him. And here the elaboration game starts. We should not omit to observe (p. 69, 20f.) that of the Moon's attendants Venus is in her exaltation and Mars in his terms and triplicity and in evening rising in the sign just before. The Sun, who also attends the Moon, has his attendants also together: Saturn in his house with Mercury, both in their morning rising.

Moreover, Antigonus feels compelled to mention a bright star (p. 68, 27–p. 69, 2) in front of the Moon and Ascendant at 20° Aquarius. The only bright star in the region was said by Ptolemy to be at 7° (*Almagest* 8.1). But belief in the existence of a regal star at 20° Aquarius was obviously based on at least one tradition, for in Firmicus (6.2.3) it is one of a canon of four such stars. For it to operate in this case, however, Saturn should be on the Ascendant or in trine, which it is not. But, anyway, this canon is undermined, since the *Mathesis* has another set of regal stars, in a later book, that require more conditions to be fulfilled. One is at 1° Aquarius, Hadrian's Ascendant:

> Whoever has that star on his Ascendant and the Moon well-located, with Mars and Saturn in favourable aspect, will be a great king, glorious, just, pious and long-lived. As life goes on, the greatest possible powers are conferred on him. (8.21.9; cf. 8.29.1)

Unluckily for Hadrian, one of these conditions is not fulfilled: Saturn cannot be said to be in any aspect, so Firmicus would cancel out the prediction for him.

3.3.1 offers a compromise. With Jupiter exactly on the Ascendant: "He will make the native high-born, famous, always ruling great states, perhaps the first ten of the great states." The force of this prediction is apparently lessened by Jupiter's not being in his House, terms, or Exaltation.

There are two more promising passages to suggest that Firmicus might have concurred with the verdicts of Hadrian's great-uncle and the Lower Moesian. The first is 4.17.10. The ruler of the Part of Fortune, the ruler of his terms, and of the Moon's are well located, which makes "emperors whose rule extends throughout the whole world." Even so, one might quibble about the exact definition of "well located." Otherwise, there are ascriptions of infinite riches and good fortune beyond all measure (6.23.7), weakened by its being a nocturnal chart.

The best Dorotheus can provide is 2.21.1–5, suggesting that "the native will be powerful, a chief and a commander," or 2.29.1: "he'll be wealthy and gain no praise or honour for it," and 2.30.2: "he'll be friendly to kings."

Once again with this question of imperial power, as with the question of the length of life and the number of children, though in this case scattered through the pages, there is elaboration worthy of Daedalus in its labyrinthine quality. Not for nothing was Daedalus seen as one of astrology's "founders."[246] More and more complex specifications of arrangements of stars are added to the list of imperial horoscopes. This elaboration is there even in Antigonus, where flexibility is unnecessary with such a striking horoscope.

Now is the time to see the effect of this procedure on any conclusions the other two astrologers might make, for we cannot leave Hadrian there:

> But [we are] not able to explain the whole chart entirely unless all the data are brought together, the combinations and aspects of the stars as you remember we often have said. For the cold of some stars is opposed to the fire of others, the ice of cold is tempered with burning heat, and a mixture of temperaments is accomplished. (Firmicus: 8.32.1)

As will become obvious from a few other predictions, in the same way as the material on the length of life or on children, the data obstinately resist blending into homogeneity. When brought together the predictions cancel one another out or produce such a mass of details that they build up to present a life whose ups and downs far surpass the reversals of fortune in the contemporary romantic novels. Peter Brown's apprehension of the influence of the stars as baffling rather than ineluctable, and formative of a tension-ridden identity, is borne out. Clement of Alexandria talks in appropriate terms when he refers to the Fate written in the stars as a "concourse of opposing powers," a στάσις (contest) and a μάχη (battle) from which Christ rescues the baptized.[247]

It is time to add the hot to the cold, as it were, and look at some of the opposing powers' influence:

> He will be small of body, depressed in mind, weak, always subservient, and will lose all initiative in business. (Firmicus 4.22.5: Ascendant empty)
>
> Whatever he attains will be lost and ruined, whatever he seeks he will lose again, but what he has lost he will regain easily. He will do favours for many . . . but they will always be ungrateful. He will be in great danger so that his life is despaired of, but he will be freed by the gods. Many men will attack him with fierce hatred. He will work with religious writings. (Firmicus: 5.1.29: Ascendant in Aquarius)

At a pinch this might be squared with an emperor, and even with one of Antigonus' retrospective predictions, but the following forecasts are less easy to fit in: soldier or athlete, admininstrators or notaries, designer of important crafts, something noble to do with iron and fire, something to do with water, a traveling merchant, authors of false writings, criminal, malevolent poisoners.[248] Presumably, for this "the native will be condemned justly to exile, gladiatorial combat or the mines" (7.24.2–3).[249] As if this were not enough, 7.25.4 adds insult to injury:

"In an evening rising in feminine signs in a man's chart, with Saturn in aspect, Mars and Venus make perverts (*cinaedos*) who sing in temple choirs."[250]

Dorotheus also offers predictions that do not square well with his other forecast of Hadrian's being "a chief or a commander," let alone with an imperial horoscope. "He will be in difficulties or thwarted from work, dull in mind and body, disgraced." "He'll be dumb, lisping or deaf, silent and contemplative, and excessively curious; some of them will be learned in religious books, an astrologer or an augur." Alternative life trajectories are: a scribe, an orator, perhaps a steward for women and wealthy on that account, or a pimp.[250] He will not cease being a slave or servant to the end of his life,[252] though Jupiter will manumit him or at least lessen the pains of this condition (1.10.34), and he will not aspire to power and praise (2.29.1). On the subject of occupations I have made here a selection from the enormous number of predictions available in these two writers.

It is more than a question of a battle between benefic and malefic planets for his fate. For specific qualities of the stars come into contradiction with one another to produce this set of different options. One could, with difficulty, accept the sort of contradictions of character that the astrologers provide for him—oddly enough, his biographer describes him as only consistent in his inconsistency.[253] But when the predictions are for concrete events we are truly left baffled. What is the point of the exercise? I propose that there are several factors involved in the building up of so many variants in "ineluctable fate."

Astrology as Initiation

The first issue to consider is that I have taken the point of view of the neophyte pupil. An essential feature of ancient didactic practice is the teaching of ignorance and humility. This is clearest in the dialogue form, from Socrates to Hermes Trismegistus. The pupil is presented as remaining in no position to take over the teaching role.[254] The realization of inadequacy is seen as in itself an important achievement. I think that this lies behind the bewildering assault on certainty in our texts.

Plato, at least as constructed under the empire, is an important influence here. In their article on the consequences of literacy Goody and Watt point to Plato's objections to writing.[255] First, it fails as a mode of education. In the Seventh Letter[256] it is perceived as inherently shallow in its effects, leading to contempt or pride, whereas the dialectic method is an essential process in which the old pass on their knowledge to the young, and the long personal relationship may transcend the inherent incapacity of mere words to convey ultimate truths. In the *Phaedrus* Plato implies that writers and readers of manuals are wasting their time if they expect them to provide anything reliable or permanent: "Written words seem to talk to you as if they were intelligent, but if you ask them anything about what they say, from a desire to be instructed, they go on telling you the same thing for ever" (275c).

What is more, they may get into the wrong hands. Knowledge, as far as Plato is concerned, should be restricted. It is perhaps particularly characteristic of ancient education that the knowledge gained draws its value primarily from its esoteric nature. From a Platonic point of view these texts are thus products of a literacy that is only a poor substitute for the oral medium. And, of course, it was aspects of Neoplatonic thinking that became very closely bound up with astrology. Plato is specifically mentioned by Firmicus, in his prooemium to the eighth book, in the context of initiation. There Plato is put in company with Orpheus, Pythagoras, and Porphyry, as demanding oaths from his disciples so that they will not reveal to the profane what they have been taught. It is the mystical, Neoplatonic reading of Plato's works which must be seen as important. The account of the ascent to knowledge, in which the soul leaves the body, is taken in a more literal sense. Firmicus echoes these themes: "And so my dear Mavortius, look with wide open eyes at the heavens, let your soul contemplate the most beautiful fabric of the divine creation. That is the way to free our souls from the depraved snares of the body and to put off the dangers of mortality" (8.1.6). This model of learning has surely left its mark on astrological texts. The apprenticeship cannot be dissociated from the ascent, which is, above all, hard and full of reversals. The mystic quest leads the neophyte toward a goal that seems unattainable, the place of total knowledge, where all final contradictions will be resolved.

For the sort of Neoplatonic thought revealed in the Hermetic corpus (which included technical astrological works), the endless deferral of meaning might in fact offer advantages. The symbols thus employed would thereby retain their polyvalency and also their magical power. The book kept its secrets. Initiation into its pages revealed just enough for the neophyte to desire further instruction.[257] Firmicus offers the neatest of all examples of this mystic quest. He continually exploits the mystic model in ways that lead to contradiction. Thus, time is divided into smaller and smaller units, each successively undermining the next (2.26–28). Whatever answers came out in the first division will be canceled out by the next. The division of the chart moves throughout the book from the first crude division by the cardinal points, through the eight-house system to the twelve-house system, to the Lots and then the *Sphaera Barbarica,* where individual degrees are considered. But even this fine division is not enough. At 5.1.36 and 8.18.1 he refers to a division by minutes of degrees (sixty to a degree) in a work of "Aesculapius" inspired by Mercury (a Hermetic text) called the *Myriogenesis* (Countless Nativities) on divisions into "minutes" of degrees. He cites his first selection of bright stars in individual degrees from a work of his own on *myriogenesis* (6.2.8), but clearly a work that promises to divide individual Ascendants into minutes will indeed generate almost an infinite number of horoscopes and will demand very thorough treatment:

> But, my dear Lollianus, do not look for the theory of *myriogenesis* in this book. When our meagre talent, with the help of favourable powers, will have finished this book then I will write for you in twelve books the secrets of that teaching. For now everything must be learnt step by step, for we cannot reach *myriogenesis* by any other way except that our minds have first grasped the secrets of the beginnings of the art. (5.1.3)

"I have reserved for another time the explanation of the *myriogenesis*" (8.1.10), he observes tantalizingly. Presumably, in a sense this comment might invalidate the whole book. It was just this grading of knowledge that made it eminently suitable for the cult of Mithras, with its hierarchized initiations.[258]

Another way of looking at the operations of astrologers is to see them as working with the goal of "magical" completeness rather than in a modern Western logic based on avoiding contradictions. The association of the word *magical* I want to exploit here is given succinctly by Geoffrey Lloyd: "The criteria that are relevant to judging magical behaviour are not whether it achieves practical results, but whether it has been carried out appropriately or not."[259]

This attitude also was not confined to astrologers, as we shall see when it comes to medical prognosis. It may be also that there was something of this privileging completeness over noncontradiction in Roman jurisprudence, though much more work would need to be done to draw out similarities and contrasts.[260]

But these contradictions in the astrologers are veiled in secrecy: they are not evident to the lay public. Ptolemy's *Tetrabiblos* is remarkable for how much it conceals of the long ascent to knowledge; there seems an unbridgeable gulf between master and pupil. Here are his comments on potential contradictions:

> Such are the effects produced by the several planets, each by itself and in command of its own nature. Associated, however, now with one, now with another, in the different aspects, by the exchange of signs (houses) and by their phases with reference to the sun, and experiencing a corresponding tempering of their powers, each produces a character, in its effect, which is the result of the mixture of the natures that have participated, and is complicated. It is of course a hopeless and impossible task to mention the proper outcome of every combination and enumerate absolutely all the aspects of whatever kind since we can conceive of such a variety of them. Consequently questions of this kind are best left to the enterprise and ingenuity of the astrologer,[261] in order to make the distinctions. (2.9.19, p. 90, 1–13, trans. Robbins)

The art of the master is not lightly to be passed on.[262] Often a pupil had to take oaths not to reveal to the profane the secrets of methods learned. Vettius Valens, at the beginning of the prooemium to book 7 of his *Anthologies,* says: "Now, concerning all these things and this book, an oath should be required of all who receive them, to receive guardedly, and as if it belonged to the mysteries."[263] In the fourth book he says:

> I adjure you, most honoured brother, and all those being initiated into this systematic art, learning of the starry bowl of the heavens, and the zodiac and sun and moon and five planets, and also of foreknowledge and holy necessity, to keep all these things hidden, and not to share them with the uninitiated, except those who are worthy and able to guard and receive them rightly.[264]

Firmicus similarly warns his addressee Mavortius, at the beginning of book 2, not to communicate the book to anyone.[265]

Astrology as a Glass Bead Game

There is another factor predisposing to elaboration of this sort. In this model of apprenticeship literary and oral thinking are complementary. In another intellectual arena they are also closely intertwined. The rationale and methodology of astrology and other *scientiae* were generated in the arena of the ἀγών.[266] Written rhetoric retained the imprint of oral exchange. In the Greco-Roman world the competitive debate tended to provide the impetus toward intellectual developments that look bizarre to us. In the fourth century, according to Eunapius, a medical sect known as iatrosophists appeared. The famous story about this sect was that its best-known exponent, Magnus of Antioch, used his oratorical training, in public debates, to argue that his opponents' patients were still ill, even when they were thanking their doctors for having cured them.[267] Far from any modern Western concept of medicine as this was, it was only the logical culmination of the agonistic genesis of medical thought.[268]

Maurice Bloch's fieldwork among Merina astrologers in Madagascar is suggestive of the implications of such debate for the genesis of astrological theory: "When I went to one man of importance and then went to another for information, the second would immediately ask what the first had told me, and would then go on to elaborate further, to the admiration of all present" (1968, 294). He goes on to describe the competitive debate of two rivals over a ritual at a wedding, which was conducted not in terms of who was right and who was wrong but, instead, to show who knew the most elaborate version.

Galen's view of a dispute between a Greek and an Arabic bird diviner is particularly instructive here.[269] He is more impressed by the skill of the Greek who appeals to past experts and, above all, draws more subtle distinctions, when asked. Distinctions are the mark of a real τέχνη:

> ἔγνων οὖν ἀδιόριστον μὲν τὸν Ἄραβα, διωρισμένον δὲ καὶ τεχνικὸν τὸν Ἕλληνα.
>
> So I knew that the Arab was lacking in distinctions, while the Greek was full of them and proficient in his craft. (*Vict. Acut.* pp. 129, 33–130, 1 = K.15.444)

Similarly, Artemidorus in his work on dream interpretation offers advice to his son: "If you give a bare, simple explanation, you'll appear to be inexperienced" (4.20). He himself claims to have made subtle but irrefutable distinctions (4 pr.)

Bloch's point is that the astrologers cannot possibly use all these ornate explanations. He would seem to be backed up by Artemidorus' advice to his son (4.23) to use the technique of the anagram, when he wanted to seem wiser in competitive debates with other interpreters, but never for actually interpreting dreams, as it does not work. Aristandros the "excellent" dream interpreter put in his introduction but never employed it, he claims.

This strategy of recommending techniques that were not for use persisted in the written medium. In Firmicus' polemical introduction to the ninetieth degree he says:

> The use of this degree seems unknown to many, and is only lightly treated by a few writers. The tract of Petosiris on the subject seems to me to betray a hostile prejudice and an attempt to conceal the concept. From this degree can be discovered the nature of death for the native, his misfortunes, dangers, good fortune, the whole essence of the chart.

He never mentions it again.

Yet the only original (nonliterary) horoscope in the collection of Neugebauer and Van Hoesen (1959) to provide more than one prediction might suggest that this sort of elaboration left its mark at one level of practice, at least (1959, no. 95). *Papyrus Londiniensis* 98 must be one of the most significant finds in the historiography of astrology, if it is, as I believe, a horoscope with interpretations. Griffith (1900) conjectures that the papyrus may have been found originally with wooden tablets containing Demotic planetary tables for the years A.D. 71–132, since these were also in the collection of Stobart from his visit to Egypt in 1883–84. So this might be the nearest thing to an astrological "kit" so far found.[270] The editors date the horoscope to A.D. April 13, 95: hence, the papyrus is from the second century.

After dicussion of the Lots, the cardines, and the ruler of the nativity, the writer moves on to the interpretation. From line 83 onward (col. 3) the papyrus clearly discusses the periods of life. The Greek may be freely translated, as Neugebauer and Van Hoesen have done:

> The first period Venus rules up to 6 [years, 9 months, 25 days. Its position in Lot 1 Agathos Daimōn, indicates well-being and abundance] of pleasure. If he is a slave [he will be set free; if he is poor he will become] rich; if he is rich he will become richer and [whatever slaves] he is master of he will increase, as the nativity indicates; and [his crops (?) of whatever sort they are] will do well; and the children from whatever union born will have inborn in them a fine nature like their parents. And he will have excellent associations extending everywhere. He will suffer from cold or fevers or other illnesses; such are the things that Mars portends. . . . Venus is in Epanaphora. And Saturn is in trine to Venus (and portends that) he will be cold as regards women. He will be tried before the magistrate for unspeakable accusations . . . he will suffer miserably and will live a miserable life abroad. For the first lot is a separation [?], the second likewise a separation [?] and the third likewise a separation [?].

At line 118 a new hand takes over in Old Coptic, a language that presents many difficulties. There are also severe problems of legibility. It is clear, however, that the Coptic continues discussions of the periods of life. Indeed, each announcement of a new period is written in Greek, in a different hand from the rest. The first period of life from lines (col. 3) 83 to 115, extending from birth to 6 years, 9 or 5 months, and 25 days, was ruled by Venus. The second probably began from lines (col. 4) 116, just before the Coptic started, and continued to 125. It went up to 25 years, 2 months, 25 days, and was ruled by Mars (?). The third, from lines (col. 5) 125 to 134, extending to 34 years, 5 months, and 24 days, was ruled by Jupiter. The fourth, from (col. 5) 134ff., extending to 54 years, 10 months, four days, was ruled by Mars (?). This division does not prove sufficient, however, as at line 167 year 30 is mentioned, and at lines 144ff. an interval from years 42 to 92 occurs, and at 152f. and 178 there is again discussion of year 42. The editors comment that they do not know how these data were determined, but they remark that such detailed divisions occur in the literary horoscopes of the fifth century, such as the compilation of "Rhetorius."[271]

Neugebauer and Van Hoesen have used the work of Černý, Parker, and Kahle (1957) on the Coptic. These scholars' equation of the Coptic word *afcōpe* with the Demotic *'iw-f hpr,* makes them translate it as a conditional: "if there were" throughout. It is unclear, however, why they decide to assimilate it to *ecōpe* (which appears in the text at line [col. 5] 142), and is more certainly a conditional,[272] while *afcōpe* would normally be translated as an imperfect, simply "there was." Griffith's earlier version certainly takes it as such. Old Coptic is so rarely found that there is little room for certainty; still, it would seem that there is no need to translate with conditionals throughout, as that only creates problems. The difficulties become clear in Neugebauer and Van Hoesen's discussion. It is clear that the text from (col. 3) 83ff. is a continuous discussion of the periods of life. Also, line 111 ties the discussion firmly to the preceding horoscope, referring to conditions obtaining: "with Venus in Epanaphora and Saturn in trine." The editors recognize that both in the Greek and in the Coptic "the specific numbers assigned to these intervals require specific data for their computation and it is natural to assume they are the data of the horoscope" (1959, 37). They decide, however, on the basis of the conditionals and on the grounds that "the predictions are held in an extremely vague form" that this "would fit much better a general astrological treatise than an individual horoscope." Once it is realized, first, that the conditionals are of dubious status and, second, on the basis of my research so far, that contradictory or vague predictions are to be expected, we can conclude that we are dealing with the interpretation of a horoscope.

Here I offer a translation of the Coptic that follows Griffith's line on αγσωπє but otherwise relies on the work done by Černý, Parker, and Kahle, with some help from E. G. Turner (1957):

> The sun became to him as a friendly star, (and) Mercury, and they were at enmity to this st[ar . . .], it shall not be effective (?) . . . as hostile star. The two gods . . . (are . . .) during his life. They were in *akhelo;* they shall make 24 evils against him . . . of his life (and) his occupation, . . . after 35 (evils) from it. He had M[ercury itse]lf as his *krahtouot* [col. 5 begins]: (so) his growth (?) shall be established in its likeness, whether (?) it be against his good or evil. There was an evil star as his *krahtouot* (so) he will go to . . . man (?) or god, ⟨or⟩ he shall go into misfortune, or (he shall) see a man's death. It shall come to him through him or through his snake.
>
> *Third period: Jupiter decides. From year 25, month 2, day 25 until year 34, month 5, day 24, Jupiter decides.* It happened that Jupiter (was) a hostile star on the ⟨day⟩ of his birth, perhaps he will pass by (= neglect) his wife, or be at enmity to her, or his children will misbehave in turn, or he will part (from them) on mercantile business. There was an evil star . . . , a wife will not make a term for him ⟨for ever⟩, a child will not come to him for ever. Evil will happen after him. They will . . . hireling . . . and [t]hey will cause the S[un] to come again, it shining forth there opposite Jupiter, and a wife will burn to (the) hair. It happened that a good star gave to him an omen . . .
>
> *Fourth period: [Mars] decides from year 34, month 5, day 24 until year 54, month 10, day 4.* It happened that the Moon was a friendly star to him on the day of his [birth] . . . will . . . upward. After closing as a friendly star on the

d[ay] of his birth, (it was) (?) a friendly star to him again. The said man, the half of his . . . shall . . . against him. His evils shall multiply. A woman of . . . [will] . . . him, and his heart will ⟨become good⟩ through her. He will take a name(?) . . . in the service of kingship . . . his relatives, he causing them to appear as those who take a wreath of gold to their head(s) in the years named, and he shall speak and they will act at his voice and he will see a law which is great to his heart. If an evil star was coming up after them, against his good and for his evil, a woman will cause him to take shame, or he will be hunted(?) from year 42 upwards. A woman will be to him. He will take one until year 94. He will see a [wife's] death or shall be parted from her and ⟨they⟩ will examine him while he . . . and . . . of his will make his evils or . . . of his. A good star was . . . , he will escape his place of confusion . . . to them . . . and they will cast 31 winters on them(selves). He will take counsel from a woman and [she] will take counsel from him. He had a good star take closing on the d[ay]of his birth, perhaps he will see (the) death of a man who is close to him ⟨or⟩ (the) death of a relative (and) he will not make new profit with him (but) his heart will become good for a wife (and) send to him a child from year 42 {from year 42} again and according to the way with him which . . . before it is decided for his good (or) his evil, and his ⟨heart⟩ will become good for his life and he will not have died in a past hour (but will) see . . . child . . .

So ends column 5, the best-preserved part of the document. Clearly, it is full of contradictions. There may well be more. It is certain that there are at least three further references to women, at least one being a wife who leaves him in what follows.

Neugebauer and Van Hoesen, as noted, are not certain of the ways in which the data were determined. They also remark on the "great number of discrepancies between [the] text and orthodox doctrine" (1959, 35), citing, first, the determination of the Lots "according to principles unknown to us" and, second, the reference to two sorts of decans (one sort called "the 36 horoscopes"), both with some names corresponding to the Egyptian names of decans known elsewhere (1959, 36). They decide that this may be because so little of astrological doctrine is known before the second century (1959, 35). But it may also be that the idea of "orthodox doctrine" is too rigid.

This document is unique as evidence for astrological practice. First, it shows that quite unfamiliar doctrine was used, which fits in with the picture of a certain amount of improvisation. Second, it offers predictions that are equivocal, complex, and contradictory in just the same manner as the unabridged compilation I have been reconstructing by following the texts. Whether or not it was a rough draft rather than a finished horoscope is a question I shall touch on later. Certainly, it would hardly seem an appropriate form in which to present it to the client.

Astrology and Religion, Science, and Magic

Yet, beneath all this elaboration the core doctrines were kept in sight. The planets always retain their genders and general character, whether beneficent or maleficent. As J.-C. Hébert noted on the subject of Merina astrology, the fundamental elements might serve as mnemonic devices.[273] For practicing astrologers we must imagine an important role for the memory, a further characteristic of oral thinking. Bouché-Leclercq notes that the mnemonic qualities of Dorotheus' original verse insured the triumph of his version of the ὅρια (terms) rather than Ptolemy's.[274] And Firmicus warns: "You should note attentively what we say and commit it to memory. Otherwise you will not be able to interpret the fates of men" (5.2.1).

It is also notable that the astrologer carried out his *bricolage* [275] with some basic, familiar building blocks. Firmicus refers to "obvious and clearly-defined facts, facts which we not only discern with our reason, but perceive with our senses and our very eyes" (1.1.1). The Moon's effect on the tides is a simple example. But astrology drew on fields of inquiry such as physics, geography, numerology, philosophy, and biology (to use anachronistic terms) as well as on common sense and, thus, established connections that offered familiar categories in a new light. For example, the symbolic associations of the Moon with femaleness, change, growth, birth and death, and humidity were intuitively satisfying, given existing categories, without being obvious.[276] Stoic physics, working on similar principles, formed a suitable basis for astrological "influences." Thus, Cleanthes drew an analogy between the renewal of the human ψυχή (soul) with exhalation from the blood and the sustaining of the heavenly bodies by exhalation from the oceans and other liquids of the world's "body."[277] Ptolemy draws on Aristotelian physics in referrring to the δύναμις (*dynamis* [power]) emanated from the ether, causing changes in the sublunary realm and to the four elements (hot, cold, wet, and dry).

Yet Favorinus, whose attack on astrology is preserved in Aulus Gellius (*Attic Nights* 14.1.1ff.), attacked the weakness of the link between obvious physical effects of the Moon and detailed predictions (e.g., of the outcome of a lawsuit). It was also to divert attention from this that astrologers concentrated on detailed elaboration on the bases beyond the link, or rather gulf. Richard Gordon (1990) suggests that a new religious cult must combine "cannibalizing upon a range of banal and customary beliefs" with an ever-greater elaboration of the "absurd" (1980, 23). Gordon expands on this notion of the absurd with reference to Ernest Gellner. Here Gellner depicts the master-pupil relationship:

> An intelligible belief-system, once mastered, leaves the disciple the equal of his master. He too can draw further consequences, check the master's steps etc. No such danger arises if the system contains a decent dose of absurdity. It will paralyse the learner's power of independent movement within the system. . . . Moreover, unintelligibility leaves the disciple with the secret guilt of not understanding, or not avowing it, or both, which binds him to the master, who is both responsible for it and seems untainted by it. (Gellner 1974, 54, 55).

Gellner describes as absurd those beliefs and practices that people outside the culture would deem absurd and refers to religion as a general purveyor of the absurd in this sense. This is one plausible way of understanding the success of astrology. In the same way as for a new cult a successful strategy for the astrologers in establishing their art, which Firmicus still calls a "new discipline" (8.33.1), was to combine reliance on accepted knowledge with ever-greater elaboration of their basic principles. This elaboration led to absurd contradictions, which made it ever harder to learn and, thus, paradoxically, more likely to be believed.

In noting the connections between astrology, mysticism, and cult, I am by no means divorcing it from those areas more conventionally designated as intellectual activity. As previously emphasized, I find it more helpful to question the siting of frontiers between disciplines. Certainly, in antiquity there was a blurring of distinctions between fields of knowledge regarded as incompatible today. Thus, when the author of a biography of the emperor Alexander Severus describes what has been interpreted as a reorganization of the Athenaeum, he lumps together rhetoricians, grammarians, physicians, haruspices, astrologers (*mathematici*), engineers (*mechanici*), and architects. Severus Alexander, according to him, paid them regular salaries and assigned them lecture rooms and further arranged support for poor but free-born students.[278]

It is, then, no surprise to find that one can discover many principles in common between different *scientiae.* Simon Price (1986) compares the principles of the Empirical "school" of medicine with those of dream interpretation, and Pack (1941) notes that an Empirical tone pervades the physiognomist Polemo, whose work I shall be considering in the next chapter. The triad Price notes of "tradition," "practice" (πεῖρα/τήρησις), and "analogy" (μεταβάσις τοῦ ὁμοίου) would transfer easily enough to astrology, although it is not clear that astrologers have specifically Empirical leanings.

For Bouché-Leclercq, who perhaps contributed most of all to explicating it, astrological theory was a morass.[279] I think a helpful label to describe the process that leads to this "insane complexity" and to "explain" it by comparison is the anthropologist Alexander Goldenweiser's concept of "involution" (1936). He describes the initial reaction to activities as diverse as Trobriand matrimonial etiquette, Plains Indian sun dances, and Bach fugues: "we are overwhelmed, almost shocked, often bored by what seems an excessive heaping up of unit elements and the total effect of what seems to the novice bewildering complexity" (1936, 103). The important feature of these activities is that, while a limiting frame is set, within it change is permitted, even invited. Perhaps the most vivid of his examples is that of Maori decorative art, for which the entire object is pervaded by the decoration, every corner minutely covered. In art originality takes the form of combination, repetition, or juxtaposition of relatively uniform elements; in writing it manifests itself in progressive hairsplitting. Ancient astrology might also be seen in such a light. We shall see that involution is not confined to astrologers.[280]

To recapitulate briefly, then, I have revealed a problem here—a problem only apparent once you cast a horoscope: Why this absurd accumulation of contradictory answers to questions about the future? And I have suggested various factors that help to explain, or make sense of, this nonsense. First, I have suggested two "sociological" factors—the influence of the institutions in which the body of knowledge is built up—the master-pupil relationship on the one hand and the ἀγών (agon) on the other. Both tend to privilege other aims over avoidance of contradiction. I have touched on the way in which this complexity is simple to generate from memorable elements, which fit with existing knowledge, and I have suggested that the elaboration might work to divert attention from premises that might seem dubious. Finally, I labeled this elaboration "involution," suggesting that it is not after all particularly bizarre or unusual but, rather, widely found and indeed understandable. At the end I come to the question of astrological practice outside the texts, to consider if there is a further answer to my problem there.

Astrology as Craft

The reflex answer to the problem that I have posed might be that interaction with the clientele was the reason for the number of possible answers and, indeed, for the complexity of the system. It was just mystification, in short. Certainly, one must imagine that there was a practical point to the diversity of interpretations possible at this level of the consultation. Apart from the rhetorical impact of this technical complexity in justification, if necessary it afforded the leeway for varying answers in accordance with the facts that were known about the client.

Astrology was not only a cult and a science; like medicine, it was also a craft. The mass of undigested predictions in the Old Coptic Horoscope was surely only one stage in the process. No doubt, the expert astrologer would be able to cut through the knots of involuted natal astrological theory to suit the client's needs, as Ptolemy assumes.[281] The fact that astrology was a craft also contributes to the lack of clearly spelled-out connections between theory and day-to-day practice. The first book of Firmicus, in which he presents astrology within the frameworks of inquiry into nature and the doctrines of Fatalism, seem quite separate from the following seven. Neither has much connection with daily practice. Like the Divine Mind to which Firmicus appeals, they serve to legitimate the craft; they are the basis of its rhetoric. Hence, the recourse to them in the face of critical attack. One scholar has even, controversially, suggested that the connection with astronomy that Ptolemy sees as the other part of the science (*Tetrabiblos* 1.1.1, p. 2, 16ff.) is by this period largely a mirage, to the extent that the stars are rarely observed and traditional tables used instead.[282]

It is probably the case that, as has been argued by one scholar with regard to the seventeenth century, astrologers accepted the aims and questions of their clientele without seeking to impose any esoteric problematic on them.[283] This was clearly true of catarchic astrology, which was brought into fashion among the elite on the coattails of natal astrology.[284] We may assume that this simpler form of astrology was the limit of what was offered to poorer clients. It was available in the villages as well as in urban resorts such as the Circus. The fifth book of Dorotheus is entirely devoted to it.[285] It discusses questions such as when to build, when to demolish, when to buy slaves, land, animals, or a ship, when to make a request, marry, write a letter, perform an exorcism, make a will, or begin to row at sea. There are trickier ones: What's in that letter? How long will I stay in chains? Will I have a miscarriage? Where are the stolen goods? What does the thief look like? Here involution was trimmed to allow a decision.[286]

But are the constraints of interaction with the clients in consultations sufficient explanations of my problem? First, I do not find the need for leeway a sufficient explanation, though doubtless it is one factor. The differences among the three horoscopes indicate that there was some limit to adjustability to fit known facts, at any rate: not all Antigonus' predictions can be confirmed by the other two, despite their great flexibility. There were surely more straightforward ways of making the astrologer's task easier. Besides, this explanation underestimates the extent to which astrology took itself seriously as a discipline. Nor is this simply a tale of "secondary elaboration," in which a previously unmentioned variable is brought into play, once a prediction has proved incorrect, in order to explain away the mistake. Secondary elaboration, such as we find in the reinterpreted fifth-century horoscopes discussed by Pingree, is less important than the ability to tolerate anomalies, when the consensus is that astrology is the best way of finding the answers. As Pliny says: nobody should be surprised at astrology's success. I hope that the account I have given offers a more nuanced picture than the automatic dismissal of astrologers as being merely charlatans.

We have seen, in the first part of this chapter, that the battles of the stars above for control over individual destinies are mirrored in struggles below to appropriate knowledge of the truth they offered. Emperors, their friends, and their enemies were set at odds by the very possibility of absolute knowledge on the part of the astrologers. So the latter were wooed, taken as mentors, commanded, and ejected in turn by different parties. The second part of the chapter tells a different story: despite the astrologers' frequent appearances in our sources in a passive capacity, they were in the best position to exploit their knowledge, and they actively competed with one another to establish their answers as the result of true knowledge in the eyes of the lay public. The most convincing, most contemporary, style of argument ground specific truths exceeding small. But then this left room for the secret, virtuoso exercise of power.

I have here looked at the peculiar style in which astrologers sought to persuade their public. In the next chapter I look at another discipline in which a similar elaboration may be found but in which the principles according to which the art might be practiced were locked more closely into the moral universe on the one hand and into the rhetorical theory of the Second Sophistic on the other. In the following case study, rather than looking at the role of the body of knowledge at the point at which the stakes are highest, as in the case of astrology, I examine its role in political battles for lesser goals, for victories in provincial politics. There are interesting similarities with astrology, but I shall be concentrating on the differences, in order to avoid traversing much of the same ground again.

Chapter 2

Physiognomics: *Voir, Savoir, Pouvoir*

> She had a dark skin, black eyes with a tinge of red in them, and a very pointed nose. Her hair was parted severely down the middle and one half of it was black and the other white—rather unusual.
>
> "Why that's Cruella de Vil," said Mrs. Dearly. "We were at school together. She was expelled for drinking ink."
>
> —Dodie Smith, *The Hundred and One Dalmatians*

Introduction

Physiognomics[1] is the discipline that seeks to detect from individuals' exterior features their character, disposition, or destiny. That is a general definition for a phenomenon that appears in varying guises in different cultures. It seems, as Martine Dumont (1984) observes on Lavater's physiognomics,[2] that it is an art that has to be constantly reinvented; the desire to codify our pragmatic understanding of appearance as a clue to character surfaces again and again. That desire, however, appears one of few constant features in the history of the discipline.

Certainly, it is true that in recent scholarship, where physiognomics has been enjoying quite a vogue, many different accounts have been given of its significance. For those who are primarily students of literature or of art the hope is always that reading the treatises will crack the code and reveal the latent meaning of the work studied.[3] Physiognomics is here merely an interpretative tool. But the critics may go a stage further; this code may itself be examined for historical significance, as when Jeanne Fahnestock (1981) draws out the implications for contemporary women of the conventions of heroine description in the nineteenth-century novel. Alternatively, the very popularity of the science may be taken as a clue to the essence of the culture that fosters it. Roy Porter's (1985) article on physiognomics and fashion in eighteenth-century England posits a shift mid-century from the "age of the mask" par excellence, when physiognomics met with skepticism, to the age of the Romantic sensibility and concern for the truth of

"Nature Unadorned," when it returned in triumph. And Judith Wechsler's *A Human Comedy* (1982), a study of nineteenth-century Paris, which relates physiognomics to theatrical mime and political caricature, makes this new self-consciously scientific discipline a response to the new urbanization. According to her understanding, physiognomics is a way of sorting out the unfamiliar urban mass and should be seen as part of the broader exercise in social mirroring and modeling characteristic of the period.

This latter approach looks promising for a cultural historian. But, before adopting it, one needs to assess the importance of the phenomenon. I think that in the Greco-Roman world, while it is clear that physiognomical thinking has very deep cultural roots, far deeper than those of astrology, the discipline as we find it in the treatises is less culturally salient. It appears as a pale shadow of astrology in nonphysiognomical sources. The corpus of treatises is much smaller; they are less varied, less elaborate, and not so refined in the heat of debate, though the basic intellectual style is similar, as we shall see. And the physiognomist does not have the high profile of the astrologer. The Roman Empire never had its Lavater, while it had plenty of candidates for its William Lilly.[4]

Nevertheless, astrology furnishes a model for a first line of inquiry: that of treating the discipline as divination and examining its relationship to the state. Why not look for parallels in antiquity to the Elizabethan physiognomist, "liable to be whipped openly untill his body be bloudye" on the grounds that his art was potentially treasonable?[5] We do have plenty of evidence of the authorities' expulsion or punishment of all sorts of diviners for making trouble in antiquity.[6] Unauthorized physiognomical divination did go on in high places, as we know from tales like Suetonius' of the metoposcope summoned by the imperial freedman Narcissus to tell Britannicus' destiny from his face, who picked out Titus instead as the future emperor.[7] Unlike astrologers, however, such people do not significantly figure in our evidence at the intersection of high political power and knowledge.

But there is another possible line of inquiry. Several scholars have been fascinated by the more sinister uses of physiognomics for social control, such as its role in nineteenth-century Europe in classifying the insane and the criminal.[8] It is in fact this last view of its significance, as a coercive codification, that has most relevance for my project, though it is not a model I transfer wholesale, since I am not depicting a new disciplinary technology put at the disposal of the establishment.[9] In examination of the physiognomical texts I turn the gaze down from state power, from the imperial court, to make them yield information about the construction of knowledge at smaller nodes in the power network, in more localized confrontations. Here this body of knowledge operated as a taxonomy of control.

For Polemo, the second-century Sophist from Asia Minor, who wrote the most influential of these works,[10] physiognomical theory served as a classificatory grid to contain his political and intellectual opponents. In a sense it was a sophisticated development of the magical use of invective in the *tabellae defixionum,* or curse tablets.[11] The appreciation of the magical power of rhetoric appears as a theme at least as early as the fifth century B.C. It is a leitmotif in Platonic discussions of rhetoric, where rhetoricians are often confuted as conjurers.[12] Plutarch's *Life of Pericles* contains an early expression of this power: Thucydides Melesiou, when asked by King Archidamus whether he or Pericles was the better wrestler, replied that, whenever he threw him, Pericles would persuade everyone that he had not been thrown. Magnus the iatrosophist was associated with similar powers: he would win medical competitions by persuading the audience that his opponent's patients were still ill, even as they were thanking their doctors for having cured them. Sophists of the Second Sophistic, the most successful rhetoricians, such as Dionysius of Miletus, Hadrian of Tyre, and Apuleius were associated with sorcery.[13] But Polemo created a new magic of old elements, a new ψυχαγωγία (winning of souls).[14] Rather than actually making wax images of his opponents to burn, with physiognomics he constructed their bodies so as to destroy their characters. And destroying the ἦθος (*ēthos:* moral persona) of a rival deprived him of the moral claim to persuade.[15]

In an extended systematization of the common understanding of the physique as a collection of signs of the character, Polemo evolved a treasury of condensed meaning for rhetorical use. It was technically persuasive because of the form of systematization he used. Thus, it was methodologically in line with contemporary intellectual style, conforming to the model of the τέχνη (*technē*) as we have seen it in astrological writing. I mentioned in chapter 1 (sec. 11) the various links beween different *scientiae.* Physiognomics shared concerns with oneiromancy: both drew on the treasury of learning about animals, for instance. Physiognomists also drew on some of the learning common to geographical, astrological, and medical writing, in particular the ideas about the influence of the stars and the climate on physical and character types of different races.[16] For instance, the Ptolemy who wrote the *Tetrabiblos* was also the author of a *Geography,* and there was a certain cross-over in subject matter. I shall be discussing the passage in the *Tetrabiblos,* which dealt in detail with different κλίματα, zones of the world ruled by particular groups of zodiac signs and planets and the effects on the physical appearances and mores of the people, and comparing it to physiognomical ethnography (pp. 120–22). The medical interest in the physical and moral effects of the physical environment goes back at least to the Hippocratic *Airs, Waters, Places,* a work on which Galen and probably Rufus of Ephesus wrote commentaries in the second century A.D.[17]

The physiognomical gaze, "lo sguardo fisiognomico," as Sassi (1988) terms her chapter on the art, is particularly intimately associated with the image of the diagnostic gaze of the doctor, the subject I shall be discussing in chapter 3. Hippocrates was credited with founding the art, and, indeed, it is difficult to draw the line between the two types of examination of the body at times.[18] Some of the amazing deductions that Galen recounts in the *On Prognosis,* such as when he diagnoses a woman as being in love with a dancer, and a slave as worried about being caught having lost some of his master's money, are just like Polemo's spotting the women about to elope, or the man who is only pretending to have lost his goods in a shipwreck.[19] Both medicine and physiognomics establish lists of signs or symptoms, from which they infer the state of mind or body. Both often rely on common causes, either the humors, or the blood,[20] and they sometimes seek out the same phenomena in the cases of madness, epilepsy, apoplexy, and deafness.[21] The pseudo-Galenic work devoted to prognosis through astrological calculation, based on the time the patient took to bed, illustrates one kind of combination of astrology and medicine. The author quotes Hippocrates approvingly: "In those who practise medicine without a knowledge of the subject of physiognomy, the judgement goes to seed, wallowing in darkness."[22] (It also observes that the physiognomical part of astrology is the greatest part). There are other pieces of evidence that illustrate the connections between medicine and physiognomics. Loxus was a Hellenistic doctor who was one of the three sources of the Anonymous Latin author of a fourth-century physiognomical treatise (henceforth Anon.), while Adamantius, the fourth-century author of an epitome of Polemo's physiognomical treatise, is probably the author of some Sophistical works on medical subjects drawn on by the emperor Julian's doctor, Oribasius. Furthermore, Polemo's teacher of rhetoric for four years, Timocrates, was well versed in Hippocrates. Indeed, for the second-century Clement of Alexandria there are only two sorts of physiognomists: doctors and seers.[23]

It was Galen, building on Aristotle and Hippocrates, who was to provide for physiognomics the causal footing of humoral theory,[24] which lasted as long as Galenic medicine held sway. Only later in the medieval period were the two firmly linked by humoral theory in the simpler, more rigid views of the body propounded by Galen's successors. Yet Galen's treatise on how the faculties of the soul follow the mixtures in the body (Ὅτι ταῖς τοῦ σώματος κράσεσι αἱ τῆς ψυχῆς δυνάμεις ἕπονται = *Quod Animi Mores*), while hardly a "handbook on the theories of the physiognomists," as described by Evans,[25] does deal with physiognomical observations in Aristotle and Hippocrates and incidentally offers the humoral framework for such observations. Galen is certainly aware of the physiognomists proper. In *On the Temperaments,* after discussing how different parts of the body exhibit different mixtures (of the humors), so that it is a mistake to think, for instance, that because someone is bald, they must be generally of a dry mixture, he says that the physiognomists do not simply pronounce on the basis of one sign but, rather, are taught by experience to look at the different parts (a major theme in physiognomical writings). They know that if someone has a hairy chest he is spirited or that if he has hairy legs he is lustful. They do not give the first cause, however, saying only that these relationships exist because the lion is spirited and the goat lustful, facts that themselves need explaining. They can be accounted for by the mixtures, as Aristotle has explained: the hairy chest is a sign of heat from the heart, for instance.[26] In *On the Doctrines of Hippocrates and Plato* he mentions τὰ κατὰ τὸν φυσιογνώμονα φαινόμενα (the observations of the physiognomists) as apposite to Posidonius' critique of Chrysippus on ideas of how children acquire vice. He cites the observation that men and animals who are broad-chested and warmer are all by nature more given to anger, while those with wide hips, who are colder, are more cowardly, and mentions the effect of climate on παθητικὰς κινήσεις (the affective movements).[27] An example of how difficult it is to separate the two disciplines comes in the *Ars medica,* which includes a discussion of the influence of heat in producing angry, rash types with shaggy thoraxes.[28]

Physiognomics was one subject that was exempt from Sextus Empiricus' skepticism, along with his own profession of medicine: he refers to the φυσιογνωμονικὴ σοφία (the science of physiognomics) with apparent respect.[29] But, of course, it suffered from the double image of these "mantic" disciplines; Pliny has harsh words to say about the physiognomical calculation of years of life that he attributes to Aristotle, though elsewhere in his *Natural History* he endorses some basic physiognomical observations,[30] and Artemidorus also chooses to put it in the group of divinatory practices he designated as untruthful, as opposed to his own dream interpretation.[31]

Physiognomics, then, drew some of its credibility from its links with other τέχναι (*technai*); more important, the basic elements of the system were morally persuasive. The methods of physiognomics reveal themselves in this chapter as developments of some traditional τόποι (topoi, commonplaces) of praise and blame, which worked to persuade the audience to identify with the speaker against the categorized Other. The audience for our Sophist's speeches remains a shadowy crowd, whose lower social limits are uncertain. Philostratus, the chronicler of the Second Sophistic, a term he coined, refers to a variety of contexts for Sophists' speeches, occasions in which whole cities are present, the semiprivate contexts of lectures for pupils, and the private gatherings before the patron and connoisseurs. Some took place at public games and festivals; the largest audiences not in the open air required theaters accommodating thousands, normally the council chamber, lecture hall, or auditorium would be enough. Doubtless, Philostratus exaggerates the extent of Sophists' popularity, though the numbers who were prepared to suffer considerable discomfort is inexplicable unless Sophists provided good sport.[32] Such was the public context of intellectual life of the period. In looking at the physiognomical texts, one glimpses some answers to the question of what was persuasive to such audiences, in a sense some clues about its ideal self, given that ancient rhetorical theory demands adaptation to audience consensus.[33] It was only with the audience that the rhetor-intellectual could construct the fragile web of knowledge and power, after all.

The Background

The discipline of physiognomics was not invented by the Greeks. In Mesopotamia, from the first half of the second millennium B.C. onward, have been found fragments of manuals detailing the prophetic significance of aspects of individual human bodies.[34] Some examples indicate the form and variety of these observations, which would not all be described as strictly physiognomical:

> If a man with a contorted face has a prominent[?] right eye, far from his home dogs will eat him.
> If a man's face is marked by yellowish[?] lines, the state treasury will take all that belongs to him, or only his good furniture.
> If a man has curly hair on his shoulders, women will fall in love with him.
> If a man laughs while sleeping, he will be really ill.
> If a man, when he lies with a woman in a state of impurity, ejaculates too early every time, he will die in the prime of life.[35]

Physiognomics is here one of many techniques for divining the future; few examples reveal the character.[36] In Greco-Roman physiognomics the emphasis is reversed: the focus is on nature and mores, and the few predictions are generally dependent on a "pathognomical" analysis (careful judgment of the emotions from outward signs).[37] This is interestingly in contrast to the astrology of the period. Whereas today's clients of astrologers are interested in a character analysis, the ancients were far more eager for predictions, preferably of success in all areas of life.[38]

This focus on character gives us a clue to the essential nature of the physiognomical enterprise—it is for the practitioner, not the subject. In our sources the physiognomist is either hired by someone other than the person examined, as with Britannicus, or he gives the result unsolicited. So the magus Zopyrus, after inspecting his physique, kindly tells Socrates in one version that he is bound for a violent death, in another that he is stupid, thick-witted, and addicted to womanizing.[39]

The ideal type, which fits with the tone of the treatises, is of the physiognomist as sage. We are told in sources contemporary with the later treatises that such figures as Socrates, in the case of Plato at least, and Pythagoras as a matter of course, selected their disciples physiognomically.[40] An epigram usually ascribed to Leonidas of Tarentum describes such a physiognomical sage, named Eusthenes: a σοφιστής / δεινὸς ἐπ' ὀφθαλμοῦ καὶ τὸ νόημα μαθεῖν (a Sophist, clever at knowing the mind at a glance).[41] This awesome figure's gaze penetrates all attempts at deception[42] and sizes people up to the admiration of all. The third-century B.C. Stoic physiognomist Cleanthes makes it his business to unmask cowards, charlatans, effeminates, and adulterers. He spots the effeminate lurking behind the disguise of a hairy rustic brought to test him, just by the way he sneezes.[43] This wise man also writes books for others to admire and to glean a few ways to categorize for themselves. The serving girl in Petronius' Satyricon finds physiognomics her favorite divinatory procedure. She gathers people's habits from their faces and knows what they are thinking from watching the way they walk.[44] This fantasy Polemo exploits in his self-presentation as physiognomist, allowing the audience to enjoy vicariously the power of being a secret voyeur.

Physiognomical Treatises

Hippocrates was credited with founding the discipline, and the first appearances of the verb φυσιογνωμονέω (physiognomize) are in the Hippocratic *Epidemics,* in which elements of the kind of teaching found in the treatises first appeared, such as: "Those with a large head, large black eyes and a wide, snub nose are honest."[45] There was a treatise written around the end of the fifth century B.C. by Antisthenes, head of the Cynics, according to Diogenes Laertius.[47] Some systematization had taken place, for Aristotle mentions a physiognomist who had reduced his system to one of analogy with only two or three animal types. And in the first extant treatise there is criticism of three existing methods, with the implication that physiognomists tend to use only one of the three.[47]

The surviving treatises and some relevant quotations from Greek and Roman authors are presented with important prolegomena in Foerster's two-volume Teubner edition of 1893, under the title of *Scriptores Physiognomonici Graeci et Latini.* The first treatise joined the ranks of "Pseudo-Aristotles." Though Pliny and Diogenes Laertius clearly believed that Aristotle had written a physiognomical treatise, and the earliest extant was attributed to him,[48] it has long been generally agreed that what we have is an epitome of the work of two Peripatetic authors of the third century B.C. following up his interests.[49] It sets the form for all that come after, right up to the sixteenth century. The first author (chaps. 1–34), after criticizing previous methods, concentrates on twenty-two characters, listing the signs by which they may be recognized. Examples are the Flirt, the Debaucher, the Well-Born, the Irascible, or the Merciful. The second (35–74) spends more time on detailed aspects of the body, as a whole and in individual parts, listing with the signs the inferences about character. They offer an eclectic solution as regards method, the first allowing analogy with different races and animals and examination of the physical signs of known character types, and the second stressing the importance of male and female types and the principle of moderation as the ideal.

The treatise with which I am mainly concerned is the work of Polemo, written around A.D. 133–36, according to one estimate.[50] Only one sentence survives in the original Greek.[51] Fortunately, however, we have one Arabic transcript made in Damascus in 1379,[52] which was translated into Latin by A. Schmoelders and revised by G. Hoffmann in 1884 for Foerster's edition (F.1.lxxxii ff.). There are naturally problems with such a source. There are the usual additions of "God willing" and some obvious substitutions, such as the Slavs and Turks mentioned in F.1.250, which replace Scyths and Celts. The translation into Arabic has also played havoc with the syntax, removing the connectives. Worst of all, it is not infrequently dogged by lacunae or incomprehensible, where the Arab translator or the scribe has misunderstood his text.[53] Nevertheless, it seems to give a tolerably accurate picture of the Greek in conjunction with the epitomes.[54] The most important of these is by the Sophist Adamantius,[55] probably of the fourth century. The inclusion of a preamble (largely Polemo's), the systematic suppression of examples, and the pruning of variations make it the most orderly work of the major treatises as they have come down to us. There is also the work of the Anonymous Latin author (Anon.), which relies mainly on Polemo but draws also on parts of the Peripatetic *Physiognomonica* not previously known and on the lost medical physiognomist Loxus.[56] Though once thought to be from the pen of Apuleius, it has been persuasively dated on grounds of Latinity to the fourth century, a period of relatively intense activity in translating and adapting Greek technical and scientific works.[57]

Antonius Polemo lived from about A.D. 88–145.[58] In the slim book of declamation that bears his name (Hinck 1873), only a short dispute between the fathers of two heroes at Marathon over the honor of delivering the funeral speech seems to be his. It is considered a tour de force of its type by Reardon, in its ingenious pushing of an antithesis to its limits, and he believes it fits the improvisatory style for which Polemo was famous. Indeed, he thinks it reflects closely the Polemo of Philostratus, in his boldness and his desire to assume an impressive pose at all costs.[59] Boulanger, while deploring the bad taste and excess, is tempted to excuse the audience their enjoyment: "It is a fire-ball of word-combinations, of paronomasiai, anaphorai, chiasmoi, apostrophes and prosopopoeiai," he exclaims, though he has to admit that it is not easy for the modern audience to appreciate.[60] Whatever the merits of his extant rhetorical work, in Philostratus he appears as a uniquely great orator: Dionysius of Miletus is cited as saying that some of his admirers compared his mouth to a fountain with twelve orifices; others measured his tongue by the cubit, like the Nile.[61]

And his career was undoubtedly illustrious. For the details of his life we are mainly indebted to Philostratus, the author of *Lives of the Sophists*. Polemo has to be seen in the context of the political role the Sophist, as rhetorician, plays in the Roman Empire, a role first illuminated by Bowersock (1969). Recently, Bowie

(1982) has cast doubt on the importance of the rhetorical abilities of the Sophist for his political role, arguing that Philostratus is an untrustworthy witness. While Bowie is right to point to Philostratus' desire to set the Sophists in the most glorious light possible, to back up his argument he has to downplay considerable evidence suggesting that the orator's skills were crucial, in a context in which the ambassador had to meet the exacting requirements of Greco-Roman culture under the constraints of the water clock that measured out the precious minutes of the emperor's time.[62]

With due attention to the likely exaggerations of Philostratus, I want to consider some aspects of Polemo's career in detail here; their relevance to my argument will become apparent. He was to use his oratorical skill most effectively in the service of the city of Smyrna, where he learned his trade, studying under Dio Chrysostom. He first was sent on an embassy in place of the famous orator Scopelian ὑπὲρ τῶν μεγίστων (about the most important matters), in which he impressed Trajan enough to be granted the right of free travel by land and sea. But it was Hadrian who gave him the greatest honors, extending this right to his descendants, enrolling him in his Museum, and choosing him to deliver the oration in A.D. 130 when the temple of Olympian Zeus was dedicated after five hundred years. Philostratus also records the rumor that it was Polemo who prepared the final statement on the empire for Hadrian, in the context of the emperor's desire to protect him from Antoninus. He tells the story of how the emperor valued him so much that, when the Sophist turned the heir apparent Antoninus out of his house where he found him lodging, he let it go by. But even Antoninus himself forgave him, we are told, to the extent that he allowed Polemo's rhetoric to work on Smyrna's behalf posthumously.[63] Here, clearly, one must allow for exaggeration.

Smyrna also gave him the supreme honors, allowing him to board the sacred trireme. Philostratus says that he actually administered the city's affairs (in addition to those of his native city of Laodicea). His achievement in uniting the factions of local politics behind him in Smyrna can certainly not have been unconnected with his success in turning Hadrian's favor toward the town and away from its old rival Ephesus.[64] It was a coup that not only brought the city the new Olympic games (over which Polemo naturally presided) but also funds to enhance its prestige to the tune of ten million drachmas. An inscription testifies to what was obtained διὰ 'Αντώνιου Πολέμωνος (by means of Antonius Polemo).[65] Personally, his role as ambassador to the emperors on the city's behalf clearly brought him great wealth and influence. Consular families took sides in his quarrels, the opulence of his entourage excited much irritated comment, and his imperial *amicitia* (patronage), as we have seen, was manifested in many prestigious privileges. One is given to understand from numerous anecdotes in the *Lives of the Sophists* that both his ability and his arrogance were legendary.

An interest in physiognomy was natural in a rhetor, for whom delivery was an important part of the training.[66] This part of the art was devoted to teaching the would-be orator to use his physical presence to present his case most effectively; thus, stress was laid on the ways in which the character of the speaker, his ἦθος, was revealed by his body. It was vital to master this language of the body, and Polemo was an apt pupil. During his speech he would get up from his chair and stamp the ground like a horse—even, apparently, when crippled with arthritis.[67] The works of his teacher Dio seem to reflect some of the tenets of physiognomics—Dio's *Oration to the Rhodians,* in its praise of their gait as a sign of dignity, is in fact a significant precursor of Polemo's work—and to a lesser degree this is true of his contemporary Maximus of Tyre,[68] but Polemo took this interest much further. He saw the possibilities of an entirely new variant on the themes traditional in the oratory of praise and blame, in which body and soul were considered in turn.[69] What economy and force if treatment of body and soul could be combined!

Polemo's practical interest insures that, while there is little change in fundamental doctrine, the spirit is quite different from that of the Peripatetic treatises. Particularly in the second Peripatetic, there is a background interest in the causal relationship between ψυχή (soul) and body that follows up Aristotle's own researches into the vital functions and faculties. For instance, in his explanation of the signs of movement the Peripatetic offers a theory on the effect of the body's size and temperament on the ψυχή (813a, 10f.). The nearest Polemo comes to physiological speculation is exemplified in the section on the area from the navel to the chest: "When this area is longer than from the bottom of the chest to the neck, judge appetite of stomach and greed; the space for food is increased, but the instrument of the mind and intelligence is squashed" (F.1.210, 18–23).[70]

Another concern inherited from Aristotle is with the arguments relating sign and signified in physiognomics. Aristotle in the *Prior Analytics* discussed physiognomical method (of the zoological type) in an illustration of the way in which syllogistic can be used, not only in the case of dialectical and demonstrative arguments but also "to test the logical validity of an argument the discussion of which is abbreviated for rhetorical purposes"[71]—the enthymeme (2.23.68b, 8ff.). An enthymeme, he explains elsewhere, is a rhetorical mode of reasoning as opposed to a dialectical or a demonstrative mode of reasoning; it offers rhetorical proof that does not have the same validity as the proofs provided by the other modes of reasoning.[72] He remarks that the enthymeme works from εἰκότα (probable propositions) or σημεῖα (signs) and proceeds to discuss physiognomics as an illustration of inferences from signs, inferring causes from effects. A sign, he says, affects to be the demonstration of the existence past and present of a thing it accompanies. He begins with the statement that physiognomics is practicable if it is granted that "the body and soul change together in all natural affections," and then it is granted that there is one sign of one affection and that we can recognize the πάθος (property) and σημεῖον (sign) proper to each class of creatures. He takes the example of a lion—with the sign of its πάθος being "large extremities." It is important to check that lions have only one πάθος peculiar to them as a class. If they are also, as a class, generous, how would one know whether to infer courage or generosity? By comparison with members of another class, he answers, such as "Man." "If a man is brave but not generous, and exhibits one of the two signs, clearly this will be the sign of courage in the lion as well" (trans. W. D. Ross).

The first Peripatetic starts with a similar general premise[73] and also with the proposition that no animal has existed that has the form of one animal and the disposition of another—an illustration of the interaction of body and soul (805a 11–14). He says that this is the basis of the method of the physiognomists who use animals to judge humans, who assume that each class of animals has one εἶδος (form) and one διάνοια (character: 805a20–22). Then, presumably encouraged by his master's strictures on physiognomical method, he proposes serious limitations on inferences from animals, after criticism of the other two methods used by physiognomists (805b10–806a9). Courage, he says, is not confined to the lion. So, he suggests considering all brave animals and asking what properties belong to them and not to other animals. A large number is required, and they should have no other mental characteristic in common. Such rigor seems by no means a feature in the way the Peripatetic actually uses the zoological method, but the point is that he considers such logical justification necessary. At 807a9–10, he makes reference to the kind of reasoning from premises appropriate to philosophers; he clearly would like to be included in their number.[74]

This is far from the concerns of Anon.; he, however, phrases the process of inference by the ethnological method in a manner reminiscent of an abbreviated syllogism, with its conclusion suppressed:

> Hic Aegyptio est similis, Aegyptii autem sunt callidi, dociles, temerarii, in venerem proni.
>
> This man is like an Egyptian; Egyptians are cunning, teachable, rash and keen on sex. (sec. 9 = F.2.14)

(The conclusion is obviously that this man is cunning, teachable, rash, and keen on sex.) This manner of argument can best be defined as an enthymeme. While the relation of the enthymeme to the syllogism in Aristotle is currently the source of controversy,[75] it seems clear that Aristotle did regard a compressed form of the reasoning process as advisable for rhetoricians, as it was more assimilable for unlearned audiences.[76] It also seems clear that later rhetoricians' understanding of enthymemes commonly includes the idea that not all stages of reasoning are represented clearly, at least from the first century A.D., when Demetrius wrote *On*

Style. Demetrius describes the enthymeme as being οἷον συλλογισμὸς ἀτελής (like an incomplete syllogism), while Alexander Numenius, of the second century,[77] and Quintilian regard suppression of the conclusion as a feature.[78] The Peripatetic syllogism may, however, have slipped beneath the rhetoricians' horizon; Burnyeat concludes that the technical notions of a formally valid argument presupposed in rhetoricians' understanding of enthymemes are of Stoic origin. Admittedly, the rhetoricians' notions are vague; what is important is that, even if it did not conform to Aristotle's rules, the reasoning used in physiognomics might well recall the enthymeme, or indeed the syllogism to those educated in rhetorical theory.

Polemo is probably even less interested than Anon. in formal logic, but he inherits the enthymematic form I have been discussing; indeed, it may be that the Arabic translation obscures the Anon.-style formulation. With the text of Polemo that we have, one is left with this sort of statement: "A wide mouth and thick lips signify gluttony and voracity as well as viciousness and real impiety, for such a mouth is like the mouths of sea-monster" (F.1.226, 7–10).[79]

No need to say that the sea-monster has all these qualities and physical features or to consider whether they are peculiar to it. The animal provides a neat elision facility in the logical sequence; it encodes the vital premise.[80]

The form of reasoning that is capable of restatement as a syllogism (in the looser sense) comes with the terminology of signification, which is a Greek innovation. It intervenes between the simple protasis and apodosis of the Babylonian format, as in: "If he has curly hair on his shoulders, women will fall in love with him." Between the evidence, bent hair, and the conclusion, lovable, intervene the processes of analogy with ideal types (of animals, of the sexes, and of races). Hence, there is a reason for signification—in the example above the analogy of a sea-monster—that allows the construction of the frame of the syllogism by furnishing the two premises. So it could be recast as the following "syllogism," along the lines of Anon.:

X resembles a sea-monster.
Sea-monsters are gluttonous, voracious and impious.
X is gluttonous, voracious and impious.[81]

As we shall see, the appearance of the enthymematic style is not the only rhetorical influence on the analogical process.

In Adamantius' preamble, which probably preserves Polemo's, there is the minimum of legitimation for his craft. It is cast in more mystical than logical terms:

> . . . having been trained, I know it should be used like holy shrines, as a worthy gift to pass on through writing, as it will be a great help to others . . .

> the answer comes from things which are mute . . . it speaks as if with signs, Nature announces the ways of each person, from some god-sent, unerring divination, the physiognomist knows the habits and inclinations of all men, so to speak. (F.1.298, 6–11; 298, 13–299, 2)

Rhetorical proof, as opposed to the mere rhetorical assertion of the above statement, can work by example.[82] Polemo persuades by his claim to personal observation of examples. His statement that he took the maxims of Aristotle (meaning the Peripatetic treatise) and found them true is, he tries to show, no idle claim to autopsy. When he heard of a man with eyes like a crab, he tells us, he went round to sound out his character (F.1.144, 4–16). The anecdotes about Polemo's contemporaries are not just light relief: they turn out to be the point of the work, as we shall see.

Organization

In further contrast to the Peripatetic treatise, the demands of order are subordinated to the goal of introducing examples. Polemo's digressive style works to lead up to them. This lack of concern for order actually fits well with the style of his surviving rhetorical piece. Reardon comments on the latter: "It is one long antithesis, pursued through all possible avenues, with innumerable nuances, and with no concern for order—the concept of order hardly enters into it."[83] Here, too, in the physiognomical treatises there are "innumerable nuances," and simple procedures are pushed to their limits. There are plenty of subdivisions in the work, but he follows no obvious order in setting out the rules. He does not proceed through the parts of the body in any particular direction. He does not even use the hierarchy of signs that he sets out as an ordering device. He begins with the eyes, breaks off to recapitulate, continues with more on the eyes, and then halts to consider male and female types and animal comparisons. Abruptly, he moves on to other parts of the body, beginning with the nails. Even more suddenly, at 236, 8, he stops to consider the "nations of the world and their signs." Then, using these as a way in, he moves on to complexion, hair, gait, breathing, and the voice. From 268, 19ff., he sets out character types' signs, shifting to signs of people's destinies for the last three chapters (see sec. 1).

The subdivisions, following the distinctions, are minute within the sections, particularly in the immensely long chapter on the eyes, which makes up a third of the work. Here is involution on the basis of even simpler unit bases than astrology. But, as we have seen, absurd as it may seem to us, this is the mark of the τέχνη (*technē*). That is to say, minute subdivision is one of the hallmarks of the intellectual method. I have mentioned in chapter 1 the way that Galen, for instance, is persuaded by one of two bird diviners, and Artemidorus advises piling up subtly different options in dream interpretation to impress, even where they are worthless. Polemo certainly will not fall short of the ideal on this count. Take one subdivision, the movement of the eyes:

> Eyes which move quickly indicate distress, low suspicion, lack of sincerity and something between cowardliness and bravery. When you see both the eyelids and the interior of the eye agitated, judge that the owner is timid; if indeed you see them hardly agitated except in the interior, know that the owner is bold and brave. . . . Anyone with eyes somewhere between rest and motion is moderate in everything concerning him. . . . But an eye whose gaze darts everywhere indicates love of sexual crimes and shamelessness. From a blinking or trembling eye which is also big, judge the owner as lazy [lustful or greedy], slow, apoplectic [timid?], inclined to sexual crimes and drunkenness. . . . When you see the whole eye agitated, as if a mote were in it, be sure that the owner is devoted to sex.[84]

Here I have left out consideration of the alternative in this category, that is immobility, and of all entries which mention other variables, in order not to confuse, so I am already simplifying. The minuteness of distinctions is illustrated by a typical entry on the color of the eye, which runs: "If in amber[?] eyes you see mingled red and black, with the red not apparent from a distance and not a very strong red . . ." (F.1.124, 19–126, 2).

In consideration of the eyes—in addition to mobility and color—clarity, size, texture, humidity, prominence, shape, and the direction of the gaze are all relevant factors. These variables jostle in seemingly endless permutations for thirty-two pages in the Arab version. Polemo remarks that the common man cannot even recognize one sign, however distinct. Then, in the style of the astrologers, who refer always to a further stage of knowledge, he observes that no one could include all the material in one book.[85] He sets out how he claims to suppose his book will be used:

> . . . after you have learnt all the signs and made trial of all according to what has been described for you, this will be the base for the knowledge of physiognomics, as when a boy is gradually taught his letters. (F.1.120, 9–12; cf. Anon. sec. 3 = F.2.6).

Similarly, he promises: "If you keep in your memory [the rest of what I have explained and decribed to you] you will be able to know other things physiognomically by yourself."[86] He refers to his own great zeal and long experience (F.1.192, 16–18) and later to fools who despair and deny the truth of physiognomics: for those who really try, the *scientia* does not seem very long (F.1.292,

24–27). These, however, are no more than the usual encouraging remarks. Polemo will keep his monopoly of knowledge of a τέχνη (*technē*), which seems initially based on far more straightforward methods than astrology.

Method

Thus, the basic principles in Polemo are generally left implicit, and they are remarkably few. Most interventions, as in astrology, are to emphasize a particular point as all-important or to remark on the necessity for combining signs carefully.[87] Nevertheless, implicit throughout is a high regard for proportion, or moderation, as he puts it. Associations already present in the language and culture are unpacked and used: blinking is cowardly, paleness is an indication of (feminine) feebleness.[88] Or the physiognomist may use value-laden adjectives in assumption of a common understanding: "When the nose is rightly and temperately joined . . ." (F.1.228, 11–12). Many associations are common to our culture, such as that of flabbiness with overindulgence, stupidity, and inertia or blinking with timidity. But sometimes we know that peculiar cultural conventions are involved, such as those in the codes of comic masks. For example, the Πικρός, or misanthropic type, in Anon. (sec. 99 = F.2.124) and Polemo, chapter 60 (F.1.276, 8–12), must surely take his pale, grimacing face, arched eyebrows, and lined forehead from a mask. The irascible type, with his reddish complexion, rounded forehead, bristling hair and eyebrows, and snub nose (Anon. sec. 108), is also a familiar stage persona.[89] But the rationale cannot always be followed, and one remains unsure whether any common opinion lies behind assertions such as: "A thick, flattened end of the nose indicates brutality" (F.1.228, 6–7).[90] It is possible that in such cases it is rather the interpretative work of the physiognomist that has left its mark.

Polemo is more explicit about the use of analogy in the case of the ideal types of the two sexes, of the animals, and the different races.[91] He is also quite explicit about synthesizing the data. There is a hierarchy of the signs' importance (F.1.168, 1–9). The eyes[92] are followed by the eyebrows, brow, nose, mouth, and the general shape of the head. After the face come the neck, the chest area, the shoulder area, the stomach, back, arms and legs, and the feet. The general color, the voice, breathing, and gestures are also important, but their place in the hierarchy is uncertain. He is not, however, as clear as Anon., who faces up to the problem of signs' opposing one another with more precise advice: "Pronounce according to their number or degree of clarity and prominence." The latter then enjoins memorizing the hierarchy of the signs and provides an example of how to synthesize the data, as follows. When a man has the lashes of a loquacious man, the forehead of a thinker, and the eyes of a madman, his forehead will not have complete sway, but it makes the loquacity less disagreeable and the madness into mere ebullience."[93] This by no means solves all the potential problems if one really takes all the signs into account; as with astrology, the "handbook" turns out not to give many straightforward answers.[94] But Polemo is even less serious about teaching his readers: in the examples throughout his work the signs are enumerated and the characteristics set out, but with each side of the equation in an undifferentiated mass. If the boy-pupil succeeds in "learning his letters," he will hardly be in a position to read a coherent message from the bodies set before him as a result of reading Polemo's book.

Characterology

It is noticeable that the use of the rhetoric of the τέχνη (*technē*) involves ever more subtle distinctions on the physical side of the equation, while the character traits supposedly indicated remain hopelessly inaccessible to such fine drawing. Characterization stays broadly within the stereotypes familiar from Theophrastus, comic drama, satire, and oratory. We have already seen the connections with some of the comic dramatis personae. Lists of "psycho-social" types, as Bompaire (1923) calls them, are increasingly common in Middle and New Comedy and their Latin successors. Terence lists a few in the Prologue to *The Eunuch* (runaway slave, matron, courtesan, parasite, braggart soldier [36–37]); Quintilian enumerates the cast in generic terms: slaves, pimps, parasites, rustics, soldiers, prostitutes, maidservants, stern and mild old men, upright and luxury-loving youths, married women, and young girls.[95] Bompaire contrasts this comic heritage with the "Aristotelian tradition," obviously older, the origin of which is less analysis for the pleasure of analysis than the wish to put at the disposition of the rhetorician portraits drawn in advance. From Aristotle onward, he claims, one sees the indissoluble link between rhetoric and the study of characters and passions.[96] There were many imitators who produced lists for rhetorical use; we know of the lists of Heraclides, Ariston of Ceos, and the Epicurean Philodemus, of which fragments remain. Quintilian recommends *ēthologia* as a school exercise and refers to such studies—of rustics, pimps, and misers—as developments of the *ēthos*. The schools of rhetoric were given to practicing such character sketches, exercises entitled χαρακτηρισμός or ἠθοποιΐα (*characterismos, ēthopoiia*).[97] In Theophrastus' list we find a few coincidences. The εἴρων (dissembler) and the δειλός (fool) reappear.[98] Perhaps the lists in the physiognomists were derived entirely from some lost imitator of Theophrastus. But, if there are developments within the physiognomical field specifically, they only follow on in this tradition. Yet there is no explanation of what the coward, for instance, is like. The type is simply named, and all the characteristics can be taken from the common rhetorical treasury of "characters." Only with individual examples are the κοινοὶ τόποι (commonplaces) brought into play. The focus of contemporary rhetoric was on the use of these to develop an agreed point. The author of a rhetorical treatise that came down to us under the name of Hermogenes explains:

> The so-called commonplace is the amplification of a thing admitted, of demonstrations already made. Once agreed, that so-and-so is a temple-robber, there are many and various ways of developing the import of this theme: e.g., . . . beginning with small offences, he went on to this one last, so that you have before you in the same person a thief, a house-breaker and an adulterer. . . . It is called commonplace because it is applicable to every temple-robber. (pp. 11, 21–12, 5; 13, 23–14, 1; trans. T. Burgess)

Quintilian refers in the context of commonplaces to the denunciation of vices such as adultery, gambling, and profligacy (2.4.22). Polemo similarly amplifies the number of vices, to a point that puts the rhetorical theorists in the shade.

Take the man from Lydia, his longest case study (F.1.126, 4–32, 28). He had dark, fiery eyes with a reddish tinge, as if drunken or angry, his eyelids wide open, with an effeminate mouth, fastidious speech, a long nose and chin, and cheeks some way from his eyes. He was fat, with a short, thick neck, a huge stomach, plump legs, short digits on his hands and feet, fleshy hands, and a harsh, distorted voice. His gaze was that of a wretched, accursed, and dangerous man. He ground his teeth like a wild boar after the hunter's blood. He had a high-pitched laugh. "So," says Polemo, "I knew he was full of evil," a theme he reiterates, with specific mention of ingratitude, violence, murder, and sexual crimes with adolescents and women. "He was more malevolent to friend than enemy, as eager to harm friend as enemy, free man or slave, he found innumerable new forms of evil. It was amazing no one realized" (F.1.128, 15–18).

He goes on to relate how, on a festal day, this man sent a party of his neighbors a basket, apparently containing dishes of oysters. Beneath was a man's head. He used to get people to fall asleep by getting them drunk and then shave off their beards or suffocate them. He was a sorcerer versed in every vile art, especially poisoning. He killed his father and mother by a poisoned drink and by drowning, respectively. Even his sacrifice was unacceptable to the gods.[99]

The Oratory of Praise and Blame

All in all the description of the unnamed but doubtless then identifiable Lydian is a tour de force as a piece of invective. The commonplaces of the tradition of διαβολή (slander, invective) are very much in evidence.[100] This is no accident: Polemo is often explicit about his use of physiognomics for praise and blame: "If you see (in the side of the head) a depression, and in the middle (of the head) a cavity, then a full, ample occiput while the head is upright, omit nothing in your praise. "I don't praise a concave mouth," he says (for it indicates envy, love of carnage, sex mania); "Never praise a small, short nose" (as it shows thievishness and a mean spirit).[101] Despite the appearance of plenty of theoretical physiognomies worthy of praise, only one of Polemo's contemporaries is the recipient of an encomium, the owner of a pair of clear, shimmering eyes: "Certainly Hadrian's eyes were [are?] of this type . . . full of beautiful light and bright, sharp in gaze. No one with a more luminous eye was ever seen."[102]

Due homage to a patron, traditional panegyric of the emperor, it has also an original touch. Such eyes are praiseworthy not only as beautiful but also as virtuous. They are the opposite of those that scatter rays, that reveal the betrayers of friends, fickle people, involved in prostitution and so on. As perceiver of his virtues Polemo sets himself up as virtuous,[103] constructing his ἦθος (ēthos) or claim to persuade in ancient rhetorical theory. And whose virtues better for the construction of the ἦθος than the emperor's?

In an anecdote about his tour of the East with Hadrian[104] he again aligns himself with the emperor and virtue, but this time he takes up his usual stance of reprobation. People said that Polemo handled invective more skillfully than any other Sophist, according to Philostratus (*VS* 1.25. [542]). Here the Sophist attacks a man from Corinth from the intimate circle of Hadrian at that time. This Corinthian, he claims, was secretly an enemy of the emperor. The man has somewhat optimistically identified with Lusius Quietus, a conspirator against Hadrian known from other sources.[105] Though the Corinthian was obviously recognizable immediately at this time, Polemo is too carefully vague about the nature of his crimes for us to know now. It is a tribute to his rhetorical skill that scholars have accepted his picture of this figure at face value. His evidence should be taken with as much caution as Cicero's on his political enemies. Indeed, Cicero offers in his invectives against enemies some examples of precursors of Polemo's procedure. In *On Behalf of Quintus Roscius* he ridicules the idea that Roscius could have cheated Chaerea. He demands that those who know them compare the characters of the two and that those who do not look at their faces to find out.

> Nonne ipsum caput et supercilia illa penitus abrasa olere malitiam et clamitare calliditatem videntur? non ad imis unguibus usque ad verticem summum, si quam coniecturam affert hominibus tacita hominis figura, ex fraude, fallaciis, mendaciis constare totus videtur? oculi, supercilia, frons, voltus denique totus, qui sermo quidem tacitus mentis est, hic in fraudem homines impulit. (7.20)

> Don't that head and those eyebrows so closely shaven seem to reek of evil intent and scream out sharp practice? If a person's silent face allows any conjecture, doesn't Chaerea's whole body, from the tips of his toes to the top of his head, seem to unite in showing him made of cheating and trickery. His

> eyes, brows, forehead, in sum, the whole face, which is the speech of the unspoken mind, has brought people to commit crimes of deception.

Piso's servile coloring, hairy cheeks, and rotten teeth are also singled out against him.[106] Polemo is following in a well-established line of political invective here. Such invective worked by exciting laughter against opponents, creating solidarity with the attacker. For almost all rhetorical theorists the chief source of wit was in bodily as well as moral defects.[107]

Looking at Polemo's treatise in its political context illuminates the real point of the work. The examples are not just anecdotes casually thrown in to spice up a dull theoretical treatise; from a political point of view they are what the work is written for. In physiognomics he found a new resource for attacking rivals and enemies.[108] The odd feature noted by Anon. (sec. 44 = F.2.61), that there are more negative than positive physiognomical signs, is explained by the fact that Polemo needs more often to assert his dominance over his opponents than to align himself with superiors and allies. The predominantly judicial terminology, inviting a verdict on moral status—"When X . . . judge Y . . ." (with the signs metaphorically cast as witnesses or informers betraying the truth)[109]—may spring from the background of forensic speeches of praise and blame. Looking at the literature of invective suddenly sets physiognomics in a framework that makes sense. The τέχνη (*technē*) is used to elevate these potentially undignified assaults on opponents. The methods on which it is based are not just arbitrarily selected for elaboration; they too coincide with τόποι (topoi, commonplaces) of invective.[110]

There are three methods to be considered here, all based on commonplaces: "Three things are lucky: to be born a man and not a beast, a man and not a woman, a Greek and not a barbarian," say the old sages.[111] Accordingly, within physiognomics we have three methods of comparison.[112] Fraenkel notes in his commentary on Aeschylus' *Agamemnon* that to ask "What or whom does so and so resemble?" was a question more natural to the Greeks than to us.[113] There was "a popular old game probably played all over Greece" that consisted of one player asking "Do you know what you seem most like to me?" and characterizing the other δι' εἰκόνος (by means of a likeness). The latter then replied with an ἀντεικάζειν (a likeness in return). Aristotle connects this game with physiognomics, in the context of a mention of physiognomists' using animal comparisons; he says: διὸ πολλάκις οἱ σκώπτοντες εἰκάζουσι τῶν μὴ καλῶν ἐνίους τοὺς μὲν αἰγὶ φυσῶντι πῦρ, τοὺς δ' οἰῒ κυρίττοντι (often those who are mocking them compare some of those who are not so good-looking to a fire-breathing goat, others to a butting ram [*Generation of Animals* 769b18–20]).

Perhaps it is better to talk of a relation of metaphor in the broadest sense (as master trope), comparison with an awareness of difference. One is inspired to metaphor, as Aristotle notes, for purposes of adornment or disparagement. To adorn, one borrows from things superior, to disparage from things inferior.[114] The three methods here involve borrowing from the inferior: the Woman, the Foreigner, and the Animal,[115] though within these broad groupings more positive metaphors are available. The *Rhetoric Addressed to Herennius,* a treatise from the eighties B.C., connects the trope *imago* (εἰκών) specifically with the oratory of praise and blame (4.46.49):

> *Imago* is the comparison of one figure with another, implying a certain resemblance between them. This is used either for praise or censure. For praise, as follows: "He entered the combat in body like the strongest bull, in impetuosity like the fiercest lion." For censure, as follows: "That wretch who daily glides through the middle of the forum like a crested serpent, with curved fangs, poisonous glance, and fierce panting, looking about him on this side and that for someone to blast with venom from his throat—to smear it with his lips, to drive it in with his teeth, to spatter it with his tongue." To excite envy, as follows: "That creature who flaunts his riches, loaded and weighed down with gold, shouts and raves like a Phrygian eunuch-priest of Cybele, or like a soothsayer." To excite contempt, as follows: "That creature who like a snail silently hides and keeps himself in his shell, is carried off, he and his house, to be swallowed whole." (trans. H. Caplan)

Here we have examples using animals above all,[116] but also in the penultimate case combining the other two topoi. It is particularly interesting to note the explicit focus on the effect of these comparisons on the audience. Modern theorists of the social uses of metaphor have also been concerned to note the way in which it moves the audience to action. While Quintilian remarks that metaphor provides a name for everything (8.6.5), Kenneth Burke elaborates the concept of "entitlement" in order to explain what metaphor does. Language, he says, is not to be viewed directly in terms of a word-thing relationship but, rather, indirectly, by thinking of speech as the entitling of complex nonverbal situations, as the giving of names. Christopher Crocker (1977) follows Burke, observing that metaphors "entitle" by shifting domains, by redefining, not through generalizing but, instead, through specifying. This explains their social use: rhetorical entitlement is "that process by which actors attempt to provide a linguistic truth about a social situation which summarizes its essence in such a way as to define possible action." This naming is not automatic, though it draws on stereotypical answers for a general class of situations: what it does is to codify social opinion on particular matters, so that possible action is defined.

As we shall see, Polemo's selection and use of metaphor/comparison deliberately excludes much available in preexisting commonplaces. He tends to exclude more positive connotations of his chosen domains of comparison. What he presents is designed to elicit a specific reaction—that of scorn, often by means of laughter. Everybody knows the range of responses to an effeminate, a beastly, or a barbarian man; once someone is cast in this role, the responses are brought into play. Most important, as has been mentioned, you must not believe such a man. The process works by "staining" the victim, to use Richlin's (1983) term: some of the mud thrown will stick. This entitlement is an attempt to mobilize social opinion, to make it solidify around a particular situation. Metaphors are performative strategies.

Topoi

The Woman

The first topos involves a male perception of gender difference. Women, like animals in Lévi-Strauss's phrase, are "bonnes à penser"; they are "good to think with." They may be set up as a type, which then defines its opposite male type. Hence, they can be used to categorize men—with the time-honored accusation of effeminacy or androgyny. Ortner and Whitehead in their introduction to *Sexual Meanings* observe that: "very commonly the same axes that divide and distinguish male from female (and indeed rank male over female) also cross-cut the gender categories, producing internal distinctions and gradations within them" (1981, 9). They go on to comment that this shows that gender systems are prestige systems, with all the patterns of deference and condescension that go with them. Now it is interesting to note here that the picture is not always so straightforward. In Anon. we have a fragment of Loxus' work, which presents a more flattering picture of the female type. He notes, for example, that there is no good character that does not borrow from the courage of the masculine and the wisdom of the feminine.[117] But in Polemo the ideal type of woman appears in an almost entirely negative light. The physical description is stained by deviation from the male norm; in comparison with the male she has:

> a small head and mouth, softer, black hair, a narrower face, bright, glittering eyes, a narrow neck, a weak, rather sunken chest, with weak ribs, big, very fleshy hips, narrow calves and [knock]-knees, dainty fingers and toes, the body otherwise moist and slack, with soft joints . . . a weak voice. [Her strides are smaller and more frequent, her limbs less rigid (καμπτόμενα), the movement more fluid (ὑγροτέρα)].[118]

Thus, she has the opposite properties of man, being "quite undaring, most deceitful, of bitter disposition, concealing her thoughts, stubborn, unfair;[119] she really loves an argument." (F.1.192, 23–194, 1). As a good orator, Polemo wants a clear antithesis.

This orator is not interested in real women. While he mentions that male signs may be found in a woman, he henceforth ignores it as unnecessary to his project. There are only male actors in his political arena. He concentrates on scrutinizing them for feminine signs. The art of spotting an effeminate man was not foreign to the authors of tragedy, Old Comedy, Greek and Roman oratory and poetry, and even graffiti.[120] Many of the signs were matters of physique or physical movement. Curly hair, smooth skin, a soft, high voice, and general softness, weakness, and tremulousness are frequent themes. Gestures such as scratching the head with the little finger and a limp and fluid gait were also giveaways.[121] It was a frequent theme in Sophistic quarrels of the period, an insult that flew in every direction. Dio Chrysostom refers to "those who violate nature's laws in secret, but whose true character is revealed by their voice, glance, posture, hairstyle and gait, shifty eyes, receding neck, and by certain upturned gestures of the hand" (*Orations* 33.52), while Lucian in the *Professor of Rhetoric* (17) casts the teacher of the easy way to success as an effeminate. A key association of the effeminate man, the κιναιδός (*kinaidos*), or *mollis* (*soft man*), was that of sexual passivity.

The ultimate effeminate is the eunuch; thus, intellectuals insult one another as eunuchs. Dio Chrysostom has the sage Diogenes, in conversation with Alexander the Great, explain why Sophists should be compared to eunuchs: they pretend to virility, but their unions with women are unproductive (*Orations* 4.35). Aristides compares those who abandon the classical tradition to eunuchs, who are as unconvincing in their declarations that their physical deficiencies are not the fault of nature or fortune but, rather, of deliberate policy (34.11).

Lucian, in *The Eunuch,* satirizes Sophistic rivalry. The competition is for a chair of philosophy at Athens, in which one Diocles challenges one Bagoas (a standard—Persian—name for a eunuch). Having thrashed out the philosophical doctrines with his opponent, Diocles moved on to Bagoas' mode of life (5). At length he said that it was not at all permissible for Bagoas to lay claim to philosophy and the rewards of merit in it, since he was a eunuch and should be excluded from places of public assembly and worship; it was an ill omen to meet such a monster first thing in the morning (6). Lucian allows Diocles the more convincing case. Ultimately, he catches his rival out, by reminding him that he secured his acquittal for adultery by claiming eunuchism (10). Bagoas is unwilling to come out either as eunuch or adulterer. In the second century, at least, it can actually be seen as the job of a physiognomist to spot effeminates and adulterers.[122]

Effeminacy, this favorite topos of Greek and Roman invective, was a gift for physiognomists. The unknown abbreviator of the Peripatetic *Physiognomonica* abused Dionysius of Miletus by inserting οἷος ἂν εἴη Διονύσιος ὁ σοφιστής (Dionysios the Sophist would have been like this) in the description of the κίναιδος (*kinaidos* [808a16]). For easy reference all the treatises from the Peripatetic *Physiognomonica* onwards offer Κιναίδου / Ανδρογύνου σημεῖα (signs of the *kinaidos* or androgyne).[123] The androgyne in Polemo represents a summary of the signs listed under the female type:

> (. . . You see him really flashing) and rolling his eyes [looking around] with a [brazen,] moist gaze; with a narrow [screwed-up] forehead [and cheeks] (he moves his cheeks) and eyebrows (excessively), with his head cocked, [his loins mobile,] he (often) moves his back and limbs [all his parts] (as if they were loose) [and he trips along with little jumping steps, his knees knocking; his palms are upturned, he looks about him. His voice is thin, grating(?), shrill and very languid.][124]

When Polemo was young he took sides in a quarrel between two of his teachers, Timocrates, a physician turned Stoic philosopher, and Scopelian. He chose the masculine model of his own precepts and supported the lionlike Timocrates against the depilated (and thus effeminate) Scopelian.[125] When he was of an age to fight his own quarrels the lesson was not lost on him. But, as usual, he wanted to improve on his teachers.

The topos is taken to its limit in Polemo's attack on the Sophist Favorinus of Arles (F.1.160, 6–162, 21). Though, like the rest of the targets of Polemo's assaults, he is not named, the identification is supplied by Anon. "The Celt," as he is here identified, was a famous rhetor, philosopher, and "eunuch."[126] He was a friend of Plutarch and Fronto, who lived in Rome under Trajan, Hadrian, and Antoninus. His speeches were apparently so dramatic that Philostratus claimed that people came to hear him even without understanding Greek (*Lives of the Sophists* 1.8 [491]). An almost exact contemporary of Polemo, he was soon his rival. Both were pupils of Dio Chrysostom, and both won imperial *amicitia.* While Polemo represented Smyrna to the emperors, Favorinus represented Smyrna's eternal enemy, Ephesus. This famous quarrel began in Ionia but moved to Rome, where consular families took sides in it, according to Philostratus. That author censures the pair for the speeches they wrote assailing each other and remarks that Polemo's teacher, Timocrates, also did so.[127]

The emperors were sensitive to the effeminacy of orators: when Philiscus came to court he gave offense by his gait, by the way he stood, his clothes, his effeminate voice, and his indolent language. The emperor (Caracalla) exclaimed: "His hair shows what sort of man he is, his voice what sort of orator." Again, the emperor reacted adversely to Alexander Peloplaton: "You are the fellow who is always arranging his hair, cleaning his teeth and polishing his nails, and always smelling of myrrh!"[128] Polemo certainly knew how to exploit this topos to good effect: no effeminate could effectively represent his city. And Polemo clearly won his quarrel, as Smyrna gained the imperial favor and Favorinus dramatically lost it: it seems he was eventually exiled to Chios, though he returned to Rome under Antoninus.[129]

Polemo must admit to his popularity, which he puts down to sorcery, and his learning (162, 8ff.). But overall it is an attack with no holds barred, quite different from the bons mots of other Sophists on the subject of Favorinus' eunuchism.[130]

> When the eye is open with a shimmer like marble and a sharp gaze, it indicates little modesty. This is the type of eye found in men who are not like the rest, like a eunuch born without testicles rather than castrated. I doubt whether you could find anyone of this type apart from the one who was from the land known as that of the Celts. He was lustful and dissolute beyond all measure, for his eyes were those of the worst type of man, just like that description . . . he had a puffy(?)[131] forehead, soft cheeks, a wide mouth, a long, thin neck, thick legs and fleshy feet. His voice was just like a woman's, and all the rest of his limbs and extremities were soft; and he did not walk upright, but with slack joints and limbs. He took great care of his person, [by nourishing] his thick hair, and by rubbing medicaments into his body, in short, using anything to arouse desire for sex and coitus. He had a voice like a woman's, thin lips. In the whole human race, I never saw anything like him or his eyes. (F.160, 6–162, 7)

Favorinus is most importantly a *monstrum,* or prodigy, having become a eunuch naturally. Polemo claims that this has far worse implications than the ordinary eunuchism resulting from castration. The Romans in the second century B.C. actually used to drown such *androgyni* with solemn ceremony. *Androgyni* were also to be found in the traditional catalog of the "Monstrous Races." And "monster" (*monstrum, prodigium*) was a term of insult.[132] The presence of monstrousness as a term of invective is the linking theme between the three main topoi here. Androgyny is monstrous, and the races become increasingly monstrous with distance; while the "*monstre par excellence,*" in Claude Lecouteux's (1980) phrase, is "*l'homme animalisé.*" Clement of Alexandria illustrates the associations between one set of category crossers and another when he refers to effeminates as amphibious and lecherous beasts (*Paedagogus* 3.3.18) and notes that the more refined and luxurious effeminates keep Indian birds and Median pea fowls, reclining with peak-headed creatures, playing with satyrs, delighting in monsters (ibid. 30). At some level the three topoi connect, and the three main physiognomical methods are designed to diagnose any divergence toward the incorporation of these Monstrous Others. The physiognomist will sniff out any hint of monstrosity in the subject's body, ever alert for signs of the woman in the man, the foreigner in the Greek, or the animal in the human.

The Alien

Whereas the sexual difference in the ideal types used by the physiognomists is a binary opposition, allowing straightforward rejection of Other by Self, ethnic differences offer the opportunity for variations on a theme as well. The old theme of the simple division (favorable to Greeks) between Greeks and barbarians is still fundamental to the ethnography of the Greco-Roman world, as to the classical Greek.[133] In physiognomics the binary opposition occasionally surfaces, for instance: "Hair covering the upper forehead running back towards the head bespeaks an impetuous and imprudent spirit; for it recalls barbarian peoples" (Anon. sec. 14 = F.2.23).

But following the usual geographers' model of κλίματα (*klimata,* zones of the world),[134] the main section on the different races in Polemo offers a variety of different Others for moral reflection (F.1.236, 9f.). The subject of climatological influence on physical and mental differences between the races is the most common of all in Foerster's selection of quotations relevant to physiognomics from the ancient world (F.2.237–52). The inbuilt value structure can perhaps best be illustrated by the relocation of the center of the world in Vitruvius, who moves it from Greece, where it was set by earlier Greek scientists,[135] within a few lines to Rome, where it serves once again as a justification for rule: "And so by its policy, it curbs the courage of the Northern barbarians, by its strength the imaginative South. Thus the Divine Mind has allotted to the Roman State an excellent and temperate region to rule the world."[136]

Ethnic characterizations are doxic knowledge, part of accepted understanding of the world: Galen seems to treat them as demonstrated knowledge in his *Quod Animi Mores.*[137] Cicero is one rhetorician who exploits such commonplaces. He considers the scientific background in his philosophical works, but in his speeches he simply exploits the tendency to accept the idea that the ethnic groups supposedly represented by his opponent(s) are widely known to be untrustworthy, ignorant, and so on.[138] Quintilian, in his treatise on rhetoric, in consideration of the kinds of proof relating to persons in a legal case, refers to the fact that each nationality has its mores (5.10.24). It is a tradition at least as old as Old Comedy and the Attic orators.[139]

There are, of course, more positive assessments of foreigners, usually in terms of the "noble savage" topos.[140] One of the "*progymnasmata,*" or elementary rhetorical exercises, involved retailing the customs and peculiarities of particular countries; it was a topos particularly suited to encomia and diatribes.[141] The more positive associations of other countries are not much in evidence in Polemo.

In his division of the world Polemo follows in a long literary tradition. This tradition is related to more technical schemes to be found in geographers, astronomers, and astrologers, and doubtless derives some authority from them.[142]

Astrologers needed the world divided into zones, or κλίματα (*klimata*), to simplify calculation of rising times and usually opted for seven zones, one for each planet.

The astrological material furnishes interesting comparison with the physiognomical: Ptolemy, in his *Tetrabiblos,* offers by far the most complicated schema. Some astrologers simply divided up the Earth, assigning areas to the zodiacal signs, while others subdivided relentlessly on this basis.[143] Ptolemy begins with a simple threefold division (2.2.2, p. 58, 22–23). Those who live under the more southerly parallels (latitudes), from the equator to the summer tropic, since they have the Sun over their heads and are burned by it, have black skins and thick, woolly hair. They are shrunken in stature, hot by nature, and have savage mores, because they live continually oppressed by the heat. The animals and plants of the region are similarly the result of baking in the heat. Broadly speaking, these are known as Ethiopians (2.2.2–3, pp. 58, 23–59, 10). Polemo observes, in his section "On the Shape of Southern Peoples," that these people are black, have curly hair, narrow ankles, metallic-colored eyes, black hair, and thin flesh. Their corresponding features are as follows: they are kind [?], ready of wit and memory . . . and [take?] pleasure [in learning?], but they are always thinking up lies, they are greedy and inclined to theft (F.1.238, 14–20).

In Ptolemy those living under more northerly parallels, with the Bears over their heads, since they are far from the zodiac and the heat of the Sun, are cooled but more nourished by moisture. They are white-complexioned, straight-haired, tall and well-nourished, and rather cold by nature. These people, too, are savage in their habits, because they live constantly in the cold. These characteristics are reflected in the size of the plants and the wildness of the animals of the region. Broadly speaking, these are Scythians (2.2.4, pp. 59, 10–60, 2). Polemo observes, on those who live under the Bears in his section "On the Shape of Northern Peoples," simply that they are tall, white-complexioned, with red hair, *glauci* (gray-blue) eyes. They are rough to the touch, with thick legs, dense, plump bodies, soft flesh, and huge stomachs. Their corresponding characters follow. They are quick to anger and quick in debate, and they are rash, honest, and find it hard to learn (F.1.238, 6–12).[144]

In Ptolemy those in the middle, between the summer tropics and the Bears, enjoy equable temperatures. They are of medium complexion, moderate stature, in nature even-tempered (2.2.6–7, 60, 2–10). They live close together and are civilized in their habits. He goes on to consider East and West, before coming to the pure Greek (not the Argive or Corinthian) and returning to bodily signs in general via the color of the skin: a black skin indicates timidity and long trouble and sorrow, as in the case of Abyssinians, Zingae (?), and Egyptians (meridian types).

Ptolemy, too, begins to subdivide the peoples of the middle: those more to the South are shrewd, inventive, and inclined to astrology; those more to the East are more masculine, with more strength and vigor, thanks to the influence of the Sun; those more to the West are more feminine, softer, and more secretive (2.2, 8–10, pp. 60, 10–61, 3). He is careful to note that there are exceptions (2.3.2, p. 61, 17–19) and that special conditions of character and customs are influential (2.3.1, p. 61, 6–8). Interestingly, the astrologer Firmicus Maternus (1.10.12) rejects zonal determination of character and habits, though he allows determination of physique, for just these reasons; you can find sober Asiatics, serious Greeks (!), quiet Scyths. Ptolemy argues that this general astrology must be taken as the base of individual nativities (2.1.2, p. 57, 5–18). Presumably for him, too, the ethnic topos had a persuasive function: here he could explain anew what people accepted as knowledge about racial character and appearance and thus gain apparent backing for his astrological perspective.

At 3.33 (p. 62, 1ff.), Ptolemy seems to start afresh, with a complex arrangement of triplicities of signs and pairs of planets governing the four quarters of the world, with further subdivisions. Here the effects on the bodies of foreigners are largely ignored in favor of detailed discussions of racial characters.[145] His concerns also lead him to produce a different model from the physiognomical. Ptolemy's chief problem is to match up the planetary patrons with the protégés. The resulting complication allows considerable detail in the ethnic portraits; many are recognizable topoi (the incest of the South-East quadrant, the Persian homosexual tastes), but others seem dictated by the logic of the scheme, given the associations of the planets. Obviously, in the cases of both astrologers and physiognomists there is plenty of room for creativity. Indeed, Bompaire remarks on the ease with which the ethnic groups may be exchanged in literature in general: "This flexible representation took on a very strong rhetorical colour: the descriptions are interchangeable, running from the Scyths or the inhabitants of Taprobane to the Jews and Germans."

Polemo, unlike the Peripatetic, does not dwell on causation; he merely exploits the learned associations of the division of the world in describing the different physiognomies of North and South, East and West, and the corresponding character types. There is no direct link between gender types and the extremes in Polemo, since for his purposes the ideal medium type must not be a mixture of female and male as it is in Loxus. Instead, the "pure Greek type" has the physical characteristics that link him with the ideal male in the first topos and the Lion in the third.[146]

Polemo actually starts off on the subject of the races immediately after a discussion of the signs of the head, introducing them in the context of skin color and hair type (236, 8ff.). The proposition follows: "As often as you judge from these indications about any people or nation in the world, you'll judge correctly" (236, 13–15). It is followed up by some cautionary remarks; signs and dispositions may change, for the worse or for the better (236, 15ff.). The initial list of examples of ethnic types in Polemo is short, and the Constantinople epitome has a longer, more exotic list.[147] The list in Polemo has doubtless lost a great deal in translation. It appears obscure at points; furthermore, where races appear elsewhere in the text, their identification may be problematic, since the Arab translator may have had difficulty with the names as well as his own ideas about equivalent groups. Clearly, in some cases later substitutions have intervened, when Slavs and Turks appear instead of Scyths and Gauls (250, 11). One cannot be sure, for instance, whether there was a Greek original for the region of Thrace that extends to Constantinople, where all the natives' eyes roll and twitch, a sign of malice only restrained by fear (F.1.110, 12–17). Adamantius is unfortunately not inclined to detail on the races; even Anon. lists only Egyptians, Celts, Germans, and Thracians, apart from an even briefer discussion of the northern and southern peoples (Anon. secs. 9, 79). The form is clearer, however, as we have already observed: Celts are recalcitrant to teaching, strong, savage (*feri*), and so on, so, if a man looks like the Celtic stereotype, his character may be deciphered.

The association of remote peoples with the animal world is a natural development of such characterizations. This association is so widely found that the structuralist anthropologist Edmund Leach (1983) claims that it constitutes a human universal. In the ancient world people, like animals, are judged by physique, voice, and sexual and dietary habits, and those found wanting are classed as beastly. ὠμότης and θηριώδης (rawness and beastliness) are the qualities Strabo finds at the edge of his world.[148] From Caesar to Ammianus Marcellinus barbarians are *feri,* or wild beasts. The animals of the country are sometimes considered at the same time as the people (see Ptolemy). But at the margins of the world categories become confused; norms are flouted. India and Ethiopia, often conflated in earlier worldviews, are the haunts of the most extraordinary wild beasts and people.[149]

This sort of material seems to offer promising material to the structuralist anthropologist. Leach (1964) again suggests a candidate for a human universal: the use of markers like animals to divide up the human continuum. His example is a scheme that, he claims, represents British culture. He sets a series of pairs along a spectrum running away from Ego, the perceiver, each pair consisting of an animal and a class of person defined according to the sexual relations possible with them. Thus, the pet, belonging in the house, is inedible, as the sister is unavailable for sex; farm livestock are edible if castrated, and premarital relations are possible with a first cousin, but not marriage; game is edible if hunted, and a neighbor may be married; remote wild animals are not considered for eating, nor is a stranger marriageable. Whatever problems there may be with this particular scheme, the logic is clear. There are traces of this transformational logic, which pairs up elements from different classifications, in the physiognomical literature.

We have already seen how masculine and feminine categories can be mapped on to the races and how a particular animal can be transformed on to the pure Greek and the male types. But, crucially, it is always a strategic move. Structuralist concerns with revealing universal mental structures have been justly criticized. It is surely more justifiable to look at the particular contexts in which markers are set along the human continuum and the relations set up between these markers. For instance, the neatest example of this transformational logic outside physiognomics is in the orator Isocrates (436–338 B.C.), who compares the superiority of Athens over the rest of the Greeks to that of Greeks over barbarians and humans over animals in his *Antidosis* (293–94). Here he was not articulating fundamental conceptual categories in the Greek (or even Athenian) mind; he was arguing in a particular context (a fictional defense of his life before an Athenian court). In his *Discourse,* perhaps in the interests of uniting the Greeks to conquer Persia, there is an absolute opposition between Greeks and barbarians. Indeed, here he represents geographical conditions as producing an aptitude for slavery. In the *Nicocles* (5–9) and in the *Evagoras* (66–67), however, his account of human evolution seems to exclude such an opposition. It is rhetoric that clarifies oppositions; they are not given.

The structuralist concern with category confusion has, nevertheless, been a fruitful one, in focusing attention on the role of the taxonomic anomaly, in particular its role as "*bon à penser.*" The original position, which seemed to rely on the assumption that the boundary crosser universally aroused automatic fear and loathing, has been refined. Dan Sperber (1975, 11) pointed out, in discussion of the structuralist work of Mary Douglas (1966), that it was odd that people actually created taxonomic anomalies in legends, if they were so disturbed by the ones that they met. Yet it is again necessary to stress the importance of the rhetorical context—that the boundary crossers are not just good for organizing mental categories but also may have a persuasive function. Claude Lecouteux implies that theriomorphs, or animal-man monsters, are in a special moral category (1980, 264–65). Whereas monstrous races such as the Sciapods, with their exaggerated feet, which double as sunshades, or the Blemmyae, with faces on their chests, are in a sense known, expectable kinds of monster, being recognizably human, the half-beasts are not and, thus, in myth are subject to justifiable purges. Justifiable, for it is a moral issue. It is the moral issue at the heart of physiognomics: appearance is made to function as a moral indicator. While there is a certain erudite delight in the elaborations and rhetorically heightened descriptions of the Monstrous Races in contemporary paradoxography (collections of wonders),[150] at base the fascination comes from the potential of all such category confusion to offer material for symbols of great moral import. In descriptions of the theriomorphs such as the Cynocephali (Dog-heads) or Hippopodes (Horse-feet), their physical appearance is most obviously an expression of moral judgment on their lack of human qualities.[151] The old legends offer material for the allegory hunters of a later age, particularly in the Christian era. But from Homer onward the Centaurs, despite the good qualities of Chiron and Pholus, are overwhelmingly associated with unbridled animal instincts, for drink, sex, and violence.[152] Thus, the Centaurs, as other theriomorphs, become a resource for invective, as is clear from Suetonius' collection of insults.[153] But there is a moral issue in all monstrosity. Interestingly, Anon. comments explicitly on this: "there are also legends which imagine and create from different bodies hydras, chimaeras and giants, to make known the diversity of evil" (Anon. sec. 44 = F.2.62).

Physiognomics had learned precedent, of course, for its idealization of the moderate, in Aristotle's *Nicomachean Ethics* and its followers, in which excess and deficiency are a mark of vice.[154] Monsters are the vivid illustration of extremes of excess and deficiency, at the opposite extreme from the perfect body. I have already suggested that the three main specified methods of physiognomics scrutinize the ordinary man for traces of the monster. It is clear that the implicit principle of moderation that operates throughout physiognomical writings springs from the same concern.

The Beast

The particular association of physiognomics with animal comparison, which seems to operate in Aristotle's time, is revived in the sixteenth century with Della Porta, in the seventeenth by Le Brun, and in the eighteenth by Lavater.[155] This third topos is also the most striking in Polemo's work.[156] For him some part of everyone is comparable with some animal (F.1.190, 12–14; 170, 26–172, 2), and apart from the general remarks on the zoological method, and its frequent application in the body of the text, we have a list of the characters of ninety-four species.[157] This may, however, originally have been a separate treatise (Misener 1924). Animals had long been used for various divinatory practices, and their symbolic associations varied, while retaining a family resemblance, in each tradition. In the work of Polemo's contemporary Artemidorus on dream interpretation, for instance, there are different developments of similar themes (Pack 1941, 330). Also in astrology[158] animal symbolism is there to be exploited in the signs of the zodiac. The crudest kind of astrological method will simply declare that someone born under a certain sign is bound to share the character of that sign, and here, too, the bull, the lion, and the ram will have other associations as well. Interestingly, the use of animal comparisons in physiognomy was, like astrology, threatened by the rise of Christianity.[159] As Dagron notes, Adamantius, writing in the fourth century, puts more emphasis on masculine and feminine types, to which he adds types according to age, and is careful to limit the resemblances between humans and animals.[160] Like Polemo, in fact, he concentrates on resemblances at the level of parts of the human body, rather than comparisons of the whole form. Since Man was created in the image of God (*Genesis* 26), finding resemblances between humans and animal species was blasphemous.

The recent academic fashion for analyzing human constructions of the animal world,[161] that "uniquely rich field of reference and source of symbolic expression," to quote Robert Parker (1984), is doubtless not unconnected with the detachment of animals from humans in the industrialized world, as John Berger has argued.[162] It has found inspiration in the discipline of anthropology. The nineteenth-century interest in totemism and the work of Durkheim and Mauss on "primitive classification" in the first decades of this century laid out the lines of inquiry. But the most influential single author must be Claude Lévi-Strauss. His work (1969 [1962], 1974 [1962]) focused attention on humans' use of animals in an effort to order perceptions of themselves. For the physiognomist their special value is as "raw nature," incapable of dissimulation. Their role as "*bons à penser*" is illustrated by the crucial proposition in the Peripatetic treatise: "No animal has ever existed such that it has the body of one animal and the disposition of another" (*Physiognomonica* 805a12f.). Anon. expands:

> It is besides quite certain that the study of humans is made difficult by the effort each makes to conceal his flaw. But also culture and social life often mask the true character of humans, and often matters are as in this case: the character of an individual man presents several aspects, whereas animals are simple, naked, take no precautions and show their nature out in the open. (sec. 132 = F.2.144, 7–14)

Lévi-Strauss emphasized the importance of the mental operations performed with animals. Dagron (1987), in his discussion of animal physiognomics, takes up Lévi-Strauss's work on the use of animals for classification. He points out that the relationship between men and animals implied by this physiognomical method evokes "totemic" thinking as described by Lévi-Strauss, first in that the analogy with animals allows definition of psychological categories in humans in the same way that the "totem" allows characterization of socially defined human groups, with the same equivocations. Second, he refers to the importance of the general homology between two systems of diffentiation as opposed to particular homologies between human categories and animal species. Third, he follows Lévi-Strauss in quoting Bergson's remark that it is the immediate perception of the genus through the individual that characterizes the relation of humans to animals. "For the physiognomists too, posing an analogy between men and animals is the easiest way, perhaps the only way, to pass from individual differences to specific differences, that is to say to classify," he concludes (1987, 73). Certainly, for the Greeks in particular, there was a long-standing concern with this kind of relationship between humans and animals, which was an obvious area for the physiognomist to exploit.

The most important precursor of the physiognomical enterprise, as it appears in Polemo, is mainly based on analogies with animals. It was a clearly rhetorical use of the preexisting treasury of thinking about them. Semonides of Amorgos' *Invective against Women* (Ψόγος γυναικῶν) of the seventh/sixth century B.C. divides the "race" of women into "tribes." Eight of the ten tribes are associated with an animal. The poet takes each woman in turn to censure her for her reprehensible characteristics as a wife, characteristics summed up under the heading of the animal concerned. Only one, the Bee-Woman, is the subject of an encomium;[163] the ratio of praise to blame is not dissimilar to Polemo's. The relation of each woman to her animal, including participation as well as analogy, can best be described as metaphor, argues Loraux.[164] The similarity of this early invective to the physiognomical enterprise is obvious and offers further support to the idea of the closeness between the rhetoric of praise and blame and physiognomics as well as pointing to the centrality of animals to physiognomics. The *Rhetoric Addressed to Herennius,* as we have seen, offers the very germ of the physiognomical method, and here too we find the same focus. The primary vehicle of *imago,* a particular type of comparison, is the animal.

The rhetoric of praise and blame is part of the process of moral instruction, and animals inserted into the same framework as people are not only good to think with but also good to teach with.[165] It is striking that Pliny, Aelian, Plutarch, and the rest of the writers on the subject clearly find Aristotle's writings on live animals and their mores richer in interest than his work on their biological structures and functions, based on the dead animal.[166]

The animal kingdom in physiognomics is divided up strategically along the lines of a logic with which we are now familiar. As with invective,[167] first one finds the wholly negative picture of animals as a group, which corresponds to that of barbarians. So:

> a dry eye cast down, [lacuna], a rough[?] forehead, a fixed gaze, hair hanging down and an eyebrow with bristling hairs are signs of absolute coarseness[?], as of beasts
>
> Copious . . . leg-hair, because it brings beasts to mind is a sign of ignorance and depraved habits.[168]

Impudence and lack of discretion are seen as typical of beasts in general in one passage (200, 8–10), while stupidity and insanity(?) or at least viciousness, are detected from similarities with animals, though the following lines suggest that only some animals are meant (280, 6–11).

Next we find the binary division mapping on to the human division of the first topos. There are ideal male, good animals: the lion and the *draco* (type of snake) in Polemo (in which there is at least one animal missing from the text); the lion, the boar, the eagle, and the hawk in Anon. There are also ideal female, bad animals: in Polemo the panther and the viper, in Anon., the panther, the stag, the hare, the peacock, the partridge, and the magpie.[169] The chief representatives, the lion and the panther, go back to the Peripatetic *Physiognomonica.* The lion, physically remodeled in the shape of man, as sometimes in art,[170] takes on the features of the ideal male and the pure Greek, as we have seen. In the list of animal characters in Polemo the lion is: "brave, a bold hero, angry when hurt, long-suffering, modest, generous, great-hearted and ready to spring" (F.1.172, 5–7).

In the rest of the treatise it is often singled out for particular physical and moral qualities. First, its mane; thick hair in a man implies strength, energy, and great-heartedness. Quintilian tells us that some orators used to brush their hair backward to provide a terrifying effect, perhaps to look lionlike.[171] Similar qualities accrue when one has eyes concave in the middle, a wide mouth, and thin lips, the upper drooping, or a lionlike gait, with lowered hands, relaxed feet and shoulders moving as if slightly sloping. It is most often recreated in the shape of kingly *virtus.*[172] L'Orange detects the influence of physiognomical readings of the lion in imperial portraiture, as does Evans in the literary portraits of Suetonius and Ammianus Marcellinus, while Dagron points out that Constantine and his dynasty chose the lion as their emblem.[173] Its virtues are certainly kingly; stories of its generosity to benefactors and vengeance on enemies abound.[174] It should be stressed that alternative traditions (of the lion's lust and savagery, e.g.) have been classified out in this idealization.[175] Traces of unkingly characteristics such as lack of loyalty in friendship and impiety appear in Anon. from another physiognomical tradition.[176] Polemo, however, presumably needs his lion pure for imperial encomia.

Correspondingly, the panther becomes the perfect contrary of the lion, the ideal female type (F.1.196, 4–198, 2). There is precedent for this version: Detienne (1979 [1977]) analyzes its place in the bestiary opposite the lion in Greek iconography and legend, as pursuer of the cunning hunt and seducer. Thus, for Aristophanes and his contemporaries a courtesan was a panther.[177] In Polemo's description it has a small head and forehead, sharp eyes, soft limbs, a narrow neck, a thin chest, slender flanks, a large back, a light body, and soft hair. It is weaker, less open, more timid and vicious, and less patient in adversity (F.1.196, 2–8, 9). The positive features of this animal, whose bravery was a byword in Homer and even still allowed in the Peripatetic *Physiognomonica* (809b37) and whose qualities of magical attraction led a later age to take it as a representaton of Christ, are suppressed.

Though, as a group, tame animals are better than wild, the domestic animals so familiar from traditional invective appear as representatives of ignorance, stupidity, clumsiness, and sexual shamelessness.[178] It should perhaps be mentioned that they may draw their power to insult from their function as names of the sexual parts, a metonymy that makes an interesting parallel to the animal within in physiognomics.[179] Polemo seems to prefer more exotic animals for his examples: in them men like a seasnake, a crab, and a tortoise appear.[180] Yet even the exotic animals repeat the same failings of character, restricted by the traditional themes. But Polemo relied on the power of animals, their power as irreducible symbols. It was a power to be harnessed and driven down other well-trodden paths of other moral landscapes.

Rhetoric, Ancient and Modern

It is by now, I hope, clear how fundamental was rhetorical consciousness to the construction of the discipline of physiognomics in the period. Its underlying form of reasoning can best be described as a rhetorical syllogism; its examples are elaborated according to the traditional topoi. Moreover, one sees the influence of the oratory of praise and blame in the choice of method, the treatment of examples according to the stylistic figures of *imago,* εἰκών, χαρακτηρισμός, εἰκονισμός (*eikōn, charactērismos, eikonismos*), the old themes of body and soul, and the entire moral framework. And in the context of the rhetorical aim of making vivid the trope metaphor, with its power to translate, or literally to carry over on to its object the scorn or admiration of the orator, lies at the very heart of the physiognomical method. These comparisons are to be seen as performative strategies, as attempts to codify social opinion. Hence, Polemo can be seen to select from the common knowledge available. Crocker observes that the procedure of persuasion works best if the claimed truth is presented as a new revelation about how things are—which emerges from setting things in new relationships.[181] Here is the basis of wit. In his physiognomical work Polemo is creative in selecting carefully the material for his base and in setting it in a new context—a fine persuasive strategy.

Here also, as with astrology, the valuation of mnemonic qualities remains to show the influence of the oral in a "literary" age in which rhetoric, with its firmly oral roots, is in fact the archetypal form of intellectual activity. As Sassi notes, there is a particular association between that part of rhetoric concerned with memorizing and physiognomics.

Physiognomical descriptions are often used in different contexts for greater persuasive efficacy or in their turn use formal models of a rhetorical type: in general, first of all there is a search for images of the greatest perceptual concreteness that are best imprinted on the mind, a search carried out above all by means of the use of analogy. It is no accident that a great proportion of ancient mnemonic technique rests on visual associations and analogical approaches; this also springs from the need to find images that best fix the recall of more or less abstract concepts.

Further, the transformational logic that we have seen operating between the topoi (elaborations on the basis male-female; Greek-barbarian; human-animal), rather than being a function of mental structures, as classical structuralism would have it, would be better seen as the result of the rhetorical desire for antithesis. Where Lévi-Strauss proves inadequate is in his rigid presentation of relationships. It is the fluid nature of these analogical relations that is important. It is a matter of definitional perspective which parts are essential and invariant members of a whole. No single association of dog is primary, as Crocker has it. These codes offer possibilities for manipulation—the complexities of social relations can be set in relation to these unities—but in the process the unities are shifted in accordance with context.

In examining this discipline, I have been concerned to show the influence of contemporary rhetorical theory and practice on the ways its practitioners attempt to persuade their audience. But this is not just a matter of setting a body of knowledge in its intellectual context. The reason rhetoric is important to my model in general is because it is in rhetoric that knowledge and power meet. And, in examining rhetorical theory, one finds the most explicit confrontation with this nexus. The ancients were always aware of the dangerous potential of rhetoric, of its magical power to lead wherever it willed. Of course, most intellectuals whose writings have come down to us wanted to set certain areas of knowledge aside as independent of manipulation. (Here the heffalump trap rears its head once more.) Modern theoreticians of rhetoric, however, who always begin with ancient theories but push them further, have a more totalizing view of the presence of rhetoric. As I have argued in the introduction, the political element in communication can best be described by rhetoric, and this thesis is about science as rhetoric. Here is the crucial link that allows me to make the leap from intellectual politics to the domain of activity more traditionally known as politics.

Thus, with physiognomics I add another dimension to my depiction of the interrelations between power and knowledge throughout society. In examining astrology, I also linked intellectual politics and politics, in that case "high politics." I concentrated on the struggles for possession of the truth to be found in the stars between the authorities and astrologers, among astrologers themselves, between astrologers and clients, and between astrologers and would-be astrologers. Here was a complex interaction between two channels of power, the first running between the rulers and their subjects and the second between the wielders of intellectual power and their audience of both clients and pupils. The battlefield upon which these knowledge claims were fought out could become confused, since, for instance, astrologers were among the subjects whom the emperors hoped to persuade of their link with the stars, and emperors were among astrologers' clients and were even sometimes their pupils.

In turning to physiognomics I have looked at intellectual power working in tandem with political power at a local level. Thus, the intellectuals here are situated more precisely and unambiguously in the model, in a brokering role. Now this relation is by no means specific to physiognomics. Two cases will illustrate how astrologers fulfilled this role: first, Balbillus who, at a time when other astrologers were being expelled, obtained the right for Ephesus to hold sacred games open to the world, a privilege granted only this once in Vespasian's reign.[182] Second, Philostratus tells us of Philiscus, who traveled to Rome and, by attaching himself to Julia Domna's circle of astrologers and philosophers, managed to secure for himself the chair of rhetoric at Athens.[183] Meanwhile, Claudius' doctor, Gaius Stertinius Xenophon, who obtained the citizenship for his native island of Cos, the less well-known Titus Statilius Attalus, and Lucius Gellius Maximus, or the doctors in power in the cities mentioned by Galen, will serve to illustrate that doctors could also be brokers.[184] But such broker positions only increased the chance of having the emperor's ear: the task of persuasion remained.

In this case study of physiognomics we have a particularly lively and detailed cameo in Polemo's quarrel with Favorinus, which stands as an epitome for the innumerable clashes of rivals for imperial favor and local political influence that have left no trace in our evidence. This story represents, in effect, an expansion of the ἀγών (agōn) that took place before the emperor in the case of disputes.[185] In it I wanted to depict the power of the seer-sage using all the resources of scientific rhetoric to make it a matter of knowledge that his opponent was morally unfit, as he himself was morally fitted, to enjoy imperial beneficence. To those for whom power still only proceeds downward from the state, and for whom knowledge connotes the certainty of a realm of Ideal Forms, my treatment of rhetorical interaction under these headings will no doubt appear as a sophistic redefinition. But, according to the model of power-knowledge interaction, it makes sense; Polemo's small victory for himself and his city is a fine illustration of rhetorical power, in the sense of "*pouvoir*" or "power to . . . ," and the phenomenally successful nature of Polemo's whole career suggests that his rhetoric was confirmed as knowledge.

Finally, there is another aspect of the game of persuasion that was only lightly touched on in the preceding case study—that is, the relationship between orator and audience, which was given so much consideration in rhetorical theory. So far I have left the implied audience undefined, since we cannot be sure exactly whom Polemo had to persuade to achieve his aim. How many intermediaries had to be involved for him to find himself in a position to sway imperial decisions? It is a question I leave for others to answer.[186] What is clear is that, whomever they are, the Greco-Roman orator must work on fundamental cultural categories as his basis for argument; there must be some culturally salient ἔνδοξα (*endoxa* [generally approved ideas]) on the basis of which he can begin to codify social opinion.

He begins with general acceptance of the principles and some of the details of physiognomics and with the common knowledge involved in the three topoi.

It is here that the whole issue of self-presentation, the ἦθος (*ēthos*) of rhetorical theory, becomes important. The Self that Polemo presents has profound implications for the nature of the audience's consensus. The mutual implication of the oratorical Self and the audience is an issue to which I return in my third chapter on medicine. In this case it is significant that Polemo elects in the last part of his treatise to align himself with the three perfect ideal types in giving the same features to the sage as are found in the male man, the pure Greek, and the lion. Aristotle, in the *Rhetoric,* observes that in epideictic exordia, one must make the hearer believe that he shares the praise in some way or other.[187] In presenting these types to the audience, Polemo confirms them in their ideal definitions of themselves, these definitions made in opposition to all the ideal-type Others. So they, too, as they join the sage on his pedestal, enjoy the power of the omniscient voyeur, the diviner of monsters within.

Chapter 3

Medical Prognosis: The Doctor as Diviner and Detective

"How did you know for example that I did manual labour? It's as true as gospel, for I began as a ship's carpenter."

"Your hands, my dear sir. Your right hand is quite a size larger than your left. You have worked with it, and the muscles are more developed."

"Well, the snuff, then, and the Freemasonry?"

"I won't insult your intelligence by telling you how I read that, especially as rather against the strict rules of your order, you use an arc-and-compass breast-pin."

"Ah, of course, I forgot that. But the writing?"

"What else can be indicated by that right cuff so very shiny for five inches, and the left one with the smooth patch near the elbow where you rest it upon the desk?"

"Well, but China?"

"The fish that you have tattooed above your right wrist could only have been done in China. I have made a small study of tattoo-marks and even contributed to the literature of the subject. That trick of staining the fishes' scales a delicate pink is quite peculiar to China. When, in addition, I see a Chinese coin hanging from your watch-chain, the matter becomes even more simple."

Mr. Jabez Wilson laughed heavily. "Well, I never!" said he. "I thought at first that you had done something clever, but I see that there was nothing in it after all."

"I begin to think, Watson," said Holmes, "that I made a mistake in explaining. *Omne ignotum pro magnifico,* you know, and my poor little reputation, such as it is, will suffer shipwreck if I am so candid."

—A. Conan Doyle, "The Red-Headed League"

Introduction

In this chapter I move into the domain traditionally reserved for the historian of science in order to show that the sociopolitical constraints that shaped the other areas of intellectual life that I have been considering are operating here too. Indeed, I shall illustrate, with regard to a topic that has been celebrated as one of the achievements of ancient science (the "discovery of the diagnostic value of the pulse"),[1] how the strategy of searching for anticipations of modern science has blinded historians to the distinctive idiom of ancient knowledge. Here we remain with the theme of the politics of knowledge but consider exclusively the level of intellectual politics. This is, first, because it presents such interesting contrasts to the politics of knowledge in modern medicine and, second, because I want to concentrate on the similarities to the intellectual politics in the previous two chapters in order to explode the unhelpful but still ubiquitous division into science and pseudoscience, itself a result of a modern politics of knowledge.

I have chosen to focus on the art of prognosis in order to set it against the other semiological disciplines' claim to tell the past, present, and future. While astrology and physiognomics, each with differing emphases, interpret the signs (in the stars or in the body) in order to tell the character and the destiny, prognosis in medicine interprets signs, as with physiognomics, in the body, to tell the past, present, and future of the patient. Carlo Ginzburg, in an extraordinarily wide-ranging article, has discussed a concept he calls the "conjectural model" for the construction of knowledge, which, he argues, "quietly emerged towards the end of the nineteenth century in the sphere of the social sciences, and still has not received the attention it deserves." Even more interesting, he expresses the hope that "it can perhaps help us to go beyond the sterile contrasting of rationalism and irrationalism."[2] He maintains that the concept of using obscure or remote clues in a speculative manner to build an epistemological model has been an essential, if largely unrecognized, component in our cultural heritage. He poses as examples of this paradigm the work of three great "detectives": Giovanni Morelli, Sigmund Freud, and Sherlock Holmes. Morelli, a nineteenth-century art historian, pioneered the method of attribution of works of art based on painters' habitual characterization of small, "insignificant" details of the body, such as earlobes, fingernails, and toes. Gathering an encyclopedic knowledge of such details, he was able to detect imitations and wrongly assigned authorship in a spectacular fashion.

Ginzburg draws parallels and indeed some connections between these methods,[3] Freud's interest in the "psychopathology of everyday life," the apparently unimportant details so revealing of the psychology, and Holmes's solution of crimes by reading the clues. He also suggests an origin for this everyday, universal style of knowledge in the primitive skills of the hunt and also, significantly for my argument in this chapter, in divination, such as that found in Mesopotamia from the second millennium B.C. onwards.[4] The word *conjecture,* as Ginzburg points out, is in origin associated with the *coniector,* a priestly soothsayer or diviner.[5] Furthermore, he draws attention to the medical connections of these three paradigmatic figures.[6] The medical art was indeed the στοχαστικὴ τέχνη (*stochastikē technē*),[7] the body of conjectural knowledge par excellence. Moreover, medical prognosis on the basis of symptoms has been hailed by others as the original semiotic art, the beginning of the process of reasoning that the Pragmatist philosopher C. S. Peirce described as "abduction," in contrast to induction and deduction.[8]

Peirce illustrated what he meant with the following schema:

Deduction: Rule—All the beans from this bag are white.
Case—These beans are from this bag.
Hence, Result—These beans are white.

Induction: Case—These beans are from this bag.
Result—These beans are white.
Hence, Rule—All the beans from this bag are white.

Abduction: Rule—All the beans from this bag are white.
Result—These beans are white.
Hence, Case—These beans are from this bag.

(Peirce 1935–66, 2.623)

His construction of abduction describes the process that occurs when the subject is faced with an observed fact that seems important. To explain the fact he or she must come up with a "known law or rule of nature or other general truth," which will explain the truth retroactively; ideally, it will reveal its relevance. So here, a "rule" is a law of nature or general truth; a result is an observed fact and the abductive conclusion, or "retroduction," as Peirce sometimes called it, is what is referred to as the case. But in the cases of deduction and induction here rule and case can both indicate an observed fact. The further difficulty with this over-simplified model is that the choice of process with which to form a conclusion would seem to depend on which bit of information came first.

Peirce in fact developed his theory of abduction in an attempt to formalize the processes of reasoning involved in scientific method that could not be subsumed under the headings of either deduction or induction. While the latter two processes could be described as tautologous, abduction was the creative part of science, providing the hypotheses for testing. In itself, of course, the abductive conclusion is invalid; it needs external validation. Holmes's use of abduction lays itself open to ridicule and parody, when, as often, the hypotheses are not tested but simply validated by the author. It is also obviously different from Peirce's scientific abduction in emphasis, since detective work involves getting back from a particular event to a particular cause, rather than to some general law or, more usually, to a rearrangement of some intermediate laws so that the particular observation fits with the general law.

Leaving aside reconstructions of the modern scientific method for the moment, here I want to concentrate on the abductive process itself. The systems of conjectural knowledge to which Ginzburg refers were developed and invested with meaning by the postulation of rules to explain the observed data before a causality was proved. A cultural or experiential knowledge is required to codify such a system, but, ultimately, however rationalized, there must be a kind of guessing involved, a kind of leaping from known to unknown by inference on the basis of clues, such as in the Arab *firasa* in physiognomics. Such a procedure is also at work in Greco-Roman physiognomics and astrology. It is possible that this form of reasoning comes under scrutiny in the ancient world. Peirce tried to read an analysis of abduction into chapter 25 of Aristotle's *Prior Analytics,* a work in which he does indeed subject physiognomics to formal analysis, as we have seen, but it may be that Peirce might have found something closer to his ideas in Stoic nondeductive inference.[9]

There is always a tension between two images of knowledge present in both Holmes and Galen. Dr. Watson's summary of Holmes's article on his "science of deduction and analysis" exhibits this potential conflict:

> It attempted to show how much an observant man might learn by an accurate and systematic examination of all that came his way . . . the reasoning was close and intense, but the deduction appeared to be far-fetched. . . . Deceit, according to him, was an impossibility in the case of one trained to observation and analysis. His conclusions were as infallible as so many propositions of Euclid. So startling would the results appear to the uninitiated that until they learned the processes by which he had arrived at them, they might well consider him a necromancer. . . . Like all arts, the Science of Deduction and Analysis is one that can be acquired by long and patient study. (*A Study in Scarlet*)[10]

There is much reminiscent of Galen's self-presentation in this quotation: most obviously, the emphasis on a science of deduction is familiar. Galen, too, was fond of citing geometry as his model for infallible knowledge and often compared his medical work with the model, though he admitted that it was not really necessary for the ordinary doctor to be versed in geometry.[11] The stress on observation is also to be found in Galen, though it does not always figure so largely.[12] While all this has often been noted by modern commentators, they have been less sensitive to the relationship between Galen's self-presentation and the model of the diviner, if I may leap here from the word *necromancer* (elsewhere Watson declares of Holmes "You would certainly have been burned, had you lived a few centuries ago"). While it is true that Galen distances himself from γοητεία (sorcery), his attitude to divination is more accommodating, as we shall see.

The use of the term *uninitiated* is also significant, in its evocation of the religious model of the mysteries. This is connected with another feature of the Holmesian/Galenic attitude. It is just because of the necessity for an "abductive leap" that the politics of knowledge enter the scene. Certainly, there are obstacles from the start, because of the difficulty of communicating such a skill. On the problems of translation Ginzburg notes: "One needs only to think of the gulf separating the rigid and schematic treatises of physiognomy from its perceptive and flexible practice by a lover or horse-dealer or card-player" (1983, 101). But we shall see that there is evidence that Galen's attitude to teaching is reminiscent of Holmes's. Despite his idealization of the autodidactic doctor and his implication that anyone who follows his example can enjoy similar fame and success,[13] he appears to relish the mastery of such knowledge more than he does attempting any real communication of it. The "teaching" offered promised initiation into the mysteries (a term Galen uses),[14] at the end of a long, hard road, but it remains questionable whether these masters wanted their pupils to attain the ultimate mysterious knowledge. Both he and Holmes, in their different ways, find the thaumaturge an image vital to their arts at the same time as they attempt to describe them as rational, logical procedures that can be communicated to discerning audiences.[15]

I have chosen to focus on Galen because he is a "hard case." No one will doubt that doctors he attacked, the Pamphiluses and Xenocrateses,[16] with their "magical"-sounding herbals, had an esoteric view of knowledge, that they dabbled in iatromathematics and won clients by their rhetoric. Galen, on the other hand, is someone who lays explicit emphasis on strict logical demonstration in his science and on the possibility of making knowledge available to everybody. His watchword is ἀκρίβεια. He refers to rhetoric only as a defect of opponents.[17] He was also the doctor who set great store by observation, the master of anatomy, who confounded his opponents by dissection. How could this towering figure in ancient science, whose systematization of medicine was to be influential even to the present day in some parts of the world, be compared to a tuppenny-ha'penny superstitious astrologer like Dorotheus or to an amateur physiognomist like Polemo?

Galen is also the best author to focus on, because he is an extraordinarily rich source for the social context; it is through his works more than those of any other medical writer that one gains an insight into the politics of intellectual life in the period, as indeed Bowersock realized.[18] Certainly, in many ways Galen was not a typical doctor, even among the practitioners at the learned end of the spectrum. The extraordinary length of time for which he studied sets him apart and suggests a bias toward the learned image of the discipline.[19] It may also be true that he was of a particularly polemical disposition, but at any rate it is not only his own activities that he reveals in his writings but also those of his predecessors and contemporaries. It is also important that one can draw parallels with Polemo, or court astrologers, in one respect: even taking into account his exaggerations, he was clearly successful by means of his rhetoric (in the broadest sense) in gaining court favor, since he treated members of the imperial family.[20]

Rhetorical Modes: Rational and Mantic

I begin with a theme that follows from my earlier investigations of the interpenetration of the religious and scientific discourses in strategies of knowledge. While this may be uncontroversial in the case of astrology, it is certainly not so in the case of medicine, in which the post-Darwinian search for a secularist ethos dictates an approach minimizing religious influence in appreciation of ancient achievements. Much has been made of the opposition between "temple-medicine" and "naturalistic," or "scientific," medicine from the Hippocratics onward, which might lead one to expect that the two will operate with entirely different methods. There is an old debate over the true nature of prognosis that tends to surface in some form whenever consideration is given to the subject, which typifies the pitfalls of such an approach. Scholars seem to feel the need to take a stance on whether it is *really* scientific and rational or merely a form of divination used for self-advertisement.[21] It is an issue that appears to be alive and demanding attention still in Vivian Nutton's edition of Galen's *On Prognosis* (1979, 232). He is among the majority of scholars who are keen not only to applaud Galen's scientific attitude in distancing himself from diviners[22] but also to take his professed desire to impart knowledge at face value and to praise it. But I would argue that this opposition between rational science and divination is a fundamentally unhelpful antithesis, which runs the risk of pandering to an anachronistic and, indeed, idealistic notion of science. It is in fact another formulation of the science/pseudoscience distinction that I want to abandon, as I have argued in the introduction. Ginzburg's work on the "conjectural model," with its divinatory roots, when associated with Peirce's arguments that abduction is a vital part of "the logic of scientific discovery,"[23] further suggests that such a dichotomous model is inadequate.[24] Here the remarks of Curry (1985), which I mentioned in chapter 1, about the pseudoquestions and radical incoherence generated by crude dualism, seem apposite. Asking why scientific doctors sometimes posed as diviners is such a pseudoquestion; the point is that this was a period in which boundaries between science and divination were fluid and negotiable.

What if, following on from the arguments and ensuing lines of investigation in earlier chapters, we rearrange the terms of the debate and ask a question susceptible to an answer that respects the peculiar character of ancient "science"? One could start off with the proposition that scientists then, as now, were in the business of establishing their inquiries into nature as bodies of knowledge and simply ask how—what were their strategies? A few problems immediately arise. One is faced by a lack of cultural consensus about what science is. Better, then, to say that numerous "disciplines" competed for the status of knowledge. But this latter term also fragments on inspection. There is first an intuitive kind of knowledge, which resists dissection, such as is exercised in divination of the traditional kind (as opposed to astrology, e.g.). Second, there is the kind of knowledge that has to justify itself in more detail. As Peirce's model indicates, the two are not necessarily to be opposed.

Here taking up the line adumbrated above of looking at science as rhetoric helps us to ask more fruitful questions. In a sense this binary distinction (divination / intuitive knowledge vs. science / justified knowledge) corresponds to the two levels at which the learned practitioner's rhetoric had to work. First, he had to establish his ἦθος (*ēthos*),[25] a self-presentation that worked at a very practical level and was pervaded by a strong moral significance. As we have seen with physiognomics, establishing the right to persuade is an essential prelude in ancient rhetorical theory. In the case of medicine all the factors leading to the patient's putting his or her trust in the doctor are involved. The second level at which the rhetoric of knowledge had to operate is the "technical." And the learned practitioner had to establish his discourse as a τέχνη (*technē*) that was more than a vulgar craft.[26] Specific strategies had to be employed to sustain his claim to knowledge of this sort. The medical writer could claim a basis in the theoretical disciplines. Thus, Galen produced a treatise entitled *That the Best Doctor Is a Philosopher.* Apart from a guide to ethics,[27] what he claimed to seek within philosophy was a body of epistemological canons, an ἀποδεικτικὴ θεωρία (apodeictic method), a method of argument that attains its conclusions by proceeding from true premises.[28] He even hoped, he tells us, to find out from philosophy answers to questions about the creation of the world and the body.[29] But, ultimately, he looked to mathematics to provide the axiomatic-deductive model. (According to him, all philosophical sects, though at odds on everything else, were agreed that mathematical methods produced certain proof.[30] And he claimed to find in "dialectic" the right way of ordering data. In the field of prognostic signs, as we shall see, the operation of διαίρεσις (diaeresis), the method of collection and division that goes back to Plato, to which he attaches great importance in general,[31] is most striking. But we shall see that this rhetoric of logical division is not unconnected with the model of knowledge as initiation.

If we go back to our initial antithesis (whether ancient prognosis was really scientific and rational or simply a form of divination for self-advertisement), we can see that, once we locate it in a rhetorical context, it dissolves. The second half, self-advertisement, reinforces rather than undermines the first: science (τέχνη, *technē*). Further, even traditional divination, the μαντική (*mantikē*), which makes no attempt to justify itself, could contribute to a claim to knowledge at this first level of self-presentation, establishment of the ἦθος (*ēthos*). Galen not only did not deny divination's success, as Nutton puts it (1979, 169), but he also exploited it to good effect on occasion. Technical justification could be kept in reserve, for the audience that challenged. It is important to see Galen's remarks distancing himself from μαντική[32] in the context of criticism from rival doctors rather than as constituting an absolute opposition between medicine and divination.[33]

The operation of his persuasion at two levels is clear from several incidents in *On Prognosis,* typified by the case of Eudemus. Galen does not object at all to his patient's announcing to everybody that "Pythian Apollo has deigned to prophesy to the sick through the mouth of Galen." Yet he calls the Erasistratean doctor Martianus' suggestion that he derived his forecasts from divination slander.[34] There is another instance that illustrates how cautious one should be before seeking a secularist ethos in what looks like resentment at being called a diviner. Galen records a conversation with one Severus, probably Marcus Aurelius' son-in-law,[35] who suggests to him that the imperial chamberlain Peitholaus may have passed on the news of Galen's latest remarkable prognosis to the emperor. Galen replies in typical fashion:

> Possibly . . . he has told him, but personally I am not bothered about my reputation with such people. I don't go around broadcasting my prognoses and cures so as to earn greater enmity from doctors and philosophers and have them calling me a prophet and other such names. But to you, my friends, who have condemned medicine because of the ignorance of men like that, I declare that this art is worthy of Apollo and Asclepius and that these doctors have abused it.[36]

It seems also noteworthy that here it is rival doctors and philosophers who call Galen a prophet as an insult. They are the ones who want a technical justification, which might suggest that it is only the ignorant layperson who takes prognosis as a species of divination. But the picture turns out to be more complicated. At the time when Galen makes his final prediction for Eudemus the latter does demand an explanation, claiming that he understands more than the doctors, and praises him for a "truly logical exposition of how he reached his conclusion."[37] But certainly it is true that on the whole Galen does not expect to have to justify himself in this way to his patients. They should regard the doctor as "a little like a god" so that they obey his orders willingly.[38] There is something in Pliny's cynical gibe that some patients have greater confidence in a doctor the less they understand them (*Natural History* 29.17). But it is clear from the following anecdote that Galen treats learned colleagues in the same way and that they may respond appreciatively to the use of the divinatory model.

Prognosis: Divining and Detecting

The most revealing case of prognosis comes not in *On Prognosis* but, instead, in the *On the Affected Parts.*[39] It is a story that is worth a detailed examination, as an example of the kind of narrative of prognosis to be found in Galen. He describes a meeting in the street with the philosopher Glaucon, who tells him that he has just been visiting a Sicilian doctor whom Galen had met a few days before who was now ill. Grabbing him by the arm, he invites him to come and see the man. It is important to stress that these protagonists are no ordinary lay observers but, rather, are from the very groups that might be expected to demand technical explanation. But the philosopher's first words confound such an expectation: he reveals that the reason he has eagerly hailed Galen was that he has been told that he was a man who made diagnoses that had more to do with soothsaying and divination than with medicine (362, 3–8). He declares that he wanted not so much to put him to the test as to see if the medical art is capable of such diagnosis and prognosis. Here one has the distinct impression that the divinatory image is one to which the medical art must aspire. Galen is worried: he has no chance to say before they arrive at the door that, while sometimes there is a secure sign, at other times all are ambiguous so that a second and third examination are necessary. It is at this point that the narrative takes on the air of a Holmes retrospective revelation at the end of the book:

> As we entered the house we fell in with someone carrying a bedpan from the bedroom to the rubbish-dump, which contained a liquid looking like the water in which freshly-slaughtered meat has been washed, a very clear bloody serum—the certain index of a bad liver. I made as though I had seen nothing and entered with Glaucon. (362, 14–18)

Galen put his hand to the patient's wrist to see if he had inflammation or just weakness in the liver. The patient, clearly not ready to resign the medical role, eagerly asked Galen to judge whether the frequency of his pulse had been increased by his getting up to relieve himself. Ignoring this sally, Galen decided that there was inflammation. Next he had the kind of luck typical of the detective story:

> Then, having seen near the window a small pot containing hyssop crushed in honeyed water [*was it labeled?!*], I deduced that the doctor believed himself attacked by pleurisy because of the pain in the false-ribs which happens sometimes in liver-inflammations . . . and because of his fast, shallow breathing and the small coughs which irritated him. Knowing that chance had given me a means to shine in Glaucon's eyes, I guided the patient's hand to the false-ribs on the right-hand side and pointing to the place declared that it was there that he had pain. He agreed. Glaucon, who thought that I had discovered the source merely by taking the pulse, was full of admiration. And to make him even more astonished I added: "In the same way as you admitted that the pain is there, you can now tell me that you have an urge to

> cough and that from time to time you cough a little, drily, without expectorating. As I was speaking it happened that he coughed in just this manner. (363, 7–364, 8)

Naturally, according to our narrator, Glaucon was mightily impressed and launched into a loud eulogy, but Galen, ever the true showman, stopped him: there was more to come. He continues:

> Don't imagine that these are the only things the medical art is capable of divining [μαντεύεσθαι] on the subject of ill people. There are other things besides these which I shall now mention to you and the patient will confirm it. When you breathe deeply you also notice, I imagine, that the pain gets stronger at the place I pointed to and that you get a pain in the right hypochondrium. (364, 10–17)

At this point the patient himself begins to shout in admiration along with Glaucon (!). But Galen still has not finished. He almost ventures to say something about the collarbone, thinking that it seems to be held in a low position. But he knows that this may be complicated by the severe inflammation and induration of the liver and so does not have the courage to speak, for fear of making a mistake after all this praise. So he thinks of a careful way of putting it and says that the patient will soon notice a drawing sensation in his collarbone, if he has not already. In view of the further astonishment that greets this last announcement he offers to give a final prophecy (μαντεία) to astonish them completely—the opinion the patient has of the nature of his own illness. Glaucon made it clear that he was waiting eagerly, while the sick man, left in a stupor at this incredible promise, could not take his eyes off Galen, in his anticipation. And, naturally, his supposition that the patient thinks he has pleurisy is quite correct. The patient is awestruck, as is the man who had been attending him, who had just before been applying hot oil to his chest against pleurisy!

In all this account Galen never seems to reveal to the patient and audience what the illness actually is and certainly gives no clue about a rational method. It is only long afterward that he lets out, in the Holmesian manner, the signs that led to the prognosis. And, as we have seen, they turn out to have nothing to do with the index on which he has given the appearance of relying: the pulse. It was a unique combination of circumstances that presented him with the clues: first, in that his arrival coincided with the servant bringing out the bedpan, and, second, there was the fact that the patient was a doctor. This obviously gave a special significance to the last piece of luck; when Galen spotted the medicament on the shelf, he was able to conclude that the patient had selected it for himself. No matter—Galen is proud to announce that from this moment the philosopher held not only Galen himself but also the τέχνη (*technē*) in high esteem. He does not appear to worry at all that he might have shown the art in a bad light. On the contrary, this is a triumphant celebration of the persuasive force of the dramatic. Holmes, too, though he liked to refer to his method as that of rational deduction[40] open to anyone who took the trouble to gather the encyclopedic knowledge he possessed, was fond of dramatic gestures that made his knowledge appear miraculous.[41]

There is a further question to be considered in relation to this episode, that of its value as instruction. Galen claims after this account that he reported the story to make the reader understand

> that there are some symptoms specific to each disease and others which one disease has in common with different diseases, and in addition to these, there are always symptoms which are connected with either type, but which represent sometimes frequent, sometimes doubtful and rare signs. (366, 6–9)

He adds that this serves as an example of how the student should seize opportunities and elaborate on the basic symptom. Actually, the only straightforward piece of information that the student can use is that in liver disease the excretions appear like water in which freshly slaughtered meat has been washed and that there are other symptoms (he names) that, though not peculiar to liver disease, may be associated with it. Simply knowing these facts would not allow the reader to imitate Galen's achievement here.[42] Watson never learns from Holmes either.[43]

The problems posed for teaching by strategies designed to persuade a wider audience that the practitioner is a master of knowledge will become evident in my discussion of Galen's doctrines on the pulses. I shall be considering the tensions inherent in combining two strategies of knowledge: the claim to be able to teach, via a framework of explanation, the kind of knowledge that leads to successful treatment and the claim to be operating a superior διαίρεσις (diaeresis), with regard to the two major prognostic signs (pulses and urines). But before that I want to look at the importance of self-presentation generally in Greco-Roman medicine. I shall be considering the claims, first, to technical competence and, second, to moral competence in theory and practice. I go on to discuss the involvement of the audience in the construction of the ἦθος (*ēthos*), which leads to examination of the implications of the agonistic arena for presentation of the self in contrast to others and thus to the question of tradition and originality.

The Foregrounding of the Self

In modern academic works on medicine the ethos of objectivity demands a depersonalization of the authorial role. Certainly, the author would not set him- or herself up as an exemplar in an overt way. In the ancient world, however, the personal experiences of the doctor were regularly discussed as such in works of medical theory. This might come under case histories or illustrate a particular disease but often would simply set the moral tone. Scribonius Largus' preface to his *Compounds,* discussed by Deichgräber (1950) in his study of the ideal of the medical profession, is a typical instance of the genre, with his own work set against the decline in pharmacological learning. Similarly, Marcellus Empiricus justifies his own writing on herbal remedies on the grounds that contemporary surgery is barbarous (1.8–10).[44] Galen's *On Examining the Best Physicians* sums up the way Galen sets himself up as the example to follow, in his constant devotion to medicine, as opposed to attendance on the rich: "He who can say that his performance is comparable to mine, provided that he is endowed by nature with intelligence and can quickly understand this great science, he should be trusted even before he is examined" (9.3, p. 103).

Now, certainly, like this latter treatise, *On Prognosis* lays less claim to expounding theory than much of Galen's work, but it is best to see it as lying at one end of a whole spectrum of shades of self-presentation rather than as being kept in a separate category. *Therapeutic Method* is a typical example of a technical work in which the self frequently obtrudes. Here he contrasts himself with other doctors who spend their time in the trains of the rich, who only care about seeming wise; he has always spent his time searching for the truth (K.10.609, 3–16). It is also true that Galen's personality obtrudes in his writings more than those of other medical writers in theirs, but again it is a question of degree.

The first priority of *On Prognosis* is to establish Galen's competence from a technical point of view. According to his work *On Examining the Best Physicians,* the complete physician foretells the nature of the disease at its onset, when it will reach its culmination, and the occurrence of its crisis (5.5, p. 71). Indeed, if Nutton is right, he is reestablishing this competence in response to challengers who charge him with being a mere λογίατρος, or "doctor of words." Nutton connects the composition of the work with the return of Marcus Aurelius to Rome in late A.D. 176, after eight years' absence, when he brought with him other doctors who had obeyed his request to accompany him on his German campaigns.[45] But self-justification of this sort is normal in Galenic writings; *On Examining the Best Physicians* is very similar and cannot be connected to any such circumstances. But in such works, since instruction is not his major aim, he refers the reader to other treatises for that.

The doctor is present, however, in very much the same way in case studies in other works of theory, as we have seen in *On the Affected Parts.* Other kinds of autobiographical sketches occur in the technical works on prognosis: most often they are accounts of his confrontations with other doctors, philosophers, or members of the general audience who failed to see his point of view. One could take as examples the amazing prognoses and following dialogues or the disputes over definitions of the heavy or the full pulse in *On the Varieties of Pulses.*[46] But we also find accounts of his problems, as in the case of his quest over many years to feel the systole (pulse contraction) at the beginning of *On Discernment of the Pulses* (1.1, K.8.770, 15–772, 7).

The confrontations that litter the pages of Galen are not just about technical competence; the distinctions he draws between himself and his opponents are infused with a strong moral significance.[47] Scientific demonstration itself is equated with virtue and opposed to laziness, luxury, the pursuit of pleasure, riches, and prestige, in Galen's presentation.[48] After all, trust in the doctor is of primary importance, especially when things seem to go wrong: in cases like that of Sextus,[49] it is vital that his audience believes Galen when he accuses his patient of deliberately delaying the crisis by his diet and bathing habits (pp. 120, 28–122, 5 = K.14.652–53). The theme of the establishment of the ἦθος (*ēthos*) is often set at the beginning of a treatise, as in the case of Largus and Marcellus. This theme of moral decline runs through the technical treatises. Thus, Galen begins *On the Varieties of Pulses* with a rejection of the modern sophistic, useless, and contentious discussion about names and a claim to return to ancient simplicity and practicality: people come to doctors for healing, not for fine-sounding names. He starts *On Discernment of the Pulses* with the warning that no gain will come from the study of his book, as long as it lacks truth lovers as readers, while pleasure rules, and honor is of no account.[50] But it is in the less-technical works in which the full treatment is required. The canvas is broadened in *On Prognosis,* in which his usual righteous indignation at people who disagree with him becomes a full-blown diatribe directed at the whole of Roman society. He begins with the doctors:

> For since those who are eager for the semblance of ability rather than the reality have come to predominate in medicine as well as the other arts, the finest aspects of these arts are now neglected and attention is lavished upon what may bring them a high reputation with the general public—a gratifying word or act, a bit of flattery, a toadying salutation each day of the rich and powerful men in the cities, accompanying them when they go out, staying at their side, escorting them on their homeward journey, amusing them at dinner. (Trans. Nutton, p. 68 = K.14.599–600)[51]

But then the moral failings of the rich and powerful men themselves also come in for attack, in particular their venal nature, which serves as a neat foil for the ideology of the *medicus gratiosus* (the doctor who does it all for love) described by Deichgräber.[52] This picture of the corrupt rich and their corrupt physicians forms the backdrop against which the emperor's praise of Galen as first among physicians and unique among philosophers gleams all the more brightly, "for he had already met many who were avaricious, quarrelsome, proud, jealous and spiteful."[53] Like Polemo, he aligns himself with the best patron, from a moral point of view.

After the passage cited above Galen goes on to criticize the doctors' attempt to persuade the unsophisticated that they are important by their ostentation in clothes, jewelery, retinue, and equipment. This is a subject long thought suitable for discussion by the medical writers: how the doctor should present himself.[54] It, of course, finds its counterpart in satire and its antecedents. Not only dress, but also the haircut, the state of the nails, and body odor are matters for serious consideration.[55] In this, together with the concern about the gait and whole bearing, one sees the self-consciousness of one trained to be aware of the physical element of the persona in rhetoric. And the key terms in the ideal persona to present are heavily invested with moral overtones: dignity and moderation. Pride and haughtiness, on the one hand, and humility and an effeminate air, on the other, are to be avoided.

A rhetorical education also instilled a constant awareness of audience. In fact, Galen tells us that he actually wrote a work on the relations between orator and audience, which has unfortunately not survived.[56] In the same passage on the doctor's self-presentation Galen warns against solecisms and barbarisms in discussion with the cultivated man. He also claims (in contrast to Archigenes and others) to write a clear Greek prose, uncontaminated by the solecisms of the marketplace or by hyper-Attic refinements: other people, in contrast to Hippocrates' good style, can even make two mistakes in one word.[57] A good style is one of the factors that can help to instill trust in the doctor, where a discerning audience is involved.

The implied audience can itself help to construct the ideal persona of the speaker. Again there is an important contrast with modern academic work, in which the implied audience is specialist and lay people are conventionally viewed as ignorant and irrational. Popular appeal counts against the academic writer, as the inadequate audience entails an unscientific persona. Obviously, in Rome the divide between experts and laypeople was not so sharp; in Aulus Gellius it is assumed that it is disgraceful for a liberally educated man to be ignorant of health and medicine (18.10.8).[58] Favorinus can deliver a eulogy of the quartan fever (17.12) and quote Erasistratus in discussion at the sickbed of a friend, while Gellius himself quotes Hippocrates and his commentator Sabinus on eight-month-old children (3.16.8). Gellius describes with delight the occasion when Calvisius Taurus the philosopher puts his physician to shame by teaching him the differences between arteries and veins (18.10).[59] The important divisions were social, as far as credibility was concerned.

In the works in which Galen concentrates on presenting the "*alto profilo*"

(Vegetti 1981) of medicine, making it more than a craftsman's art, the φιλόκαλοι (lovers of elegance) are ever present.[60] They dictate the line on the one hand, and they are made obtrusive to define Galen as one of their number on the other. For them, where possible, all the arts of literary and rhetorical cultivation are on display. Nutton (1972) suggests at least four genres as influential models *On Prognosis:* the diatribe, the *pinax* (list), the autobiography, and the *commentarii* (memoirs). As he comments, nowhere else does Galen display better the value of his expensive education. The very variety required for an impressive style contrasts with the rigidity of style expected of medical writing today. Now the triumph of science over the arts is symbolized by this deliberate impoverishment, while then a τέχνη (*technē*) elevated itself by participation in literary culture.

Another audience is present in Galen's writings to construct his successful persona: the Roman political elite.[61] Of course, it is not in his interest to distinguish too much between them and the previous group, but they do have a cachet of their own. They are far more prominent than their status as medical cases would ever justify in *On Prognosis.* Obviously, the emperor Marcus is not included in the work as an interesting case of indigestion.[62] It was these people who made you or broke you as a doctor. In assessing one of his rivals, Galen tells us that Antigenes was "considered to be the leading physician and . . . treated all the most influential people."[63] Galen got no small δόξα (reputation) as a result of Eudemus' case. He specifies who the important people were that Eudemus told: Sergius Paulus was "not long after, urban prefect" and Flavius Boethus a former consul.[64]

Galen's dramatic conquest of the social leaders of Rome does pose problems, however, in terms of preserving his ἦθος (*ēthos*), and it is no accident that, just at the turning point of his career, as he cures Eudemus, he inserts a section of diatribe continuing the themes of the *prooemium* but this time ascribes it to Eudemus himself. It is presented as coming in response to Galen's own innocent surprise at the ill will of the doctors in Rome.[65] He thus counters any suggestion that he himself might fit into the categories of doctor he attacks at the beginning of the treatise: the predicates *foreign* and *greedy for gold* might not seem obviously inappropriate.[66] To distance himself from them most effectively he expresses a wish to leave the corrupt town altogether, in conformity with the topos of moral retreat in works of moral philosophy.[67]

The Agonistic Arena

The projection of the Self is motivated in a rhetorical context, the context of the agonistic arena, the sine qua non of Galen's work. Not for nothing does his treatise *That the Best Doctor Is a Philosopher* begin by comparing doctors to athletes preparing for the ἀγών (*agōn*).[68] He must always find opponents against whom to define himself. Doctors were part of the Sophistic milieu examined in the last chapter and behaved similarly.[69] The quarrels and rivalries that were so salient a feature of Sophistic life find no better illustration than in Galen's oeuvre. In fact, Galen, like Polemo, attacked Favorinus, though it was an ἀγών conducted in the written medium and about philosophical rather than political issues.[70] And Galen himself performed in public, like a Sophist. Sometimes he was directly pitted against opponents in the way he describes *On Anatomical Procedures, On Bloodletting against the Erasistrateans in Rome,* and *On Prognosis,*[71] and once he actually refers to his performance (in dissection) at one of the medical competitions in Pergamum.[72] This casual reference to an institution obviously familiar to his audience suggests that the ἀγῶνες (*agōnes*) recorded in inscriptions from Ephesus and Smyrna were after all not isolated examples.[73] These competitions, as in the case of Galen's own initiative of speaking in public daily in his early days in Rome,[74] include the typical Sophistic challenge to treat themes given by people in the audience as well as the challenge to dissect.

But there are many examples of cases in which there is no official agonistic context, when Galen performs in a variety of venues ranging from a senatorial household to apparently open lectures, and yet the form of the ἀγών is dominant: his rivals are certainly there and waiting to challenge. In the case of his anatomical demonstrations he tells us that they sit in the front row and ask him to take on Lycus, the great anatomist, as represented by his books. In *On the Varieties of Pulses* after one "Sophist" stalks off in a rage at the dialectic that is contaminating medicine, an old man with his beard down to his chest and a scowl ("for this now is considered the dignified thing") takes on the opposing role.[75] In *On Prognosis* Alexander of Damascus opposes from the floor when Galen puts on a δεῖξις (display) of dissection for a select audience. The *Thrasybulus* gives a picture of Galen performing verbal wrestling with a trainer bold enough to suggest that Hippocrates did not know about massage in front of a less-select crowd.[76] As for disputes over pulse types, Galen describes an imaginary succession of eight people all offering their contribution, such as he has often seen in the Temple of Peace, a haunt of doctors, and at the bedside.[77] Indeed, the bedside ἀγών is something of a leitmotiv.[78]

Galen often attacks contemporary rivals through the figures from the past who are the eponymous founders of the sects. When he is in the middle of apostrophizing Archigenes, a nonagenarian follower of Archigenes rises to answer (K.8.653, 14–16). His real targets are also obviously alive in the case of the works on bloodletting against the Erasistrateans.[79] Certainly, he describes *On Bloodletting against Erasistratus* as written from a lecture given in order to attack his enemy Martianus, an Erasistratean.[80] Even when his writings are not directly based on lectures the immediacy of the polemical environment is obvious.

The element of the spectacular is very evident here. The ἀγών, after all, had its origins in athletic competition, an analogy that we have seen is present in Galen's own depiction. This is one more reminder of the different climate in which knowledge was then constructed. The ethos of objectivity that demands careful control for replicability, as in the ideal of modern experimentation, is absent. Thus, Galen advises using an animal with a loud voice for his demonstrations of the function of the recurrent laryngeal nerve, a move made in order to impress the audience.[81] True, the ἀγών sometimes would seem to fulfill modern hopes of openness to criticism, leading to progress: in *On Anatomical Procedures* (K.2.642, 3–643, 16) Galen reports that a charlatan was challenged by a prize of one thousand drachmas to prove that the arteries were empty of blood in front of a crowd of spectators and failed. But one should be cautious about accepting his portrait of the event; this is part of his polemic against the Erasistrateans about the respective roles of blood and pneuma in the arteries, to which the treatise *Whether There Is Naturally Blood in the Arteries* is dedicated. Galen's criticism of Erasistratus' theory that the arteries were filled with pneuma starts with the observation that, when an artery is punctured, it appears to contain blood. Erasistratus' answer seems to have been that, since the pneuma escapes on the puncturing, the vacuum must be filled and the only available source is the supply of blood from the veins. There was, then, no experiment that would solve this argument.[82]

It seems from some interesting comments made by Dio in one instance that, while some of the audience expressed cynicism at doctors' public displays, most did not.[83] Once more, as long as there is no challenge, there should be no shame in impressing by personal ability rather than by cultivating the audience's potential for replication. Of course, as far as the doctors were concerned, there was risk of objection that Galen was only a λογίατρος (doctor of words), but this showmanship was an essential strategy for establishing himself with his potential elite clientele. Galen observes that, when he returned to Rome at the age of forty, he swore to give no more public disputations, because such behavior only aroused enmity. But he lets slip the real reason why he could afford to do this: he had already achieved more success than he had hoped.[84] And even if he kept his promise this was simply because he turned his writings into the primary arena for his polemic.

Tradition and Originality

Commentators looking for strong commitment to original research in Galen will find grist for their mill in statements about the need to verify on the basis of one's own experience rather than just relying on what people have said.[85] Galen claims that Hippocrates is followed in anatomy precisely because research has borne him out; one should respect past authorities without blind adherence to their doctrines, he says of other sects.[86] In *The Best Doctor Is a Philosopher* the vision is of progressively building on tradition with new research. But the ideal is interestingly different from modern ideals of scientific progress, for which the achievements of the past pale increasingly with the unfolding vision of a glorious future; it is, rather, the case that scientific knowledge is seen as almost complete, and only a few problems remain to be solved.[87] Sometimes the view is even more retrogressive: in the *Elements According to Hippocrates* Galen actually claims that he does not know of anyone who has taken up the medicine of the ancients and perfected it—in fact, they have removed much that was correct.[88] Lloyd (1991, 399) has remarked on the need to avoid taking the stated reliance on tradition at face value, "exaggerat[ing] the extent to which it was in thrall to the past and correspondingly . . . underestimat[ing] its . . . originality." But what is first of all interesting is the rhetoric of dependence on tradition, whatever the other possible interpretations of the situation. The ideology in Galen is most often that of rediscovery of lost knowledge, or addition to what is essentially right, even where this seems quite difficult to sustain, as we shall see with the pulses.

The agonistic context and the necessity of a morally justifying self-presentation are the key factors to be borne in mind in considering the question of tradition and originality. The ἀγών (agōn) demanded that the speaker or writer differentiate himself from his opponents past and present, while the ἦθος (*ēthos*) entailed a degree of modesty and piety toward predecessors. As the poets presented the proper attitude to a patron in satire, so Galen exhibited a proper respect for Hippocrates, his chosen ideal doctor, and attacked others for their impiety. He accuses other medical writers of being motivated by ambition (φιλοτιμία), contentiousness (φιλονεικία/φιλονικία), and arrogance (ὕβρις) in abandoning or ignoring the writings of Hippocrates, the physicians from Cos, or the ancients.[89] Indeed, this Galenic self-presentation seems typical enough: other doctors chose different eponymous heroes for their sects, however much their readings of the heroes' work might differ.[90] The Methodists seem exceptional in their critical attitude even to forerunners in their own sect.[91]

Besides, tradition, at least in this period, if not normally in earlier medical writings, was an important source of legitimation of knowledge in an atmosphere of doubt.[92] As astrologers had to appeal to the centuries of observations by selected "Egyptians" such as Petosiris and Nechepso, so Galen gained credibility by appealing to the ancients' writings and observations before him. And, as with the astrologers, access to the earlier texts was channeled through the heir apparent.

W. D. Smith has drawn attention to the way in which Galen monopolizes the role of Hippocrates' interpreter.[93] People did need commentary to understand much of the rather cryptic material in the corpus; what were they to make of statements like the following: "Evacuate whatever must be evacuated in the direction towards which it tends, through the places from which it must be evacuated"? Galen interprets this mysterious comment: "he instructed us that we must treat superfluities which tend towards the skin by sweating."[94] Yet the relationship between Galen and Hippocrates was a symbiotic relationship, as with the relationship of orator to audience. Galen was ultimately to set up Hippocrates securely in the crowning position in the medical pantheon by his own achievements, though in his own time it was very much a re-creation in his own image that he established.

Thus, Galen appeals to Hippocrates as an earlier authority in the case of prognosis.[95] At the beginning, after discussing the doubts of many of the laity who ask the man venturing the prediction and his medical colleagues whether this sort of thing was known to earlier authorities or whether it was the personal discovery of the forecaster, he claims that the forecaster amid all this hostility dare not say that the subject was expounded by many of his predecessors and especially by Hippocrates, "our guide to all that is good." He clearly regards this as a clinching argument in favor of the practice.

Again, in the case in which he predicted a flow of blood from the right nostril, he responds to a query by showing that he learned the whole theory from the pronouncements of Hippocrates.[96] He tells Peitholaus, the imperial chamberlain, that he has written three treatises, *On the Varieties of Fever, On Critical Days,* and *On Crises,* to show that the theory by which one might predict the future course of an illness had been laid down by Hippocrates.

Smith (1979, 106) observes that Galen reduced the problem of sorting out his real technical and intellectual antecedents by elevating Hippocrates in this way and making his opponents enemies of the glorious founder of the art. One can see how this works in the writings on pulses. Clearly, as Wellmann (1895, 171ff.) shows, Galen owed much to the classification of pulses of Archigenes, the pupil of Agathinus the "Pneumatist," usually associated with the foundation of the "Eclectic" sect in the time of Trajan.[97] Indeed, Archigenes seems to be the main source of most of the treatises on pulses that remain to us apart from Galen's. But, though Galen acknowledges Archigenes as one of the best practitioners of the art of pulse interpretation (in a favorable moment in a less-technical work),[98] he gives Hippocrates more overt credit, as founder of the art.[99] Galen does face the problem of fairly minimal evidence in the corpus to support this claim.[100] The most detailed descriptions of a pulse are one ascribed to the carpenter Zoilus, which was "trembling and obscure," and the reference in *The Diseases of Women* to "pulses quivering, faint and failing against the hand." He was not ignorant of the art, concludes Galen, but he did not work it out fully or develop the terminology.[101] But Galen works harder to distinguish himself from Archigenes, attacking him for inept διαίρεσις (diaeresis) and taking the classificatory distinctions to even greater lengths.

This was clearly not an infrequent tactic. In *Therapeutic Method* he continually attacks Thessalus for his failures in logical distinction. The Methodist was a more obvious target on grounds of being too simplistic, as in Galen's depiction he offers to teach the art in six months.[102] It is against the background of such subversive claims in particular, as Deichgräber realized, that Galen was led to emphasize the length of time needed to learn prognosis through the pulse. Again, in *Hygiene,* Galen responds to the threat of competition from athletic trainers claiming conservation of health as their province by attacking them for their failures in diaeresis. The trainers actually turn out to have a remarkably complex system of classifying different sorts of massages and fatigues (κόποι), for instance, and Galen's system ends up no less complicated, at points more so.[103]

Archigenes, however, usually associated with the Pneumatists and their claims to exhaustiveness of classification, is even less easy to accuse of being too simplistic. But Galen attacks him more than his simpler predecessor, Herophilus of Alexandria, and accuses him of wasting people's time by his useless divisions. Nevertheless, as we shall see, he can only respond with greater elaboration for the most part, in a claim to greater precision. He even sets the varieties out in tables to explain them. We also find tables in the astrologers, setting out the terms, significant degrees, or the number of zodiac signs between each sign (used to establish whether transited planets activate climacterics), for instance.[104] Presentation by means of tables was obviously a persuasive technique and one that seems related to the headings and subheadings of rhetorical treatises. Quantification is another, though it does not appear to have quite the same cachet as it does today. As far as pulses are concerned, use of numbers is limited to the numbered tables and to ratios in rhythm. Galen chooses to follow neither the work of Marcellinus in using a clepsydra, a water clock, to measure the pulse nor Herophilus' classification of rhythms according to musical (metrical) theory.[105]

The Pulses

The use of the pulse in diagnosis goes back much further than Praxagoras of Cos (ca. 340 B.C.), the first Greek given credit. The Egyptian Papyrus Ebers of ca. 1550 B.C. describes feeling the pulse to measure the heart as "the beginning of the physician's secret." As Shigehisa Kuriyama (1987) comments: "It was the key to that knowledge which made the physicians and Sachmet priests a class of elite initiates." The description is, in fact, much older; it can be found in the Edwin Smith Surgical Papyrus, which is probably from the period of the first two Dynasties (3200–2700 B.C.).[106] For Galen, too, it was the art that he burned to master from his boyhood, as soon as he came into contact with physicians (K.8.770, 15–17). And his stories of his astonishing prognoses give the impression that others were similarly keen to know it. Marcellinus begins his treatise on pulses with the assertion that there is no layman who has not tried taking the pulse.[107]

The Greek story really begins with Herophilus of Alexandria (ca. 300 B.C.),[108] who probably wrote the first treatise devoted entirely to the pulse. Abandoning any association with a pathological state (classification under the general heading of palpitation), he sought to establish all the characteristics of pulses that could arise in any disease at any stage. Though his classifications according to metrical theory were not universally followed, his general format set out the terms of the debate that evolved after him. Kuriyama argues that it makes sense that it should have been the "Father of Anatomy" who began the systematic study of the pulse, since it was the new anatomical conception of the body that transformed the pulse from a vague, peripheral phenomenon of casual note to a vital sign at the heart of somatic consciousness.

What did the pulse mean for them exactly? The question of definition was early a subject for debate. Since Herophilus, at least, the motions of the arteries had been associated with those of the heart, though a variety of mechanisms of connection were attributed by his successors. Yet by no means would all of those that followed even acknowledge that connection, as the case of Chrysermus makes clear. Almost every Herophilean tried to improve not only on Herophilus' definition but also on those of his immediate predecessors (von Staden 1982). There were many different ideas about the active agents and parts of the process. Even the simpler handbooks, such as the *Medical Definitions* and Marcellinus' *On Pulses,* set out a number of definitions without making any attempt to choose between them. For Galen the pulse was

> that peculiar action (ἐνέργειαν ἰδίαν) firstly of the heart, secondly of the arteries, which are moved in expansion (diastole) and contraction (systole), by which a balance of the innate heat is maintained and animal (ψυχικόν) spirit generated in the brain. (*On the Varieties of Pulses* 4.2, K.8.714, 13–18)

To schematize drastically, this is within a model according to which the blood receives the natural spirits (πνεῦμα φυσικόν) from the liver (a very shadowy part of the model), vital spirits (πνεῦμα ζωτικόν) in the left ventricle after passing invisible pores in the intraventricular septum, and finally is impregnated with psychic spirits (πνεῦμα ψυχικόν) from the brain. The arteries must be seen as analogous to bellows, drawing in the air at diastole to cool the "innate heat" and to generate pneuma and arterial blood and expelling the air with the waste products of "combustion" at the systole. The causes of differences in pulses are, first, physiological need (increase in bodily expenditure of the psychic spirit), second, the amount of pulsative power (the vital spirit), and, third, the state of the organs of pulsation, the heart and arteries. Thus, subtle variations in the details of speed, size, and frequency were argued to mirror precisely the condition of the innate heat and the body's residues.[109]

There was clearly a well-established tradition of sphygmological debate by the time of Galen, as appears not only in his own voluminous discussions.[110] We also have preserved in the Galenic corpus two works including pulse lore, which appear to precede Galen: the *Medical Definitions* and *On Pulses for Antonius.*[111] The former records several definitions of the pulse, reflecting the variety of positions in the debate. The latter uses terminology reminiscent of divination: the pulse is "the truthful messenger of things hidden in the body and a foreteller of things imperceptible and a proof of things unclear, in harmonic motion and prophetic beat foretelling an unseen condition."[112] In addition, we have Marcellinus' *On Pulses,* which is similarly enthusiastic about using the pulse to see the future, seeing "further than Lynceus' eyes" (21–22). We also have a work on pulses attributed to Rufus of Ephesus, certainly from under the empire, and Pseudo-Soranus' *On Pulses.*[113] So we do not have to rely entirely on Galen's presentation of the disagreements. As von Staden (1982) comments in discussion of the Herophileans, the endless debate was not merely fratricidal eristic or sophistic quibbling but also a reaffirmation of the value and relevance of theoretical investigations in the face of skepticism. For the Empirics rejected the use of the pulse for prognosis, as being part of theoretical and speculative medicine and hence irrelevant to medical practice. Thus, as in the case of astrology, we have to see the agonistic debates as a response to skepticism, as if the elaborateness of the structure would somehow compensate for the shakiness of the foundations.

Galen accords the pulse in prognosis a leading role, as the clearest sign of vital force in the body.[114] There are more than a thousand pages in Kühn's edition devoted to the explication of this part of the medical art. In Galen's *On His Own Books,* in the fifth section on prognosis, after three books on critical days and three on crises, he lists four books on the differences in pulses, four on discernment of pulses,[115] four on the causes of pulsation, and four on prognosis through the pulse. There is also one on the use of pulses for beginners and, finally, a synopsis of the first sixteen books, which was to become one of the Galenic canon of sixteen books in the Middle Ages. In addition, he devoted eight books to a commentary on Archigenes' *On Pulses,* which has not survived. Most of these books seem to have been written around the 170s.

His work on pulses is interesting because it exhibits most clearly the way he adopts similar strategies to the "scientific" diviners of the future, the astrologers I have examined in chapter 1, to persuade his audience that he is able to know the future, that he has the key to πρόγνωσις (prognosis, foreknowledge). Modern scholars have, I believe, been misled in their attempts to understand Galen's enterprise by the imposition of an inappropriate model of science. C. R. S. Harris, for instance, is mainly interested in why Galen "failed to discover the circulation of the blood." Thus, he becomes irritated by "Galen at his pettifogging worst" in the books on the pulses (1973, 253). Vivian Nutton, on the other hand, is more sympathetic to Galen and, thus, tries to find justifications for the endless logic chopping. But, despite Nutton's best efforts to defend him from the charge of pettifogging, it is quite clear, even on a quick reading of a detailed text like *On the Varieties of Pulse,* that Galen's reaction to the work of Archigenes, far from "avoiding his over-refinements" (1979, 229), is to elaborate further. The relation of this elaboration to teaching is also more complex than Nutton allows in the following comment: "In his writings on pulses he set out his doctrines and methods at greater length than a modern physician would do, in order that his readers might derive the greatest benefit and instruction from his knowledge and appreciation of changes in the pulses and their significance" (1979, 229).

Nutton shares with Harris the model of what Galen should be doing in his pulse treatises. It is, of course, related to the model Galen offers of himself. Temkin also takes Galen's rhetorical justifications at face value and talks of his "philanthropy" in relation to a passage in *On Discernment of the Pulses* in which Galen claims that he has put his findings in writing in order that posterity should spend less time and trouble.[116] But these rhetorical claims should, first of all, be set against remarks elsewhere in the treatises that are less sanguine about his achievements and, second, against the context of the arenas in which the treatises are evolved. The situation as far as communicating his discoveries goes is not so straightforward, as Galen must acknowledge in the case of pulses: he compares the practical training required by pulse readers in touch, and by sculptors and painters in vision, by wine blenders and cooks in taste, perfume blenders in smelling, and musicians in hearing (K.8.773, 12ff.; cf. 768, 15ff.). There is a problem with communicating the data of touch perception in a λόγος" (in words). Thus, in *On the Varieties of the Pulses* he admits that he knows that these books will be useless to practically everybody, except those who are especially gifted, and, in *On Discernment of the Pulses,* that, since most are only in it for money or fame, he will address himself to the "one lover of truth, for either such a man is to be found now or will appear eventually."[117] While claiming it is possible to make *many* forms understandable, this does not work for all (cf. Deichgräber 1956, 26), and in these cases one must allow him his enthusiasm for research, he says. The problems of perception are serious: in cases in which the pulse is small and weak some physicians say they can at moments perceive the pulse, others that they cannot do so at all, and the same doctor will make contradictory statements after several applications to the same artery. Therefore, it is plain that in these cases some part of the artery escapes the touch. Even a physician of the finest natural constitution, who lays his hand on the artery with the most perfect technique and has the most perfect and thorough practice, would not feel the whole of the diastole. Galen himself cannot claim to do so, even where the artery has no tissues lying above it, let alone one with fat, membranes, or skin, which sometimes form a layer thicker than the artery itself.[118] Already the airy assurances in *On Prognosis* that his pulse treatises have all the answers[119] seem harder to take at face value. And this is only the beginning.

The style of teaching as actually practiced, as with the astrologers, must have been akin to a frustrating process of hierarchical initiations, which successively invalidate the previous stages. In his book specially written for beginners he will frequently comment that further complications such as the perception of the systole must be left to a later stage. And we know something of the feeling of frustration from later readers of Galen's work. Joannes Struthius in the sixteenth century speaks of "Galen's inextricable books on the pulse, which no reader of the Latin text would understand even if he worked on them till he went mad."[120] The one thing most important for the student to learn is that the master has the key to all further knowledge. Again, as with astrology, one cannot pilot by the book, without a teacher, as Galen acknowledges elsewhere,[121] though he conveniently forgets this whenever he recommends one of his own writings. There is a constant tension between the desire to communicate enough for the initiate to feel he has learned something and the effort to insure there is always more to learn. The emphasis on attacking opponents on detail serves to distract from the underlying problems, as in the case of astrology and physiognomics. Attack is the best form of defense. Like Polemo, Galen does once refer to the ignorant fools who deny the truth of his distinctions, in his work *On Pulses for Beginners.*[122]

Galen claims it would take all one's life to categorize the pulses, even that one could go on indefinitely.[123] This apparently endless subdivision takes off from its causal base with a momentum of its own, to the extent that his claim to *use* these distinctions for his diagnosis becomes problematized, in the same way as for astrologers.

Archigenes is the main focus of his criticism. He seems to be the most important rival. The pseudo-Galenic *On Pulses to Antonius* and Marcellinus' *On Pulses* is clearly based on his primary classifications, as indeed is Galen's own *On Pulses for Beginners.*[124] Galen in fact wrote a separate commentary on this predecessor's work on pulses, which is no longer extant, in addition to his lengthy comments in the second and third books of *On the Varieties of Pulses.*[125] I want to consider, first, what the criticisms are and, second, how Galen actually develops his predecessor's classifications. There are naturally problems with trying to reconstruct what Archigenes said, since none of his works has survived except in quotation and in doxographical excerpts. It may well be that Wellmann's effort to derive such a reconstruction mainly from Galen is overoptimistic, but the pseudo-Galenic "Pneumatist" treatises also provide clues. We can certainly get an idea of what Galen's criticisms are, so long as we exercise a certain caution about his initial claims.

I concentrate on the work *On the Varieties of the Pulses* here, since Galen suggests that the categories are the first thing that must be learned. He claims at the beginning of the first book that he is not interested in sophistical disputes about names: as far as he is concerned one could call a σφοδρός (strong) pulse Dion or Theon! (K.8.496, 15–19). Rather, he is concerned with the phenomena themselves (4–7), which lead to diagnosis and prognosis for the sick. But this turns out to be no more than a *captatio benevolentiae,* and his claims to value brevity in this area become more and more hollow from the second book onward. Naturally, he blames the Sophists' quarrelsome nature for this (493, 7–494, 2). Finally, his crucial difference with previous writers on the pulses, as represented by Archigenes and Agathinus, emerges as being over this very topic—the correctness and precision of the names: πῇ τοίνυν αὐτῶν διαφέρομεν; ὅτι κυριωτέροις ἡμεῖς χρώμεθα τοῖς ονόμασιν (how do I differ from them: in that I use names more proper to them [594, 2–3]). We all say that there are γένη (genera) according to the differences between pulses, says Galen (though there are no lack of arguments about which are genera and which are species and the precise place of each diffence in the logical hierarchy), but I use the proper names, referring to size as the quantity of distension, not as a quality (593, 17–594, 7). The correct term is not *bigness,* which is as inappropriate as describing the shades from black to white as differences in whiteness (8–10). He criticizes the mode of division as inept, as one of pseudodialecticians (629, 13–30, 17), people who announce that they will explain the designs of the names, beginning a dialectical presentation, but do not explain, only laying down the laws like Moses or Christ (578, 11ff.). We shall see that most of his criticisms involve an accusation of failure to differentiate logically.[126]

Let us examine a particular case in which he is concerned to show the correct method of collection and division. Archigenes, because he is untrained in logic, fails to describe logically separable differences, just because in reality they are never found on their own,[127] argues Galen, in language reminiscent of Aristotle. If someone says that they cannot conceive of line or surface without a solid body (612, 17–13, 2), that does not destroy geometry. Archigenes, rather than neatly dividing, badly butchered the categories (κακῶς δε ὁ 'Αρχιγένης οἷον ἐσπάραξεν αὐτό),[128] saying there were only six pairs, ignoring the other twenty-one (entailed logically [615, 18–616, 1]). Galen carefully sets out a table of nine pairs, explaining how another two similar tables would be generated. Galen accuses Archigenes of falling into contradiction by not working out all the permutations but, rather, by singling out particular combinations (606, 11–14). The expansion Galen is making here does not appear to be based on empirical findings, if indeed one can easily speak of such a thing in pulse perception, so much as on a logical development. Certainly, he does not allow for the possibility that Archigenes' classifications may have been logically deficient precisely because they were based on the limits of his empirical findings. In *On Prognosis through the Pulse* (2.3, K.9.278, 7–10) Galen comments that Herophilus treated pulse rhythms in the manner of one describing observation and experiment rather than of one expounding logical method. It is remarks with this kind of anti-empirical emphasis that lead the frustrated Harris to observe that most of Galen's criticisms seem to depend on logical technicalities rather than on physiology. But there are severe problems with the empirical enterprise here; even Galen admits that there are problems in perception in the case of these first twenty-seven differences. As mentioned above, they may be confused by the condition of the tissues surrounding the artery.

Now to examine how the frameworks of division compare. At K.8.576, 17–577, 2, Galen attributes eight modes of division to Archigenes, according to: "μέγεθος, σφοδρότης, τάχος, πυκνότης, πληρότης, τάξις, ὁμαλότης, ῥυθμός" (size, strength, speed, frequency, fullness, order, equality, rhythm). These are the ἁπλαί ποιότητες, or "main types." Herophilus had six of them, and Archigenes (or perhaps Agathinus, as Wellmann suggests [1895, 172]) added two, fullness and frequency. Archigenes refers to these eight as being in common use (διηχημέναι), and we do find them in Marcellinus. Certainly, there is general agreement on most of the categories but not on the complete list. In this section Galen is criticizing him for his notion of the full pulse: if this covers three meanings (the quality of the body of the artery, what is inside, and the pneuma within), then there are really ten divisions (577, 2–8). Galen immediately after this passage criticizes him for leaving the category of "hardness" out of account in this list, when in a later list he begins with size, strength, fullness, and hardness.[129] Galen appears to cut down drastically on the number of categories, at the beginning. In addition to the first category of size, Galen takes on board initially categories of speed (the time of movement or rest), size, τόνος, hardness (of coats), fullness, and equality (the ratio of the time of diastole to that of systole), saying that these are the only differences within one pulse (501, 2–502, 3). But, as with astrologers, it turns out that this is only the first formulation. At 502, 3–6, we learn that there are two other συστηματικαί differences, differences observable over more than one beat (ὁμαλότης and τάξις [equality and order]). Eventually, he seems to end up with nine categories, or γένη, remarkably similarly to Archigenes'.[130] Even in the book written for beginners (in which logic chopping is kept to a minimum) Galen differentiates between the moderate, the big, the long, the broad, the high, the strong, the soft, the quick, the frequent, the equal, and the ordered pulses and their opposites as well as discussing particular composite unequal pulses (K.8.455, 1–61, 17), though he refuses to discuss fullness or rhythm, referring them to this fuller version, as the matter is obscure enough already.[131] He does not offer beginners the twenty-seven differences in size, though in *On the Varieties of Pulses* (600, 9–14) he says they should know them.

But, if we go back to the first category of size, we find that Galen does not limit himself to the thirteen subdivisions apparently espoused by Archigenes,[132] let alone the twenty-seven different types he himself finds in three dimensions. In *On the Varieties of the Pulses* we find first that we must double up with a second set of permutations, taking into account the size of the systole (contraction) as well as the diastole (distension) (602, 7–9). Though we know that Archigenes was one of those who believed in the perceptibility of the systole, Galen certainly does not let us know if this involved the kind of logical extension of differences in which Galen indulged. But, before considering how one beat of the pulse is divided up, we should note Galen's extra refinements. Regretting that it is impossible to quantify exactly (in feet or cubits!) the amount of distension, he improves on the threefold division just used for the table of twenty-seven differences in size by making a sixfold differentiation:[133] First, you have the maximum size and the moderate at two extremes and the big size in the middle, and then you add two, first, between the maximum and the big and, second, between the big and the moderate. At 616–17 he remarks that it is even better to explain differences rather than give them names because it teaches more and, at 618, 3–5, suggests that such differentiations could be made within other categories, as well as the big pulse.

> καὶ γὰρ ἐπὶ θερμοῦ καὶ ψυχροῦ καὶ ξηροῦ καὶ ὑγροῦ καὶ πάντων ἁπλῶς τὴν κατὰ τὴν τέχνην τὸ διαιρεῖν ἐπὶ σμικρότητα δύνασθαι καὶ ταῖς κατ' ὀλίγον ὑπεροχαῖς πειρᾶσθαι παρακολουθεῖν ἀνδρός ἐστιν ἄλλως τε συνετοῦ καὶ προσέτι γεγυμνασμένου κατὰ τὰ τε ἔργα καὶ περὶ παντὸς ποιουμένου το στοχαστικὸν τῆς τέχνης εἰς στενὸν ὡς ἔνι μάλιστα συγκλείειν. οὐ μὴν ἔν γε ταῖς ἀρχαῖς τῆς διδασκαλίας τμητέον οὕτως. τοῖς μὲν γὰρ ἀσυνέτοις τῶν μανθανόντων ταραχὴν οὐκ ὀλίγην παρέξει, τοῖς δὲ συνετοῖς εἷς ἐκ τῶν εἰρημένων ἐπινοηθήσεται.
>
> And in the case of hot, cold, dry and wet, and in fact everything in the art, the ability to subdivide into the smallest categories and an effort to trace accurately even the smallest deviation are marks both of a generally intelligent man, and of a man trained in practice and one who makes great efforts to confine the conjectural part of the art as narrowly as possible. Division of this kind should not be made at the beginning of the teaching, for it causes great confusion for the unintelligent learners, while even the intelligent understand only one of those [distinctions] spoken of. (618, 14–619, 5)

Here is the ultimate approval for minute distinctions, which he says he left until this book. Notably, he exempts beginners from this subtlety. But this is not the end of subdivision. He says that the differences of degree are really infinite (comparing it to the number of notes the voice could sing) but that beginners could start with just the two either side of the moderate (619, 5–520, 16). With time and practice beginners will divide twice, then perhaps three times, and four times. The better you train, the smaller the differences you recognize. Here are the stages of initiation with which we are familiar.

There is in fact a fourfold division of one beat of the Galenic pulse, when the two rest periods (first, that between diastole and systole and, second, that after the systole and before the diastole of the next beat) are included. As before, he insists that the lengths of these four intervals are both perceptible and useful to the physician (514, 1–4). It is this view that makes his original categories of speed and frequency insufficient. So we get the συστηματικαί differences (over more than one beat). The differences in equality are in the mutual proportions in a single beat and those in order and rhythm over a longer period. But, again, the original twofold division in these categories is far too simple. Immediately, four divisions according to age are established, and so it continues. The category discussed in chapter 14 (528–29) may suffice to show the level to which the subdivision has proceeded. Among the "non-intermittent in distention and unequal but perpetual in motion," there are six types. Chapter 17 offers *seventy-eight* divisions in one category, in which four fingers are used to take the pulse (543, 7)! (The number of divisions is smaller when fewer fingers are used.)

Even Galen sometimes gets lost in his maze. There were various vividly named pulses, like the "anting," the "worming," the "wave-like," the "mouse-tailed," and the "tapering," which were obviously originally separate from the γένη, or "main categorizations," and aroused such interest because of their memorable nature and thus relative ease of perceptibility, despite their marginality in clinical practice.[134] (It seems that Herophilus only came across the "gazelling" pulse once, in a eunuch.)[135] It is no wonder that Galen had problems trying to fit them into his logical program. He launches into Archigenes on the subject of the "double-hammer" pulse, one of this type, for inadequate treatment of its origins and consequences. Yet in his own work it appears under two categories, and thus different causes get attributed. First, it is attributed to a defect in the arteries and then to a defect in the heart as well.[136] As Harris comments (1973, 421), the originally picturesque description of Archigenes loses its sharpness under the haze of Galen's logical distinctions.

It is not surprising that he falls back on his own authority rather than attempting to explain when challenged by doctors, in a case in which he predicts a flux of the stomach. "No one takes a single fleece of wool to the fuller," he says, meaning that they could not possibly understand this, when they did not understand "the shortest things." When asked again about how he predicted a nosebleed and tumors, he only muttered to himself words from a comic poet about not being able to strengthen bent wood or transplant old trees (656, 1–17).

One could excuse this as a temporary and unusual failure of the will to teach, in the face of particularly intransigent opponents. But the problem is that so few measure up to the standard. As we have seen, Galen needs a reader of exceptional qualities, as he goes on to say here (657, 7–8): φύσει θαυμαστῇ καὶ διδασκαλίᾳ καὶ μελέτῃ (of remarkable natural ability, teaching, and training). In fact, he admits, the reader may not exist at all, but at least Galen will be playing a learned game and preparing himself for the forgetfulness of old age, as Plato says. This is in stark contrast to his earlier references to these "technical" treatises as the source of instruction.[137] Why, then, does he make this claim? It was obviously one important way to persuade people of the correctness of one's method. Aristotle presumably articulated a general ideal of ancient intellectual activity when he said that the sign of knowledge or ignorance is the ability to teach (*Metaphysics* 1.1.981b, 10–11).

Yet even the references to other books for instruction on specific points here may turn out to be as unhelpful as a route to usable knowledge as Holmes's references to his monographs for Watson's edification, such as that on the varieties of human ears in the "Anthropological Journal." It is in the context of the young man whose pulse misses a beat naturally that Galen laments the mistakes made even by reputable doctors in differentiating pulses and declares that he wrote his books on pulses to remedy this—that they are of great practical value. The doctors asked Galen how he knew that this was not a sign of illness, and he in typical fashion recalled Isocrates' remark to one of his students: "I should like you to be able to learn in one day all you ask, my child, but I would then condemn myself for ignorance because I have studied it for many, many years" (*On Prognosis* p. 140, 28–142, 3 = K.14.670).

"You will be aware of the natural differences between pulses if you read this book," Galen continues, presumably brandishing one. Nutton here excises the reference to the first book of *On Discernment of the Pulse* on textual grounds. It was, however, clearly one of the books on pulses that he offered for their instruction. Yet none of these offered anything but pathological grounds for such a pulse; in other words, they replicated the same mistake the doctors were making.[138] Only later in his *Commentary on the Prognostics* does he report the view that an intermittent pulse is not fatal—and there can only refer to this passage itself as proof![139] His vaunted concern to communicate usable knowledge obviously takes second place to his concern to present himself as master of that knowledge here.

One can see that it is important for his claim to knowledge that he should affirm a relationship between prognosis and treatment and that he should establish a relationship involving causation. This is certainly far better developed than in the case of astrologers, and it is, significantly, Galen himself who establishes a causal basis for physiognomics in humoral physiology (Evans 1941). The causal bases, however, are lost to sight in his work on differentiating pulses. Though there are other extremely complex works, such as *On the Causes of the Pulse, On the Use of the Pulse,* and *On Prognosis through the Pulse,* it seems impossible to connect them beyond a certain stage. The variations are schematic, developed according to a logic that has no empirical basis. One suspects that most prognoses were justified in the relatively simple manner in which he explained himself to Eudemus, when, after taking his pulse, he pronounced:

> "Nothing but good. . . . Tonight you will be completely free of the whole morbid condition, and the resolution of all supervening and future symptoms will follow."
>
> I also said that this was just revealed to me through his pulse-beats by the nature (φύσις) which governed his body, which was then aroused and active in expelling from the body all that was noxious in his bodily humors. "What do you mean by 'this has been shown by nature'—for surely it did not tell you so by speaking—answer me that. For you are well aware that I follow your argument better than all those wretched doctors."
>
> "Because it has caused an upward movement of the arteries even more than a lateral expansion," I said, "which it always does when it is trying to discharge an irritant from the body." (*On Prognosis* p. 86, 5–19 = K.14.617)

He goes on to explain from other signs that there will probably be a wholesale evacuation from the lower belly. Eudemus is quite satisfied: "You have made a truly logical exposition of how you reached this prognosis," he says. Further questioning would no doubt have revealed more and more complex answers.

In summary of what I have been claiming about the development of Galen's pulse doctrine, I should say that, while there is certainly the possibility of an extremely complex empirical differentiation of pulses and our ideas of the potential of touch perception are no doubt very limited, Galen's divisions cannot but appear absurd to the student working within the paradigm of the modern scientific method. Deichgräber's reference to the subtlety of differentiation possible with the aid of modern instruments cannot in any sense explain Galen's results. Trying to map his distinctions onto an electrocardiogram (or a kymograph, as Harris [1973] suggests) would be an enterprise misconceived. Galen early leaves the basis of perception by touch, which he often admits is problematic, for schematic elaboration. Differentiations must be made somewhat arbitrarily against the background of infinite possibilities, as a temporary measure (K.8.619, 11–16), with the number of possible differences perceptible imagined to increase in stages. Galen certainly insists on ἀκρίβεια, but it is evidently a flexible concept.[140] And the schematic nature of this elaboration is understandable when its genesis is set in the two contexts of the apprenticeship and the ἀγών.

It is also illuminating to set beside Greek pulse lore in general the Chinese art of *qie mo,* as Kuriyama (1987) has done. The ethnocentric value judgments made on this art by Western physicians and historians of science[141] resulted from a fundamental misapprehension: they assumed that the two could be seen as variant forms of pulse diagnosis, as different interpretations of a common reality. But, as Kuriyama argues, there is no common reality: the pulse is not given in nature, common to all cultures, but is, instead, a cultural artifact, forged in historical circumstances. The *mo* to which Chinese physicians sensitized themselves required techniques and beliefs incompatible with the Greek vision of the pulsating artery. And the two presuppose different conceptions of how words relate to the experiences of the touch. While the Greeks relied on the capacity of the mind to conceive images, *qi,* "like minds," could not be seen. Instead, its movements had to be apprehended by the response of an uncluttered mind; its directions of flow had to be sensed. Obviously, there is more than just another model of the body involved here.

The Urines

The urine seems to have been considered the secondary sign to the pulse in diagnosis, though its use was confined to acute diseases (*On Crises* [*Cris.*] p. 88, 8–10 = K.9.579). It was firmly tied to a causal base and to use in prognosis. It was one of three forms of excretions used to ascertain whether or not proper coction had taken place, indicating whether healing was at hand (p. 85, 15ff. = K.9.575ff.). In *Therapeutics to Glaucon* (K.11.24, 6–8) Galen claims urines teach all the stages of the disease and, at the beginning, even the type of fever. The feces are a sign of the state of the lower part of the stomach, the sputum of the respiratory parts, and the urine of the venous parts (*Cris.* p. 85, 15ff. = K.9.575ff.), though, in the case of fevers, even where stomach or respiratory problems are involved, the urine is a sign (p. 88, 10–14 = K.9.580). In addition, they offer signs of the parts from which they are excreted; thus, the urine tells us about the kidneys and ureters, the bladder, and the penis (especially in the case of bad sedimentary urines, those that are acrid, fetid, and bilious) (pp. 85, 18–86, 7 = K.9.576–77; *Commentary on Hippocrates's Prognostics* [*Progn.*] 37, pp. 289, 15–290, 17 = K.18B.163–64). This was the only external caveat to be taken into account.

The best urine is the most natural, of a color verging on ξανθός or πυρρός [yellow or red] (*Progn.* pp. 279, 19–281 = K.18B.146–47; *Cris.* p. 97, 18–21 = K.9.595), and, if it has a sediment, it should be white, smooth, and even and should remain after appearing immediately (*Progn.* p. 281, 6–11 = K.18B.148; *Cris.* p. 101, 13–16 = K.9.601): the sign of coction. It should be of moderate consistency, not too watery, without signs of a particular humor (p. 99, 21–23 = K.9.598). If it veers between purity and sediment, it is only semiconcocted (*Progn.* pp. 280, 22–281, 4 = K.18B.147–8; *Cris.* p. 104, 11–12 = K.9.606). A little color (ξανθός or πυρρός) is also the sign of concoction (p. 99, 20–21 = K.9.598).

The amount of sediment varies with the quantity eaten and whether a leisurely or hard-working life-style is pursued. The more you eat, the more sediment is produced. The harder you work, the more bilious you are, and the more color your urine takes on (*Cris.* pp. 101, 17–102, 8 = K.9.601–2), and the less sediment there is. If the sediment is slightly πυρρός, this is not quite as good as if it is white.

Slightly less of a good sign than a sediment is a "suspension," spread continuously throughout, then come the "clouds" or ἐναιωρήματα (*ibid.* pp. 102, 17–103, 25 = K.9.604–5). White, moderately thick clouds are all right, but yellow and thin urines with them are indications of lack of coction. Black clouds are a bad sign (*Progn.* p. 284, 18–23 = K.18B.154–55). It is better if the cloud is concentrated below rather than from above (pp. 288, 21–289, 14 = K.18B.161–63). There is also a time dimension. When the cloudy state changes a little later to a sediment, this is better than its remaining constant, which implies that there is still strong turbulence (*Cris.* p. 98, 3–17 = K.9.595–96). The worst case is when a thin urine becomes cloudy. Clouds are a result of bad distribution, due to overheating of the blood.

Of the sediments there are three bad types, which suggest that the flesh is unequally melted (*Progn.* pp. 283, 1–284, 13 = K.18B.151–54; *Cris.* pp. 102, 18–103, 3 = K.9.603). The first is when it is thick like lumps of flour, when there is great liquefaction and feverish heat. The second is when it looks like metal leaves, wide and thin. This is when the superficial parts of the vessels are loosened. The third is scaly and branlike, thick and small. These are all excretions of semiconcocted humors. Smaller lumps are worse.

Thin, foamy, white urine is bad (*Progn.* p. 283, 21–25 = K.18B.152–53), as is any urine with a crust like soup left to cool (p. 288, 15–20 = K.18B.161), which indicates bad liquefaction. Then there is a list of very bad urines. Fetid, leaden, watery, and black urines come under this category (p. 286 = K.2.157). Green is on the way to black (*Cris.* p. 103, 16–19 = K.9.603), as are livid, rotten-smelling urines (*Progn.* p. 103, 4–11, K.9.603). Black urines, the result of too much heat or cold, are subdivided. It is worse when they are thick, unless they are naturally so (p. 286 = K.18B.157). It is less dangerous if only the sediment is black, even less if only the middle, and least of all if it is only a black cloud. The worst case, the μελανθέν (blackened), is a urine no one survives (*Cris.* p. 103, 12–15 = K.9.604).

It is a bad sign in a watery urine if it is also white (ibid. p. 99, 10–12, 9.598; cf. *Progn.* p. 286, 1–5 = K.18B.157). Whiteness indicates complete lack of coction and an origin in thicker, colder humor (ibid. pp. 286, 3–5 = K.18B.157). This prognosis is fairly damning if the urine shows no other bad signs; it indicates that one of the two faculties (alterative, not retentive) is weakened rather than both (*Cris.* p. 99, 3–7 = K.9.597). It is better if there is a bilious element making it slightly πυρρός, a sign of coction (*Cris.* p. 99, 20–21 = K.9.598). The worst case is "chamberpot dropsy" (ὕδερος εἰς ἀμίδα), or urine diarrhea, when the flesh melts into the urine and both faculties are weakened (ibid. pp. 98, 18–99, 3 = K.9.596–97).

There are also age differences. For the young, watery urines are the worst possible sign, while for the mature, black urines are the worst (ibid. p. 104, 15 = K.9.606; *Progn.* pp. 286, 20–287, 15 = K.18B.158–59), because they are the most unnatural in each case.

I have here rationalized and simplified somewhat the disparate comments made in *On Crises* 1.12, pp. 97, 12–105, 3 = K.9.594–607 and *Commentary on Hippocrates's Prognostics* 2, chaps. 26–37, pp. 279, 19–290, 17 = K.18B.146–63. There are a couple of comments on urines with specific reference to differentiating fevers in *Therapeutics to Glaucon* (K.11.24, 8–11: with quotidians the urine is white and thin or thick, troubled, and red [πυρρός], whereas with tertians it is only fairly πυρρός.) On the whole Galen follows Hippocrates on the urines. He adds some categories of his own. To the lumpy sediments he adds urine with small bits of flesh like hair, for instance. He adds a technical discussion on the differences between colors and the difficulty of distinguishing them (*Cris.* p. 100, 2–16 = K.9.600). He subdivides the watery urines, and, most important, he adds the causal framework. But the similarities with Hippocrates are more striking. Even the disorganization is a Hippocratic legacy.

What is striking is that this rationalization is possible at all. The basis of the organization is the same simple threefold division into good, bad, and moderate that we find in pulse doctrine (and physiognomics). He does refer to the differentiation within the genus that is possible (*Cris.* p. 97, 14–17 = K.9.594–95). But it is a relatively simple, unelaborated scheme, with no arguments about distinctions. The crucial question is why the urines are not subject to the same degree of elaboration as in these cases. I think the answer lies in the lack of a polemical context. Nowhere in the text I have examined does Galen refer to anyone but his ideal Hippocrates in dicussion of this section of prognostic signs. He has no need to distinguish himself from his predecessors by the process of further subdivision or rearrangement of the διαίρεσις. It is not essential to mystify the student of the text at every stage. Indeed, one might speculate that it is important that he should be able to grasp the use of one prognostic sign, in order that he should be encouraged to desire further initiation into the art. Of course, as with astrology and physiognomics, any simple method must be set against numerous other indications, so that there is no danger of the pupil's becoming a master of the science.

What shows that elaboration would have been possible with the urines is the ninth-century text of Theophilus, in which he begins by discussing his predecessors, whose work he claims to be completing. First came Hippocrates, who made scattered remarks here and there in his works but left his teaching unfinished. Then Galen gathered together his teachings in *On Crises* and left many things ἀδιόριστα (undivided) and unclear as regards γένη, εἴδη and διαφοράι (genera, species, and differentiae). Following him came Magnus (the famous iatrosophist who supposedly won contests by convincing audiences that his opponents were still ill), a doctor of words inexperienced in practice, who began a diaeresis, writing down the εἴδη and διαφοράι and the diagnostic and prognostic signs, but left much unfinished, so that subsequent doctors were unable to find the solution.[142] Theophilus then offers his own diaeresis, in careful order, which he sets out in groups reminiscent of Galen's pulse distinctions.[143] Here is a very neat example of agonistic development, with each successive writer adding his own more subtle distinctions. Where there was an area left for them to work on they took their chance.

Concluding Remarks

Generalization seems rash in the case of an author such as Galen; the sheer volume of his oeuvre forbids final conclusions from the dilettante. The pulses are doubtless an extreme case of classificatory zeal, and the urines are by no means free of a degree of diaeresis (one might speculate that this is due to agonistic pressures before Galen). Without further detailed work it is difficult to be certain about the precise impact of the polemical environment on the development of his theories. That what seems to us excessive subdivision is a frequent feature of his work seems hardly in doubt; such varied areas as the parts of the medical art itself[144]—massages, fatigues (κόποι),[145] and fevers—are subject to this literary dissection. In *Hygiene,* in which massages and fatigues are discussed, it is certainly in the context of one of Galen's favorite polemics, against his rivals, the athletic trainers, who cannot be allowed to control regimen in health (cf. *Thrasybulus*).

Subdivision of massages and fatigues has little practical correlate in terms of material for secondary elaboration, retrospective explanation of mistakes. This practical use, however, which I mentioned with regard to astrologers (in chap. 1), must be seen as a factor in the cases in which he subdivides diseases. The great number of variables allows the maximum flexibility, as with the astrologers. In *On Examining the Best Physicians* there is a case of such secondary elaboration. Galen reports his triumph over other doctors at the bedside of a patient with fever. At first Galen had diagnosed it as a tertian, but when the fever recurred the next day an arrogant young man laughed at him, thinking it was a phlegmatic quotidian, and the others joined in. Galen's reply was calm: "Had you consulted books, probably you would have learned that the patient might be suffering from two (combined) attacks of tertian fever, and not from one attack of quotidian fever." Galen then makes a prognosis, refusing to explain, since they would not understand, how it could be two combined attacks and what the significance of this is (8.5–7, pp. 96–97). Galen was certainly well known to later ages for the length of his writings on the subject of fevers. The satirical Byzantine novel *Timarion* made him a member of a committee of medical experts in the underworld. When a meeting of the committee was considered it emerged that Galen was on leave of absence working on a supplement to his books on fevers, likely to be even longer than the original.[146] Galen's *On the Varieties of Fevers* indeed offered a great treasury of varieties to choose from; it is a work that seems to present similarities to the pulse writings: once again he finds reason to disagree with his main source, Archigenes. Here was a field that had been the subject of heated debate from the earliest Hippocratic writings, with the potential for almost infinite variations.

In the context of the rivalry between Galen and others the master-pupil relationship is also significant. Autodidacts, like athletic trainers, or those who made medicine simple like the Methodists, were a threat. Kollesch (1973) comments on the important role of medical handbooks in an era when knowledge was rare and expensive and many wanted to practice as doctors. Nutton (1985) has shown that anyone could become a doctor, simply by claiming the role (and perhaps by declaring himself before the magistrate, if there were tax benefits). Such people would turn to simple question-and-answer books. But learned doctors such as Galen naturally would not approve of any such easy path to knowledge, and it is in this context that his technical works must be understood. They should not be used without a teacher: as he says, one cannot pilot by the book, though, as we have seen, he chooses sometimes to forget this.

There is, then, at least good evidence to suggest that the concerns that shaped the writings of the astrologers and the physiognomists had their effects on the Galenic oeuvre as well, despite the important differences in their aims. Neither astrologers nor physiognomists worried greatly about using a rhetoric of logic, and their interest in causal relationships was, to say the least, patchy. But there has been no lack of work on this image of Galen, while there has been much less on the parts of his rhetoric that sit less easily with the picture of the rational scientist and philosopher, in particular on those parts relating to religion. Here I have attempted to redress the balance. I have pulled together, in relation to prognosis, a variety of evidence showing the different models of knowledge that exist in his work and the tensions that are evident to us between them, stressing the role of a more esoteric conception of knowledge. I have focused on the way in which his work is shaped by the environment of the Second Sophistic, in his construction of his self-image and his relationship to his predecessors, and in his agonistic style in general. Even where Galen chooses not to engage in the ἀγών he provides plenty of evidence of others who do.

In this period we have a relative wealth of information on the politics of intellectual life. One receives a very strong impression of the way in which knowledge is constructed in the absence of any of the institutional buttresses that sustain the modern divisions of the academic edifice. In a world in which anyone can set up as a doctor rhetoric is all-important, and Galen offers the finest example of medical rhetoric at its most learned and, indeed, at its most forceful.

In my work on astrology I have set the intellectual politics of knowledge within the context of imperial politics at the highest level, while my framework for physiognomics is the arena of provincial politics. In the case of medicine I am concerning myself with intellectual politics alone. Prognosis seemed a good area for comparison, since it shared with the other two disciplines the claim to foretell the future from signs. Like the other two disciplines, it had to conform to the "conjectural model" of knowledge. It was also an area in which rhetoric was at its sharpest. Failure to persuade could result in disaster for the forecaster. Various cases I have mentioned serve to illustrate the equivocation and secondary elaboration this entailed for the doctor as for the astrologer.

In this chapter I have also pursued some of the arguments set out in the introduction on the sociology of science. Here the "strong program" is put into practice, in that parts of ancient medicine that seem to be most "successful" from a modern perspective are not simply hailed as an achievement inevitable at some stage of scientific development. Rather, their success in their contemporary context is seen as worthy of investigation. In the case of the pulse the discovery of its value for prognosis has been hailed as such an achievement, whereas I have argued that this is an appreciation that loses its force with its ethnocentricity. To the reader concerned with isolating the modern ideal of a scientist in Galen my work will appear as an entirely unfair attack; there are so many other areas in which one could praise his achievements from this point of view. I would argue, however, that, though it might involve a reconsideration of some of his conventional claims about his aims, this is a fairer picture, in one sense. It is, after all, an appreciation of the brilliance of his rhetoric, of which he was, in some senses, justifiably proud.

Conclusion

The limits necessarily imposed by a study of such wide range, which has the temerity to tread within the provinces of many specialists, are very evident. Many of the generalizations that emerge would need further citation of evidence to be accepted. Most heinous perhaps in this regard is the chapter on medicine, in which not only is Galen used to provide the bulk of the evidence for the medicine of the period, but his own vast work is by no means fully investigated. In the case of astrology there is arguably more excuse for my selective concentration on a few texts, when so much material remains unedited or uncertainly dated. Obviously, too, the subjects discussed remain a small proportion of the number of τέχναι (*technai*) available for study. I can only plead in extenuation the nature of my explorations as case studies.

But there are other self-imposed limits. I have avoided discussion of many possible connections between my three main disciplines in order to focus on a particular role each discipline played in knowledge politics. I have only mentioned in passing the role of astrologers and doctors as power brokers, intermediaries between the emperor and provincial cities, though here there is more evidence to be considered.[1] There is also, doubtless, more evidence such as that discussed by Dagron for the Late Empire, on the role of astrologers in local politics, where they find themselves ranged against holy men,[2] but here I limited myself on grounds of chronological focus. I did, however, broaden the chronological focus in order to summarize the story of astrology's rise and fall at the highest level, to substantiate my argument about the relationship of the art's epistemological status with political shifts.

I have not devoted sustained comment to considering how each discipline was regarded from the standpoint of the others. Here the limitations imposed by concentrating on a few texts are obvious. Yet some suggestive evidence has emerged in my discussion. The view expressed in the astrological-medical text preserved in the Galenic corpus that the most valuable part of astrology for medicine is physiognomical serves to indicate the potential links between all three τέχναι. There are links implicit in the interest in chorography between astrology and physiognomics, which may have been formalized. Futhermore, the origins of physiogomics were partly medical, in the Hippocratic corpus, and in the work of the doctor-physiognomist Loxus. So physiognomists offered ways to diagnose epilepsy and apoplexy, for instance. Sextus Empiricus, a medical man, exempts physiognomists, unlike astrologers, from his skeptical scrutiny. Galen's attitude, however, is more complicated. On the one hand he ties together the threads in Aristotle and the Hippocratic corpus in order to provide a medical framework for physiognomics and appears to endorse their basic principles, but on the other he attacks "the physiognomists" for failing to address the issue of causation. As for Galen's complex attitude to the use of astrology for medicine, it is in part the result of his shifts in relation to particular polemics but is also in part the result of a division of rational from superstitious uses that does not exactly fit with modern assumptions. There is little doubt, however, that many doctors took astrology on board, and that astrologers strayed into medicine, as is obvious from iatromathematical treatises.[3] It is notable, too, that astrologers, where they offer justificatory introductions, mention medicine among other arts, to point out that mistakes are possible and bad practitioners inevitable but that these problems do not invalidate the whole enterprise. All in all, it is difficult to generalize about interdisciplinary attitudes, for which the lack of institutionalization prevented across-the-board positions in any one discipline.

In the case studies my primary aim has been to illuminate what I have called the metaphorical link between the three forms of inquiry into nature, emphasizing what they have in common, following up on my initial supposition that they stand on an equal footing at this stage of the battle in claims for knowledge. As I explained in the introduction, I have been led, as a result of looking at recent developments in theories about knowledge, to look at these ancient *scientiae* as rhetorical, to see the practitioners as attempting to persuade their audiences that they offer knowledge. This viewpoint involves an effort to abandon our culture-bound assumptions about what counts as persuasive; ancient and modern rhetorical theory demands that the contemporary audience be seen as the essential context.

An early theme that has recurred is the role of religious discourse in acting as doxic, or common, knowledge, a basis from which rhetoric can work. Obviously, those who seek in the ancient world what is scientific in any modern sense, as has been traditional in the historiography of ancient science, will tend to regard any argument working on religious belief and practice as symptomatic of the kind of obstacles present in this era to the emergence of "good science." In the Western world, since the nineteenth century, the religious and scientific worldviews have seemed so dramatically opposed that the only way in which they can be "reconciled" is to allow them completely separate spheres of operation. Any attempt to combine the two is made in the reverse direction. Thus, certain religious groups attempt to appropriate the name, the personnel, the status, and even the methods of science (in a teleological context). In our age science has mustered consensus on its knowledge status behind it more effectively than religion. Any attempts to bring religion into mainstream science would meet with ridicule.

But the picture with regard to the ancient world is far more complex. Astrology, first of all, justifies itself as inspiring a healthy religious attitude. Second, it is in astrology that the role of initiation is especially apparent. It is perhaps not surprising that this should be the case: Hermetic and Neoplatonic ideals are found in association with astrology, and it is also probable that the hierarchical initiations of Mithraic cult are linked with astrological symbolism. At any rate, astrology offers a particularly clear example of the role of the initiation model in ancient didactic practice: stages of knowledge are clearly marked in our texts. Astrology is also, obviously, a species of divination, though it is not explicitly presented as such by the authors of the treatises, and its source of information is the divine heavenly bodies.

But is astrology, then, not a special case? In my third chapter on medicine I moved on to consider the attitude toward religion in medicine. Here is a very different case, in which practitioners have set themselves up in opposition to temple medicine and might be expected to be hostile to any involvement of religion, seeing it as a political threat. I chose to consider prognosis because of its evident similarity to the procedures of astrology and physiognomics. Do we find utter repudiation of anything smacking of divination? The answer is that we find a degree of ambivalence. Galen does complain of being "slandered" as a diviner because of his amazing prognoses. Yet he equally exploits the very powerful image of the omniscient seer on occasion and often tends to conceal his methods in order to enjoy straightforward acclaim in the same way. This duality is not surprising in view of the typical double image of the diviner, which offers a dichotomy: there are good diviners, and there are charlatans. We know that Galen takes divination, as such, seriously from his remarks about interpreters of the flight of birds and on dreams. Furthermore, there is no straightforward desire to keep medicine in secular purity. The theological framework of the *On the Usefulness of the Parts of the Body* is its justification in the same way that it is for Firmicus' *Mathesis*. Indeed, Galen talks here in terms of initiation into the mysteries of anatomy. In certain contexts, then, for certain audiences, the religious arguments are to be invoked; elsewhere the stress is on the technical. As for physiognomics, divination does not seem to be such a significant model, though Adamantius' preface, which probably preserves Polemo's, does compare physiognomics to divination explicitly.[4]

The appearance of religion, often in prooemia, is part of the construction of the ἦθος (*ēthos*) of ancient rhetorical theory and its modern development (see intro.). It is one strategy attempting to guarantee the moral status of the author to the audience. There are also other recurrent themes: authors distinguish themselves from bad practitioners of their arts, in particular those who are only in it for the money, as do Galen and Ptolemy.[5] Thus, they attempt to use the double image syndrome in their favor. They also make efforts to display their culture for their ἦθος; knowledge of philosophy is paraded, whether it be Aristotelianism by Ptolemy, the impressive breadth of Galen, or the rather limited gestures toward Neoplatonism displayed in Firmicus Maternus. Style, too, is important in constructing the ἦθος: both Galen and Adamantius, again probably following Polemo, write for a cultured audience, as they take care to point out.[6]

I was also concerned to show that similar methodological strategies are being operated in all these disciplines. Here, too, we have to abandon assumptions about what is persuasive. So, I have laid particular emphasis on one of the initially puzzling features of ancient science. As I suggested, from the point of view of anyone concerned to isolate those aspects that foreshadow the ideal modern scientific attitude, the ubiquitous elaboration in our treatises, in the form of apparently endless subdivision, can only appear as a bizarre and negative element. This has usually been seen as simply taking to extremes the program of διαίρεσις (diaeresis) set out by Plato and Aristotle. But this is hardly sufficient to account for its presence in such deeply practical fields. In astrology one is immediately puzzled by the problems it poses for setting the texts to work on a real horoscope, as I have shown. How can one explain a text that purports to be a practical handbook when it generates such extraordinarily contradictory answers? I have offered several solutions to the problem. First, there is the nature of the primary arenas of intellectual activity in the Greco-Roman world. In the first arena, that of the master-pupil relationship, the most important lesson is that of humility, which is taught through lived experience, an experience akin to the hierarchical initiations of a cult. The second arena is the ἀγών, or "competitive debate," in which the protagonist with the best ability to cap his opponent's efforts stands the best chance. One of the most interesting aspects of the results of these processes is the way the principle of noncontradiction loses its privilege to the ideal of completeness. I associated this with the desire of the magician not to leave anything out of his spell; it is also a mystical philosophical goal, a quest for the finality in which all contradictions are contained.

In order to stress that astrology was not a special case I have considered the same pressures at work in physiognomics. Once again the initial impression that we have the equivalent of a handbook, or *vade-mecum,* turns out to be a mistake. Polemo manages to remain master of an art whose basic principles are quite simple and straightforward. Of course, he points out that his book is only a beginning—no one could fit all the material into one book—but the reader will learn the elements of physiognomics, as a boy learns his letters. It takes long, zealous experience to get to Polemo's stage. Despite such remarks, which at least allow hope that the beginner may make a start as a result of reading his book, he never sets out his examples in such a way as to allow imitation. The physical descriptions and the corresponding character traits are left in an undifferentiated mass. And where, in the rest of the treatise, he sets out the variety of signs and their meanings, he never makes clear how all the conflicts between signs are to be resolved. Though the Anonymous Latin treatise recognizes this problem, it gives no more than a simple example involving three signs to illustrate it. Meanwhile, the elaboration of endless distinctions does more to obscure the difficulties rather than to illuminate them, since more contradictory signs are generated.

Finally, I took a "test-case" in medical prognosis, concentrating on what could be learned from Galen, the physician who has been placed in the medical pantheon and whose emphasis on rational demonstration has found him many philosophical admirers. I considered how the model of the ἀγών influenced the way doctors regard the past, specifically where they felt compelled to innovate by this kind of subdivision and where they were happy to use tradition with its positive moral overtones of piety to the master as the primary persuasive weapon. I argued that the agonistic pressures encouraged much greater elaboration of varieties of prognostic signs given by the pulse, whereas, in the case of those offered by the urines, a faithful explication of Hippocrates substitutes for innovation until Late Antiquity. I also considered the master-pupil relationship presupposed by this style of instruction and the tension between a declared intent to teach and the apparent desire to remain master of the knowledge. The religious discourse of initiation is evoked by this educational procedure. For the student of medicine the pulse remained a mystery, into which only slow, gradual initiation was possible. But at least the urines offered a relatively straightforward start to prognosis.

There are other obvious parallels between the three arts. Some of Galen's anecdotes of dramatic diagnosis and prognosis could equally have been written by a physiognomist, while retrospective analyses of astrologers, showing where their fellow practitioners went wrong, exhibit common features with those accounts. All three disciplines are semiological; they must be practiced by experts not entirely able to articulate their methods but involved in some kind of enterprise purporting to do so. They are fine examples of the "conjectural model for the construction of knowledge," which Carlo Ginzburg isolated as an essential but largely unrecognized component in our cultural heritage. I looked at this model in particular in the last chapter, in which I drew out some surprising similarities (and contrasts) between Galen and Sherlock Holmes.

Involution, I argued, was characteristic of all three disciplines and, indeed, helped to mark them out as τέχναι though it was not pursued in precisely the same way in each discipline. In astrology new variables are constantly brought in, while physiognomics permutated a simpler set of variables. In medical prognosis a hierarchical structure was more visible. Initially simple elements could be combined and recombined to produce a dazzling complexity, though those elements allowed an important role for the memory. This was crucial in a context in which the battles of knowledge were conducted orally. The memorable nature of the basic elements allowed virtuoso display, such as was expected of Sophists; if necessary, it permitted secondary elaboration, if predictions appeared to be proved wrong. Opponents could be answered on the spot, whatever the circumstances.

Secondary elaboration, however, was not sufficient explanation for elaborate subdivision. In the case of astrology this is made clear by the introduction of extra variables even where flexibility was not needed, as in the case of Antigonus' retrospective horoscope. Similarly, it is too simple to dismiss the authors of the treatises as charlatans eager to prevent anyone from perceiving their fraudulence. Questions about sincerity are hardly relevant here, even if they were answerable. Just as the New Rhetoricians reminded us that rhetoric is not necessarily a deceitful deformation of communication but, rather, a normal aspect of it, so we should see the authors of the treatises as communicating normally, according to the rules of the ancient games of knowledge. The Malagasy audience for the astrologers described by Bloch would surely expect nothing less than more and more extravagant elaboration in the debate; Sophists' audiences were doubtless no less appreciative of the finer tactics in the agonistic arena. That, of course, is not to deny the element of power present in rhetoric, as I have stressed in the introduction. But my aim is not to pass moral judgment nor to write the ancient writers down as cynical quacks but, rather, to illuminate what their tactics were in these battles of knowledge.

I said that my primary aim was to emphasize what the three disciplines had in common. A secondary aim, related to the metonymical conception of power as capillary, was to use them in different ways to illustrate the workings of power in the field of knowledge, taking the insights of Michel Foucault in a new direction. I have just been discussing, in relation to all three, the lowest common denominator in these interrelations, the domain of intellectual politics. I concentrated on this exclusively in the chapter on medicine, because it exerts the strongest claim to scientific status today and thus offers very specific contrasts of method between then and now. This is not to deny it a political role at a higher level; it is simply that I think that physiognomics provides a more interesting power-knowledge relationship at the level of "provincial politics." It is itself forged into a political weapon, rather than simply accrediting its practitioner as a knowledgeable person. One sees here very clearly the dual role of persuasion where intellectual politics is inextricably entwined with the politics of the πόλις (*polis*).

In my chapter on physiognomics I looked closely at the influence of contemporary rhetorical theory on the discipline, attempting to link ancient and modern rhetorical theory in order to link rhetoric with politics. Physiognomics, I have shown, drew on the oratory of praise and blame, combining the traditional elements of body and soul, working creatively with standard rhetorical figures, and drawing on appropriate commonplaces. Moreover, both ancient and modern rhetorical theory allow us to see what physiognomists like Polemo were doing with their examples. They were attacking the ἦθος (*ēthos*), that is, the right character to succeed in persuasion. If Polemo could persuade people that his enemies were unworthy to play any political role, unworthy to persuade, he had won. Again, ancient and modern rhetorical theory help us to see how use of the *topoi* to "entitle" particular situations, to entitle people, could elicit the required response to an enemy.

But it was in the first of my explorations of the interrelations between power and knowledge that the mutually sustaining nature of the two was evident. In part I of the chapter on astrology I concentrated on the highest political level. Here we are dealing with knowledge that is the site of struggle of political actors in the grand imperial dramas. Yet the relationship is not one-way, with knowledge producing power: one can perceive the role of shifts of power at the highest level in the emergence of astrology as accredited knowledge and, to a certain extent, in the eventual lowering of its status in the Western empire. Power, then, produces knowledge too.

Above all, in this book, I was concerned to dissolve the boundaries between science and pseudoscience in looking at the three disciplines as rhetorics of knowledge. I tried to show how examining medicine in the light of concerns brought up by research on astrology and physiognomics allows a rather different picture of the former to emerge. Mary Hesse, in her argument for demarcating the subject matter of the history of science in accordance with the recognition of what it is in the past that exhibits causal continuity with our own science, suggests that throwing more light on a picture may distort what has already been seen.[7] I hope that this book will function as just such a distortion.

Appendixes

Appendix A

Astrological Medicine: Iatromathematics

Ptolemy claims in the introduction to the *Tetrabiblos* that the Egyptians, those who have most advanced the art of astrology, have entirely united medicine and astrological prediction (1.3.18, pp. 16, 8ff.) Iatromathematics was one of the most popular uses of astrology; fragments of evidence suggest that doctors could attract clients by co-opting astrology to their aid. Pliny refers to an astrological doctor from Marseilles who left ten million sesterces, having spent almost that sum fortifying his own and other cities (*HN* 29.9). In the *Corpus Inscriptionum Latinarum* (10.1497) a doctor boasts of his astrological ability on his tombstone (Nutton 1979, 171). Le Boeffle (1989, 68) mentions ivory zodiacal tablets found near the shrine of the healer Apollo Grannus, at Grand, near Vosges, which would imply the presence of astrological medicine.

Ways of linking the stars with health and disease were legion, and iatromathematicians were creative in proposing and elaborating alternatives. The links between the stars and parts of the body (*melothesia*) were well enough known for Pliny to allude to them in general terms (*HN* 2.108). The astrologer in *CCAG* 5.3 (p. 133) takes one possible path, in relating the type of disease to particular planets. See also *CCAG* 2.161, 19ff., 4.158ff. There was another doctrine by which particular parts of the body are ruled by particular zodiac signs (Sextus Empiricus, *Against the Mathematicians* 5.21; Manilius, *Astronomica* 2.453–65, cf. 4.701–10; Firmicus *Mathesis* 2.24; and the astrologer given the name Teukros, in *CCAG* 7.195, 19ff.). Or *melothesia* might involve assigning parts of the body to the planets, calculating as well according to the Moon and the signs as do Ptolemy, in *Tetrabiblos* 3.13–14 (pp. 148, 9ff.), and the unknown iatromathematician found in Ideler's collection *Physici et medici graeci minores* 1 (p. 387ff.). Alternatively, other astrological entities could be brought into play, such as the places or the Lots, used to find the governing sign (Vettius Valens, *Anthologies* 2.36 p. 103, 31–104, 12), or the decans. The possibilities are almost endless both for natal astrology and catarchic, in which the individual moment is considered. Simple means of calculating whether the patient would live or die were offered by schemes such as the "Sphere of Democritus" (*PGM* 12, 351ff.), combining the day of the month (lunar) with the letters of the name converted into numbers. Astrological elements are also linked with ingredients in the pharmacopoeia in the treatises preserved in the Hermetic corpus dealing with iatromathematics. Numerology, an important part of the medicine of fevers, is easily linked to astrology.

Appendix B

The Gnostics and Astrology

Astrological elements seem to have been significant in the cosmologies of several groups of Gnostics. The Phibionites had their gods of the degrees of the zodiac (Epiphanius, *Remedy against Eighty Heresies* 26.9). The Marcionites were primarily interested in "arithmomancy," or numerological speculation associated with popular astrology, and assigned letters to the numbers associated with the astral powers: the *Monomoiriai* (Single Degrees), the zodiacal divisions, including the decans, planets, and constellations (Irenaeus, *Against Heresies* 1.134, 166 [Harvey]; Hippolytus, *Refutation of All Heresies* 6.44; Epiphanius, 34.5.). The Gnostic text *Pistis Sophia* equates astrological entities with heavenly powers in a very complex schema: eons are equated with the twelve signs, the five archons with the planets, etc. (4.136–37, p. 356–57; 139–40, p. 361–66). This is, however, in description of punishments. At 1.13–21 (pp. 22–30) the second sphere is equated with *Heimarmenē* (Fate), which is overcome by Christ, who turns the "tyrants" (the celestial powers) to spend six months turned to the left and six months to the right, as they complete their spheres of influence: he has turned their quadrangles and triangles and figures of eight (their astrological aspects). When Mariam asks whether the astrologers will be wrong, Christ replies that they will still predict correctly when the spheres are turned to the left.

Less esoteric ideas about astral powers were also held by Gnostics. Basileides, a learned Valentinian, whose ideas were to be used by the church against astrologers, does take on board astrogeography and *melothesia* (the assignation of parts of the body to zodiacal signs), which were common (Epiphanius, *Refutation of All Heresies* 24.7; Gundel and Gundel 1966, 323).

Appendix C

Favorinus' Exile

Treatises on exile were often written as philosophical exercises, as seems to have been the case with the writings of Teles, Philiscus, and Plutarch (Plutarch, *Moralia* 599aff.). We have no evidence, however, that these authors laid claim to personal experience of exile; Plutarch claimed to be writing to console an exiled friend. Furthermore, Musonius Rufus (3.755, 20ff.), Seneca (*Consolation Addressed to His Mother Helvia*), and Dio Chrysostom (*Oration* 13) all wrote treatises on exile sparked off by events. Φαβωρίνου Περὶ φυγῆς (Favorinus' *On Exile*) was published in Norsa and Vitelli 1931, republished in Barigazzi 1966 (375–409), and by Mensching 1963, who all agree that it is evidence that Favorinus was exiled. Barigazzi is emphatic on the implications of the work: "It is not a case of a simple Sophistical exercise, but of a work born of a real event in the author's life." The treatise refers to the author's own exile several times (1.40ff., 4.35ff., 8.38ff., 11.8ff., 12.39ff., 14.39ff., 25.35ff., 26.14ff.); at 14.40 the place emerges as Chios. On the reasons for the disgrace the treatise is silent. Barigazzi associates the exile with the Polemo quarrel (1966, 6), arguing that several events recounted in Philostratus can be explained thus. In his reconstruction the quarrel led to Favorinus' disgrace and his repudiation by Hadrian when he asked to escape a liturgy and to the destruction of his statue at Athens (*VS* 1.8 [490]). Philostratus is admittedly vague, which may be as a result of reluctance to show the profession in a bad light; he only relates his pride in surviving a quarrel with the emperor: οὐδὲν ἔπαθεν (he did not suffer anything) is the crucial phrase. Yet this may be in the context of execution and may be exaggerated to provide a paradox: Dio Cassius says that Hadrian thought of putting him to death and that he elevated the antagonists of Favorinus and Dionysius to overthrow them (69.3.4–6). The editors date the composition of the work on exile to around 130, which fits with the date usually assigned to Polemo's physiognomical treatise.

Notes

Introduction

1. The following account is clearly not evenhanded—here I attempt to sketch out strands of thinking within what might be called "metascientific" scholarship that I have found helpful in approaching my project and the refinements I have made of them for my purposes. It is in no sense meant to do justice to the subtleties of the arguments among the variety of opponents of those relativizing scientific knowledge. The practitioners of the sociology of scientific knowledge (often known to themselves as SSKers) have done this work more successfully and thoroughly themselves.

2. Lloyd 1987, 332. See also Neugebauer 1956.

3. See appendix A on astrological medicine and chapter 2 on physiognomics and medicine.

4. There are different degrees of realism, in principle at least extending to "fig leaf realism" (Devitt 1984), which merely asserts that something exists in a suitably mind-independent manner.

5. For philosophers concerned with using science as the key to rationality, history has merely an anecdotal or supplementary role. Indeed, Imre Lakatos is concerned only with writing "rational reconstructions" of events where possible (where impossible, the anecdotes furnish negative exempla) rather than history as normally understood. Though Lakatos was an arch-rationalist, in fact his realism was modified. He tried to rewrite Popper in the light of Kuhn (see below) and thus made some concession to the community-based character of observation at the level of the research program. Cf. Woolgar 1988, 17.

6. These are the terms of Reichenbach, who separated rigorously the circumstances in which a discovery was made (the moment's enlightenment, the crucial experiment) from the public justification. A more socializing view of discovery would stress that discoveries only come into being in the public domain, when they are defined as such.

7. Cf. Woolgar 1988, chapter 1.

8. They refuse to acknowledge any successes among the sociologists' methods; see the critical remarks of Larry Laudan (1977), followed by like-minded historians such as A. Rupert Hall (1974).

9. The rudiments of a materialist history of science (coexisting with the usual nineteenth-century idolization of science) to be found in the works of Marx and Engels were mostly ignored. But the Anglo-German chemist Carl Schorlemmer (1834–92), a close friend of theirs and a supporter of Marxist socialism, used parts of materialist theory in a work on the history of organic chemistry (1879, cited in Kragh 1987, 13). Durkheim provided the kind of critical apparatus suitable for putting the natural sciences under scrutiny with his account of religion as a reified construction of social processes, whereby conventional conceptual tools become transmuted to something mysterious, sacred, and capable of

exercising power over the individual who has internalized them (Durkheim 1913, Douglas 1975). Similarly, Mannheim in his *Ideology and Utopia* offered a vivid depiction of a world of "total ideology," a war of all against all, excluding science.

10. The phrase is due to a frequently cited article from the early 1970s (Whitley 1972), which criticized this attitude.

11. Apart from Wittgenstein, Toulmin 1972 has been cited as influential (Collins 1981).

12. Bloor 1983.

13. Bloor 1976, 1983.

14. Quine 1953. Often called the Duhem-Quine thesis, in recognition of the influence of the chemist, physicist, philosopher, and historian of science Pierre Duhem (1861–1916). See Harding 1976.

15. Ziman 1978, 33, 35.

16. Kuhn 1970 (1962). It could be argued that Gaston Bachelard (1951), Alexandre Koyré (1968), and Ludwig Fleck (1935) had anticipated many of Kuhn's ideas, but it was undoubtedly Kuhn who was spectacularly influential. His ideas have not escaped controversy: see Shapere 1964, Scheffler 1967, and Masterman 1970.

17. Hesse 1980.

18. Cf. Kuhn 1970, for explicit espousal of relativism. Paul Feyerabend, if not an ontological relativist, following the way opened up by Kuhn, argued for methodological relativism in revolutionary style. He set up anarchy as a normative standard for scientists—"Anything goes" is the motto of *Against Method* (Feyerabend 1975).

19. Barnes 1969, Mulkay 1969.

20. Barnes 1977, Barnes and Mackenzie 1979. Cf. Ashmore 1989, 5.

21. Bloor (1973) was also interested in Mannheim, but the Durkheimian works are more representative: Bloor 1976, 1978, 1982.

22. Wilson 1970.

23. Collins 1981, 3–4; 1983. Pinch interviewed in Ashmore 1989, 128.

24. Collins interviewed in Ashmore 1989, 123.

25. Hesse 1980 (1975).

26. The usual form of the argument against relativism goes as follows: "Let P be the proposition: 'all criteria of truth are relative to local culture,' hence nothing can be known to be true except in senses of 'knowledge' and 'truth' that are also relative to that culture. Now if P is asserted as true, it must itself be true only in the sense of 'true relative to a local culture' (in this case ours). Hence there are no valid grounds for asserting P as true." Hesse replies that, of course, for the relativist there are no "valid grounds" in the rationalists' sense and answers: "If P is asserted it is asserted relative to the truth criteria of local culture, and if that culture is one in which the strong thesis is accepted, it is true relative to that culture" (Hesse 1980, 42).

27. As a loose association of family resemblance characteristics (such as aversion to anthropomorphism and teleology, secularism, impersonality, abstraction, and quantification), rather than as a province strictly delimited by philosophers' rules (Barnes 1974, chap. 3).

28. Hesse 1980 (1973), 25. This article was in fact written earlier than her article on the strong thesis, but she endorses both in the introduction to these collected papers, without indicating that she has changed her position.

29. In the first chapter I discuss an article on the Copernican Revolution (Hutchinson 1987), in which the author argues that Copernicus eventually triumphed because of the way

the new model of the universe fitted with the contemporary political situation and contemporary aesthetic taste.

30. Barnes and Bloor 1982, 23.

31. Hirst (1985) argues in connection with early modern Europe, where reasoning was given such weight, the construction of the credibility of a knowledge cannot be carried out merely by agreeing to agree, or holding beliefs. As a social process, it must include an element of genuine intellectual struggle, whose outcome is not pregiven. Hacking has most recently (unpub.) restricted discussion of styles of reasoning to those in existence in modern science and thus left out of theoretical discussion styles now "dead." Here I merely take a cue from his ideas, without necessarily remaining faithful to what he had in mind.

32. Hacking 1982, 60.

33. Since my original formulation of this criticism I have come across the work of what may become a new "school" in the sociology of scientific knowledge (SSK), those interested in the sociology of SSK itself. Ashmore and Woolgar, who seem to be at the forefront of this trend, have pointed out the lack of reflexivity in their colleagues that I noted and aim to write reflexively themselves. See Ashmore 1985, 1989; Pinch and Pinch 1988; Woolgar 1981, 1983; Collins 1983; Mulkay, Potter, and Yearley 1983; Mulkay 1984; and Oehler 1983 (cited in Ashmore 1989).

34. E. Littré and C. V. Daremberg, who edited the Hippocratic texts, C. G. Kühn, the editor of the Galenic Corpus, and S. McKay, the author of a history of ancient gynecology (1901), were all members of the medical profession.

35. Temkin (1977) gives an account of the aims of historians of medicine in Leipzig in the 1930s, when he worked there, who were still, like himself, medically trained.

36. Thus, even material designated as pseudoscience might be worth studying to help moderns avoid the irrational: see e.g., G. A. Wehrli's "Das Wesen der Volksmedizin und Notwendigkeit einer geschichtlichen Betrachtung derselben," cited in Singer 1993, 5.

37. Kragh 1987, 10.

38. Duhem 1905–6, 1954a, 1954b; Tannéry 1887, 1893, 1912–43, 1930; Koyré 1957, 1968; Thorndike 1923–25.

39. *Studies in the History and Method of Science* I, vi, xvi.

40. So many scholars could be credited with initiating and following this program that it seems invidious to single any out. The way was, however, surely led by the scholars who worked on medicine, where there were particularly obvious connections between medical sects and philosophical schools.

41. Vallance 1990, 717. In fact, the Marxist Farrington had paid attention to the broader social context in his *Science and Politics in the Ancient World* as early as 1939, and T. W. Africa had written on science and the state in Greece and Rome (1968), while in France, in the 1960s, the structuralists had turned their attention to the specific social influences on Greek science. J.-P. Vernant also did a short comparative study with Jacques Gernet on Chinese science (Vernant 1980 [1965], Vidal-Naquet 1967). It would again be invidious to single out recent scholarship on ancient science in its social context, though it is still less common than scholarship setting it in its philosophical context. Few, however, mention the work of modern philosophers of science, let alone sociology of knowledge. A notable exception is Vegetti 1983, which seems to emphasize the problems of translation even more than Lloyd.

42. Lloyd 1990. I have discussed the work of Lloyd in greater detail in my Ph.D. dissertation.

43. He later devoted three pages to astrology in connection with astronomy (1987, 43–46).

44. While allowing the consensus of the group some role in legitimating research programs and inhibiting deviant theories, Lloyd distances himself from epistemological relativism, rejecting Kuhn's suggestion that truth may, like proof, be a term with only intratheoretic applications (1983, 117) and the general notion that all judgments concerning truth must be relativized to a social group.

45. Lloyd 1987, 330; cf. 1979, 225.

46. Lloyd 1983, 216–17; cf. 1987, 335.

47. See Dio Chrysostom's remarks upbraiding the Tarsians for their attitudes to Sophistic performances (*Orations* 33.4), in which he compares the feelings of the spectators to people watching a horse galloping. Anderson compares the spectators to concertgoers (1989, 89).

48. Dio Chrysostom, *Orations* 33.6.

49. Similar tales are told of the iatrosophist Magnus of Antioch (Eunapius, *Lives of the Sophists* 497–98) and of Pericles by his opponent Thucydides Melesiou in Plutarch's version (*Pericles* 8).

50. Dio Chrysostom, *Orations* 33.4, on Sophists again: "When you hear him you think it would be boorish and inappropriate to scrutinize his statements, or disbelieve a wise man."

51. E.g., recently Von Staden 1990, Nutton 1991, as well as Lloyd 1987.

52. E.g., Horine 1941, Borsarello 1981; cf. Kuriyama 1987.

53. See n. 48. For a general problematization of the concept of discovery and the consequences of placing it in a social context, see Brannigan 1981.

54. In Barnes and Shapin 1979.

55. Thagard 1978, 227–28.

56. Cicero, *On Divination* 2.88–99, writing in some ignorance of astrological method (Long 1985), argues, first, from "witnesses," astronomers "eminent in all other branches of the art," who did not practice astrological divination on this basis and, second, says that, in forming judgments, astrologers base them on sight, the least reliable of the senses, when they should employ reason and intelligence; they should realize that the distance between the stars and earth is limitless; they should know that rising times vary according to place; they should allow for other influences such as weather, heredity, and education. Third, he casts doubt on their claimed records stretching back 470,000 years and points out some failures of contemporary astrologers (see chap. 1). Sextus Empiricus (*Adversus Mathematicos* 5), an "Empiric" doctor, bases some of his attacks on medical knowledge: he points to the variety of times it may take to conceive, once the seed has been sown, to show that conception times cannot be determined and suggests that astrologers need to repeat their observations of links between star configurations and destinies, as doctors have their observations of the link between puncturing the heart and death. This latter criticism seems closest of all to a Thagard criterion. Otherwise, having mentioned that others have repudiated the analogy between the human body's sympathetic connections and that of the universe and have queried the practicalities of predicting destiny (if astrologers can do it, what use is it?), he points to the practical difficulties of establishing the time of birth and observing the heavens accordingly and repeats Cicero's arguments about the impossibility of everyone born at one moment's having the same destiny. He also ridicules analogical reasoning based on the types of zodiacal sign (what is the connection between Leo and a real lion?). See *Tetrabiblos* 1.1–3, for Ptolemy's answers, allowing for interacting influences

and for differences in rising times. Much of the most repeated criticism (the same stars–same destiny argument, or observation problems at the time of birth) seems wide of the mark in relation to the practice of learned astrology.

57. Allen (forthcoming, 1) citing Heinimann 1961: "A [τέχνη] is a body of knowledge concerning a distinct subject-matter that enables the artist to achieve a particular type of beneficial result." τέχναι in which failure was permitted to occur were called stochastic, implying careful conjecture. In the nonstochastic arts end and function coincide; in the stochastic it is possible for the artist to fulfill the demands of his art without achieving its end (7).

58. Cooter (1980) cites the early-nineteenth-century attack on social and scientific elitism by radical/liberal phrenologists and the socialist attack on IQ tests. "To identify and attack pseudoscience is both to reproduce the social and ideological structures and relations of capitalist society and reproduce the process of concealment originally conducted in the seventeenth-century isolation and exploitation of pseudoscience."

59. Herbert Butterfield, cited in Geneva 1987.

60. Edmondson 1984, 8.

61. Burke 1969 (1945), 1958 (1955), 1973 (1957).

62. For considerations of the rhetoric of science, see Gilbert and Mulkay 1984; and Schuster and Yeo 1986. Gross 1990, which I came across since I wrote this, uses a neo-Aristotelian framework derived from the New Rhetoric to analyze modern science.

63. Edmondson 1984, 1.

64. Edmondson 1984, 4.

65. Aristotle, *Rhetoric* (*Rhet.*) 1, 1354a1–1355b25.

66. Cited in Veyne 1988, 23.

67. She cites Aristotle, *Rhet.* 1.2.1356a15ff. (when people are feeling friendly and placable they think one sort of thing; when they are feeling angry and hostile they think another) and 1.2.1356a22–25 (it is necessary to understand human character and goodness in their various forms and to understand their emotions).

68. Strathern, in Fardon 1985, 77.

69. Foucault, in Patton and Morris 1979, 36.

70. Foucault 1980, 93.

71. Dreyfus and Rabinow 1982, 207.

72. Nietzsche 1964, 184 (trans. M. Mügge).

73. Foucault 1979, 31.

74. Dreyfus and Rabinow 1982, 119.

75. Cf. Vickers 1988.

76. Cf. Vegetti 1983, 11.

Chapter 1

1. Though there is a note of humor in the passage cited, it serves well enough to indicate North's concerns: he limits his investigation to the history of the mathematics and physics involved in astrology.

2. Geneva 1987, quoting Herbert Butterfield.

3. For Boll and Cumont, editors of the *CCAG,* see references; for Usener, see Cambiano 1982, 52ff.; for Cassirer, see Bodei 1982; for Warburg, see Sassi 1982.

4. See below for examples and exceptions.

5. Sarton 1959, 421, 318, 319. Cf. his defense of Plato's attitude in the Timaeus (421f.).

6. Curry 1985, 299; Yates 1974. Curry cites also Pagel, Walker, Rattansi, and Rossi.
7. He cites Hall, Hesse, Westman, McGuire, and Rossi again. (ibid.).
8. See Curry 1985, 303–4, on Vickers.
9. See Neugebauer and Van Hoesen 1959.
10. An exception is Cumont's *L'Égypte des astrologues* (1933), which is able to combine the data from astrological treatises with evidence available from papyri. He takes it, however, that Egypt is the only social context for all the treatises, an assumption as questionable as that of Thorndike and Macmullen that the contemporary context is the only one.
11. Brown 1971, 63.
12. Manilius, *Astronomica* 4.931–35. Firmicus Maternus, *Mathesis* 1.1.1 and 1.3.
13. On iatromathematics, or astrological medicine, see appendix A. On the Mithraic cult, see Gordon 1980.
14. *Introduction to Aratus' Phaenomera,* 2.1.5 ff.; cf. 17.1ff.
15. Interestingly, he does not specifically attack the branch of the discipline that we would call astronomy. He also exempts the φυσιογνωμονικὴ σοφία (the skill, or "science," of physiognomics) from criticism in another work (*Outlines of the Pyrrhonic Philosophy* 1.85).
16. Valerius Maximus 1.3.3, doubtless based on Livy: the apparently superior reading states that a Cn. Cornelius Hispalus expelled astrologers from Italy on the grounds that it was a fallacious means of divination and that it exploited the gullible. We hear, however, of no further measures of this sort until the principate. Cato, *De Agricultura* 1.5.4: "Let him keep no parasite; let him not look to consult any *haruspex,* augur, *hariolus* (seer) or astrologer" is Cato's admonition on the subject of farm stewards. North (1990) points out that the prohibition indicates not aristocratic scorn for divination but, rather, aristocratic desire to keep control of it.
17. North 1990. I am greatly indebted to this article for furnishing the wherewithal to substantiate the hypothesis I had conceived about the transition from Republic to principate.
18. MacBain 1982, 8–24; pace Rawson 1971.
19. Liebeschuetz 1979, 7; and North 1989, 51, describe three slightly different groups.
20. They were actually ten (*Decemviri*) in the fourth century and are first described as fifteen only in 51 B.C.
21. MacBain 1982, 122–25.
22. Cicero, *De Divinatione* 1.12.20, 2.21.47.
23. Augustine, *City of God* 2.24; cf. Plutarch, *Sulla* 27.4.
24. Cicero, *De Divinatione* 2.53.109, refers to the rumor about a prophecy likely to be made in the Senate that the Parthians would only be defeated by a king, though he does not state what the prophecy was. See also 1.13.97–98, on Sibylline prophecies.
25. Bloch 1963, 129f.
26. Bloch 1963, 49ff. The *locus classicus* is Livy 52.20.2 (172 B.C.).
27. Cf. MacBain 1982, n. 99, on low-ranking *haruspices.* Support for North's suggestion here comes from the only relief showing examination of the *exta:* the person inspecting them, to judge from his clothes, is clearly a slave (Scott Ryberg 1955, pl. 45, 69a–b).
28. E.g., Cicero, *De Domo* 40.
29. Torelli 1975, 105–35: *haruspices* from Tarquinii are named and celebrated with divinatory *res gestae* on this monument. Torelli connects them with the sixty *haruspices* consulted by the Senate; see Bouché-Leclercq 1896; Rawson 1978, 140–46; and MacBain 1982, on the issue.
30. Cicero, *De Divinatione* 2.33–35.70–34.

31. Valerius Maximus 9.12.6; cf. Velleius Paterculus 2.7.2.

32. Plutarch, *Sulla* 9.3, 27.4; Cicero, *De Divinatione* 1.33.72.

33. Cicero, *ad Familiares* 9.24; *De Divinatione* 1.52.119; Suetonius, *Julius* 81.2–4; Valerius Maximus 8.11.2. Quintus Cicero refers to one Cornelius Culleolus (either a *hariolus* or a *vates,* seer, prophet), who operated during the war between Octavius and Sulla (Cicero, *De Divinatione* 1.2.4).

34. *In Verrem* 2.2.30.75, 3.12.28, 54.

35. See n. 29. Anonymity: Cicero never mentions the name of any one *haruspex* in his speech on their "reply" (*De Haruspicum Responso*).

36. Cumont 1960 (1912), see, e.g., 47ff., followed by Cramer 1956, 62; Liebeschuetz 1979.

37. Cicero, *De Divinatione* 2.41 = *Stoicorum Veterorum Fragmenta* (*SVF*) 2.1193; ibid. 1.82–4 = *SVF* 2.1192.

38. No texts actually associate Zeno or Cleanthes with specifically astrological divination. As for Chrysippus, in *De Divinatione* he is linked specifically only with oracles and dream interpretation.

39. Augustine, presumably following a lost work of Cicero, calls him "much given to astrology" (*City of God* 5.2) and even refers to him as "a great astrologer and philosopher" (5.5). He also attacks him specifically for an astrological explanation of the simultaneous illness of twins (*Div.* 2.47).

40. Especially Aratus' *Phaenomena,* translated by Cicero; Ovid; and Germanicus(?). Ovid's version is entirely lost.

41. Plutarch *Marius* 42.4–5. Plutarch may be projecting back the expectations of his age (ca. A.D. 50–120) in adding this embellishment to add dramatic irony.

42. Plutarch, *Sulla* 37.1. Plutarch tells us that Sulla was told by them that, after an honorable life, he would end his days at the height of his fortunes.

43. Cicero, *De Divinatione* 2.47.99: "I recall a multitude of prophecies which the Chaldaeans made to Pompey, Crassus and even to Caesar himself (now lately deceased) to the effect that no one of them would die except of old age, at home and in great glory." Cicero is making a cynical comment in his attack on astrology here, but his words reveal the new type of diviner clustering round the new great men.

44. Lucan, *Civil War* 1.639–72.

45. See below.

46. Strabo 16.1.6.739C (ca. 64 B.C.–A.D. 21) calls Sudines a *mathematicus* (astrologer); Frontinus 1.11.15 (ca. A.D. 30–104) refers to Sudines as a *haruspex,* in relation of an incident in Eumenes' third-century war against the Galatians; Polyaenus 4.20 (second century) refers to him as a Chaldean prophet.

47. *De Divinatione* 2.47.98.

48. For the *Tonitruale,* see Johannes Lydus, *De Ostentis,* secs. 39–41, 88–92 (Wachsmuth), a sixth-century text. On Capito, see *Prosopographia Imperii Romani* (*PIR*)^2 3:196, no. 463.

49. See above, nn. 32, 42. They could still be combined much later: Pliny's *Letter* 2.20.1–6 tells a story against his enemy Regulus about his consulting a *haruspex* and an astrologer as part of a legacy hunt.

50. Suetonius, *Tiberius* 63.1; *Vespasian* 5.2.

51. See *PIR*^{2} 5.1, 21, no. 109. Suetonius *Domitian* 16.1, without referring to Proculus by name, recorded the story of a *haruspex* interpreting a bolt of lightning as portending a change of ruler. Dio Cassius 67.16.2 refers to a prediction of the actual day Domitian would

die, a prediction impossible through traditional brontoscopy but rather typical of an astrologer. *CCAG* 8.4.100.28f., perhaps from an alternative version of Dio, gives the story with reference to Proculus as an astrologer and sorcerer. See Cramer 1956, 274.

52. *Scriptores Historiae Augustae* (*SHA*), Severus Alexander 27.6. On the *Haruspices*' prediction, see ibid. 13; on the astrologer Thrasybulus' prediction, see ibid. 62.2–4.

53. *Codex Theodosianus* 9.16.1–2.

54. Suetonius, *Julius* 88. *Iulium sidus* was Horace's soubriquet (*Odes* 1.12.46). See Weinstock 1971, 370–84, 194–95, for detailed discussion of this comet.

55. The anecdote is in Servius' commentary (*On the Eclogues* 9.46). Comets were most often seen as a bad omen, of civil war, conspiracy, etc., see Manilius 1.892f.; Pliny, *HN* 2.89ff.; Seneca, *Quaestiones Naturales* 7; Cicero, *De Divinatione* 1.11.18; Calpurnius Siculus, *Eclogues* 1.82; Plutarch, *Julius Caesar* 69.3.

56. On Octavian's support, see Servius, *Commentary on the Aeneid* 8.681; Suetonius, *Julius* 88.

57. Manilius 1.809–927. Ptolemy, *Tetrabiblos* 2.9.3, 92, 4–20 (Boll-Boer), Hephaestion of Thebes, *Apotelesmatica* 64, 75–76; 78 (Pingree).

58. Pliny, *HN* 2.94, Suetonius, *Augustus* 94.

59. A fuller discussion of this is available in Barton, forthcoming.

60. *Augustus* 94.12.

61. Virgil, *Georgics* 1.33–35, connects Augustus with Libra, while Manilius (4.542ff.) praises the man born under Libra in terms that can only refer to an emperor. By the fourth book he may, however, be referring to Tiberius, cf. 4.776. At 2.509 he has praised Capricorn as Augustus' birth sign. "Germanicus," *Aratea* 558–60, also refers to Capricorn as Augustus's birth sign.

62. 2.509: contra Capricornus in ipsum / convertit visus quid enim mirabitur ille / maius in Augusti felix cum fulserit ortum? (On the other hand, Capricorn turns to look at himself: for what more can he wonder at, since he shone auspiciously on Augustus' birth?) Gundel argues that the term *felix,* or "fortunate," recalls the Lot of Fortune.

63. See Lambrechts 1953.

64. Horace, *Odes* 2.17, written in the 30s B.C., with ancient commentary; cf. Propertius 4.1.86.

65. Cf. Hölscher 1965.

66. Alföldi 1966. Crawford 1985, 546, however, dates the coin to the Sullan period, but the grounds for this are not compelling.

67. Bearded Octavian: glass paste, Kraft 1967, pl. 2.1; Vollenweider 1966, 60. Octavian's head: glass paste, Maderna Lauter 1988, cat. 241. The corn and poppy refer to fertility, perhaps also to peace after civil war. Octavian as a child, dated by Vollenweider: carnelian: See pl. 36.4–6. She notes that the caplike hairstyle is the same as on coins depicting Octavian of 42 B.C.

68. Hölscher 1965, 64; Vollenweider 1966, 143, 23.

69. See Dwyer 1976. This was the name of the second "decan" of Capricorn: Riess 1892 fr. 6, 339. See Boll 1903, 211ff., who connects Eileithyia with Lucina in Virgil's *Eclogue* 4.

70. For this sort of formula, see references in Kraft 1967.

71. Woodward 1956, 152. *Cistophori* were a type of tetradrachm.

72. A Sibylline poem may have taken up this Dionysian theme, in referring to the battle between the bull (Antony-Dionysus) and the Capricorn, a contest that the author envisaged the bull as winning (Tarn 1932).

73. Referred to in the "record of Augustus's enterprises," which was inscribed on monuments spread throughout the empire: *Res Gestae* 29.

74. Hölscher 1988; see also Hölscher 1965.

75. Maiuri 1931, 123, table 38, 69.

76. Stabiae: Elia 1957, 40, pl. 14, where most of the wall painting is Flavian.

77. Bologna: Lehmann-Hartleben 1927, pls. 21, center, 20. In both these cases the Capricorns are merged with the cornucopias. Puteoli: von Mercklin 1962, 25, no. 616; cf. Fuhrmann 1941, 609, pl. 118, p. 612f: the work of Agrippa's architect.

78. Delattre 1899–1900, 25–26, pl. 5.6.

79. Ritterling 1925. Gaul: Espérandieu 1908–, 1, 7, 10, 14 s.v. In the context of the penetration of astrology into private life, it is worth noting Trimalchio's use of the zodiac in his grandiose building, not to mention in his cookery. There is an implication that he is here imitating his betters: as emperors were careful to conceal their ascendants in their portrayals of their horoscopes, so he left his own birth sign out of the culinary representations of the zodiac out of superstitious fear. In his discourse on astrology he is made to reveal a crass ignorance of the subject (Petronius, *Satyricon* 35.1–5, 39). See also Descoeurdnes 1987 on astrological themes in the wall paintings of the House of the Hunt in Pompeii (A.D. 71–79).

80. Ulcisia Castra: Cumont 1942, 229, no.11; Budapest sarcophagus: Kähler 1939, 30 n. 1; Piedmont gravestone: Cumont, ibid., 161 n. 1; Gate of the Soul: Cumont cites Macrobius *Somnium Scipionis* 1.12.2, Porphyry, *De Antro Nympharum* 22, Proclus, *In Rempublicam* 2.128, 26, arguing that the second-century Pythagorean Numenius is the source.

81. A "*wappenartig*" motif: carnelian: cat. 262, Maderna Lauter 1988. Of glass pastes after Actium, see cat. 263, which she (455–56) compares with coins commemorating the victory over Sextus Pompey in 36.

82. Eichler and Kris 1927, 50–51, pl. 5 reverse, pl. 7 obverse. Maderna Lauter, 453, dates it to the late Augustan period.

83. Maderna Lauter: cat. 278.

84. Cf. Richter 1956, no. 649.

85. Largest photograph in Eichler and Kris, pl. 7, color in Hannestad 1986, no. 501.

86. Pollini 1978, who claims that the themes are too Roman for it to have been a gift to or from foreigners, speculates that it may have been given to Augustus by Livia, as an optimistic *consolatio* for the loss of his legions.

87. Dio Cassius 56.1.1; Suetonius, *Tiberius* 17.2.

88. Kähler 1939, 419, also detects Capricorns on the Tiberian triumphal arch in Orange (of A.D. 21 [?]).

89. Rebel issues of A.D. 68: Mattingly 1923–, vol. 1, 300; pl. 51, 1–2, of Nerva, ibid., vol. 3, pl. 3, 8, on coins of Antoninus Pius, ibid. vol. 4, lxiv, cxxxi, lxxxii, of Pescennius Niger (rebelling against Septimius Severus): vol. 5, cxii, and for Greek versions, see Wroth, index.

90. See below.

91. Delattre 1899–1900, 25–26. That is, unless Crawford is right to date the Oppius coin to the Sullan era.

92. Waddington, Balsdon, and Reinach 1904, 20, nos. 20 and 20 *bis* (Augustus and Capricorn), 21 and 21 *bis* (Tiberius and Libra). The former are dated 60 of an unknown era, the latter 63 of the same era. Bayet 1939 suggests that it may have been issued in A.D. 12, when Tiberius was associated with Augustus.

93. The pictorial presentation often makes it clear that the animals are visualized as

constellations: e.g., the shield with the Bull of VIII *Augusta* (*Corpus Inscriptionum Latinarum* ([*CIL*] VII 495); cf. Ritterling 1925.

94. Suetonius, *Tiberius* 5; cf. *CIL* 12, p. 249, 10.6638, and fragments of the *Acta Fratrum Arvalium* (Acts of the Arval Brethren) for A.D. 35.

95. 4.773–6, which praises Rhodes, would seem to suggest that Augustus has been succeeded by Tiberius, though Gundel (1927) argues that this is a later interpolation.

96. Schutz 1990.

97. Buchner believes he has found the globe in the Palazzo dei Conservatori in Rome, see cat. 110, in Heilmeyer et al. 1988.

98. Le Boeffle 1989, pl. 5 c.

99. Coarelli 1984, 72ff.

100. ἐκ προγραφῆς: Dio Cassius 56.25.5. This is in a somewhat garbled passage, concerning the edict of A.D. 11 forbidding astrological consultations alone or on the subject of anyone's death: "Yet so far was he from caring about such matters in his own case that he set forth to all in an edict the aspect of the stars at the time of his own birth. Nevertheless he forbade the practice." Dio is presumably surprised that Augustus had such faith in his destiny that he was prepared to reveal the details. Septimius Severus was more cautious.

101. *Pauly Wissowa* 11.1187–8. Gundel dates the comet and omens in Dio 56.24.3–4 to A.D. 11 to make them contemporaneous with the horoscope, rather than A.D. 9 (the Varian disaster). Both passages in Dio are vague about the chronology.

102. See, e.g., Long 1982.

103. "A literary obsession": Bouché-Leclercq 1899, 552.

104. Virgil, *Georgics* 1.33–35; cf. *Eclogues* 9.46f. This might indicate that he knew that Libra was a recent innovation, created from the claws of Scorpio.

105. 558–60: hic, Auguste, tuum genitali corpore numen / attonitas inter gentis patriamque parentem / in caelum tulit et maternis reddidit astris. "It is he (Capricorn), Augustus, who carried up to the sky and took to his maternal stars your divine soul in the sign which bore you in the face of the amazed peoples." Germanicus' authorship is disputed.

106. *Fasti* 3.701 on Caesar. *Metamorphoses* 15.839–76 includes catasterisms of Julius Caesar, Augustus, and Ovid himself, to finish the poem. On the mythological catasterisms, see Le Boeffle 1989, 125ff.

107. *Odes* 1.12.46–8, 3.25.3–6.

108. Dauge (1983) argues for a greater allegorical use of astrology by Virgil in the Aeneid, but his reliance on Jungian theory will make his arguments less persuasive for most scholars.

109. Tibullus, 2.4.15ff.; *Panegyric of Messalla* 5.18ff.

110. This poem, which used to be ascribed to Ovid, may date to later in the first century.

111. *Odes* 1.11.1–2; *Epistles* 2.2.187: "companion who mitigates the birth-star."

112. 4.1.71–150: see Le Boeffle 1989, 61. On the decans, see section 8a.

113. Virgil, *Aeneid* 3.360; 10.176. Propertius 4.1.109ff.; Statius, *Thebaid* 3.358.

114. Robbins 1940, xii. As Nutton 1986, 33, observes on the question of what the Romans thought of their doctors, one can amass enough texts, with selective quotation, to support practically any position. It seems hardly in doubt, however, that astrology commanded far more serious attention than it does today, and the consequences of this need exploring.

115. Hopkins 1978, 233–34; Cramer 1956; Syme 1983, 84; Macmullen 1966, 128–141. Macmullen and Cramer, however, both think that skepticism gained ground among the educated for a short time after Hadrian on the grounds that there are treatises written

attacking astrology by Favorinus and Diogenianus and that Vettius Valens (*Anthologies,* p. 230, 26 [Pingree]) refers to astrology's being dishonored and rejected. (In this passage I would argue that one finds only the usual pessimism about the present-day typical of the prologue, as in Galen's in *On Examining the Best Physicians* pp. 41–43, and in *On Prognosis* [see chap. 3]). For historians of astrology, see chapters 2–3 of Boll, Bezold, and Gundel 1926; also Cumont 1960 (1912).

116. They seem quite unaware of the use of astronomical tables, e.g., in their arguments about establishing the precise moment of birth, or of astrological calculations of different "rising times" of the zodiac signs in different κλίματα (zones), when they complain of lack of allowance for regional variation.

117. A typical instance of the disjunction that may operate between acceptance of the truth of an art and the attitude toward its practitioners is to be found in Apuleius of Madaura (A.D. 124–80). In *On the Doctrines of Plato* (1.3.186) he includes a visit to Egypt in search of *astrologia* in the canonical Pythagorean odyssey that he assigns to Plato, and in *Florida* (15) the Chaldeans reveal to Plato the *sideralem scientiam* (the science of the stars), the fixed circuits of the wandering divinities, and their various influences on the nativities of men. He is, however, apparently scornful of individual astrologers in other contexts: *Apologia* (97) and *Metamorphoses* (2.12–15) (though they turn out to be right). Cf. Pliny, who, despite his frequent rude remarks about practitioners, turns to astrologers to decide the question of how long a life can be (*HN* 7.160–61). On the double image of diviners, see also Propertius 4.1.81–82; and Statius, *Thebaid* 3.551ff, 6.935–37.

118. There are many parallels between astrologers and doctors here. See Nutton 1985, 1986, on doctors. Both are uncomfortably close to the *magus,* as legal evidence suggests of doctors: Ulpian, *Digest* 50.13.1.3; accusations of sorcery: Galen: *On Prognosis* p. 70, 7–8; of poison: Pliny *HN* 29.8.20. Pliny also rails against doctors as being unnecessary, incompetent, full of oversubtle argumentation and liable to be blown along by the latest fashion: "they have brought about the deaths of the defenceless as well as the degeneration of the Roman State." Venality: Galen, *On Prognosis* p. 69, 4ff. Cf. satirical remarks of Juvenal (*Satires* 6.565f.); and Pliny (*Letters* 2.20) on astrology and inheritance hunting. As Galen promotes the image of the *medicus gratiosus,* who does it all for love (see Deichgräber 1970), so Ptolemy (*Tetrabiblos* 1.3.2, p. 11, 8–20) is careful to present astrology as a disinterested science, which leads neither to money nor fame, while Firmicus (*Mathesis* 2.30.2) demands the highest moral standards of the practitioner. Failure of practitioners / defense of divination: Alexander, *On Fate* 6.171, 7–11 (Bruns), *SVF* 2.1210.

119. The *Apocolocyntosis,* or *Ludus de Morte Claudii,* may not be Seneca's: Baldwin 1964.

120. Cf. *On Providence* 5.6f. In fact, astrologers did take the "fixed stars" into account.

121. *Meditations* 2.13, following Epictetus, *Discourses* 2.7.1–3.

122. *SHA, Commodus* 1.4. This is a story told against an astrologer who failed to foresee the early death of Commodus' twin brother; its authenticity is not even queried by Syme (1983), who is generally skeptical of the astrological stories in the Augustan Histories.

123. *Annals* 6.22.

124. Chrysippus was more rigidly deterministic: Long and Sedley 1987, 343.

125. On the chain of causation, see texts and commentary in Long and Sedley 1987, 333–43, 386–94. On the role of the stars, see Cicero, *De Divinatione* 1.117–18 = *SVF* 2.1210.

126. *Annals* 6.22; cf. Scott 1968. The introductory *quippe* seems to suggest that he continues with an example of the opinion just cited, that there are clear testimonials to the

credit of the *ars*. Tacitus seems more favorable to astrology in the *Annals* than in the *Histories*. Cf. *Ann.* 4.58, ctr. *Hist.* 1.22, 2.78.

127. *On the Temperament and Force of Simple Drugs* (*Simp. Med.*) 6 pr. (K.11.796, 8–798, 14). He attacks him for relying on books, when he has no knowledge of the herbs he describes. Pamphilus has claimed to find the thirty-six sacred herbs of the horoscopes in a treatise of Hermes the Egyptian, but this is an empty fiction. He also ridicules Pamphilus' use of incantations and spells when gathering herbs.

128. *On the Natural Faculties* (*Nat. Fac.*) 1.12, pp. 121, 24–122, 3 = K.2.29.7–11.

129. Toomer 1985, 194.

130. Cf. *CCAG* 8.2.125; and Toomer 1985, 203.

131. K.9.934, 10–936, 16. Heeg (1911) compared this to another passage in *On Regimen in Acute Diseases* (*Diaet. Acut.*) p. 372, 12–373, 8 = K.19.188–89. The Greek version is now assumed to be spurious, however, since the Arabic version has better claims to be the treatise Galen mentions having written: see Lyons 1969, 12ff. There is also the passage in which Galen says that astronomical observations in the manner of Hippocrates and Aratus are valuable in predicting the varying course of a disease (*Commentary on Hippocrates's Epidemics VI* [*In Hipp. Epid.* 6] 4.27, pp. 144, 24–245, 4).

132. *De Diebus Decretoriis* K.9.910, 16ff.; 911, 14ff.

133. No challenge to its genuineness: see Fichtner 1985. Sarton (1956, 84n.) refers to the inauthenticity of the *Prognostica de decubitu ex mathematica scientia,* included in the Galenic corpus: "this is judicial astrology, and there is no evidence Galen ever fell as low as that." Cumont (1935, 119) makes a more balanced judgment based on the manuscript tradition, which shows that Galen's authorship only came to be attributed by accident. While noting that Galen could not escape the influence of astrology, which was so much in the ascendant at this time, he regards the *Prognostica* as unworthy of him. Heeg (1911, 1003ff.) was actually led to wonder whether the *Prognostica* was genuine, on reading the astrological passages in Galen, though he ended by deciding that it was a forgery on other grounds.

134. As in, e.g., *De Diebus Decretoriis* K.9.934. In general, Galen remarks frequently that medical science must base itself on "epistemonic premisses" and work on logically from there: see chapter 3.

135. Dio Cassius 56.25.5. See Cramer 1956, 254–81. The thinking was similar in his action over the "Sibylline Books." In 12 B.C. he made private ownership of them illegal (Tacitus, *Annals* 6.12).

136. Tacitus, *Annals* 6.20.

137. In antiquity he was seen as a scholar of Pythagoras, Democritus, and Plato (Diogenes Laertius 3.56–57, 9.38). For his astrological reputation, see *CCAG* 8.4. f. 46. Riess 1892, no. 3, 354; cf. Juvenal, *Satires* 6.576, 581. Pliny cites him as a source for books 2, 9, 31, and 32 of his *Natural History* in book 1.

138. Juvenal, *Satires* 10.94.

139. In the Suetonius passage (*Domitian* 10.3) there is a list of charges that Suetonius regards as trivial but which Domitian is presumed to have perceived as threats to his sole dignity. Pompusianus not only was said to have an imperial horoscope, but he also had a depiction of the world in his hall and carried round speeches of kings and generals from Livy and had called his slaves Mago and Hannibal. The horoscope is mentioned first, however, and is also a theme elsewhere in Suetonius (*Vespasian* 14). Nerva: Dio Cassius 67.15.6; cf. Thrasyllus' deception to avert Tiberius' wrath: ibid. 58.27.3.

140. On the identity of Balbillus, see Cumont 1918.

141. Suetonius, *Vespasian* 14; cf. 25.1.

142. This desire to save the expert from errors is also found in the account of Thrasyllus' prediction that Tiberius would live another ten years. It was made, of course, to prevent further bloodshed.

143. Cf. also the Flavians: Tacitus, *Histories* 2.78, Suetonius, *Vespasian* 25. Hadrian's destiny was predicted by his great-uncle and then confirmed *a mathematico quodam* (by some astrologer) in Lower Moesia: *SHA, Hadrian* 2.3–4.

144. Suetonius, *Augustus* 94.5; Dio Cassius 45.1.3–5.

145. Suetonius, *Augustus;* Riess 1933.

146. Tacitus, *Annals* 6.21, Dio Cassius 57.19.3–4; 63 (64) 1.1. Suetonius calls Tiberius much given to astrology: *Tiberius* 69.

147. Tacitus, *Annals* 14.9.3. She was also believed to have delayed Britannicus' arrival till the astrologically propitious moment for Nero to begin his rule (ibid. 12.68).

148. Suetonius, *Vitellius* 3.2; Dio Cassius 63 (64) 4.3.

149. It is not clear whether Ptolemy and Seleucus are the same person. Suetonius (*Otho* 4.1) says that Otho conceived his hope of imperial power because Seleucus, having at first only prophesied that he would survive Nero, suddenly added the prediction of Otho's rule. The same story is told of Ptolemy by Tacitus (*Histories* 1.22.1, 3), while Plutarch blames Ptolemy for Galba's death (*Galba* 23.7), and Juvenal leaves the astrologer anonymous (*Satires* 6.558).

150. Tiberius: Tacitus, *Annals* 4.58. Caligula: Suetonius, *Gaius* 57.2. Nero: Suetonius, *Nero* 40.2.

151. Suetonius, *Domitian* 22. Brind'Amour (1981) calculated that Domitian was waiting for the Moon to pass from Aquarius to Pisces, because he had been born with Saturn in the last degrees of Aquarius. He points out that Suetonius has probably used a retrospective astrological source.

152. Gordian I in A.D. 238 was invited to become emperor at the age of seventy-nine by nobles who had revolted against Maximinus' fiscal policy. He made his son Gordian II his colleague. When Gordian II was killed in battle against supporters of Maximinus, his father committed suicide, after a reign of twenty-two days. The latter's grandson, Gordian III, fared slightly better, being saluted emperor by the Praetorian guard at the age of thirteen in the same year. He was assassinated in 244 at the behest of his successor, Philip the Arab.

153. Suetonius, *Domitian* 15.3, who mentions the actor Latinus as the witness who passed the incident on to the unhappy emperor.

154. Suetonius, *Vitellius* 14.4; Dio Cassius: 64 (65) 1.4.

155. See n. 135.

156. Tacitus, *Annals* 2.32; Suetonius, *Tiberius* 36; Ulpian, *Mosaicorum et Romanorum Legum Collatio* 15.2.1; Dio Cassius 57.15.8–9. See Cramer 1951. Suetonius says that Tiberius often pardoned astrologers, provided that they undertook to stop practicing their art (*Tiberius* 36.3).

157. On cases involving the elite, see Cramer 1956, 251–70 (he lists fourteen cases up to A.D. 205); on cases of astrologers in court: 270–75; on expulsions, 232–48. He lists fourteen possibilities till A.D. 175 and rates nine as certain.

158. Lepida, also accused of faking motherhood, adulteries, and poisonings: Tacitus, *Annals* 3.22; Lollia: ibid. 12.22; Scribonianus: ibid. 12.52; Ostorius Scapula and Anteius Rufus: ibid. 16.14.

159. Ulpian, *Comparison of the Laws of Moses and the Romans* 15.2.2–3: "But it was demanded whether the science of this type of men should be punished or its use and profes-

sion. And indeed, among the ancients it was said that their profession, not their knowledge was prohibited; later it was changed." Cf. Paulus, *Opinions* 5.21.4: "One would do better to abstain not only from [the practice of] divination, but from the science itself and its books."

160. Grodzynski 1974, 274; *Codex Theodosianus* 9.16.6.

161. *Codex Theodosianus* 9.16.1–2: only public, traditional haruspicy is allowed; 9.16.4: the curiosity of divination is to cease (here augurs appear alongside Chaldeans); 9.16.12 (A.D. 409): if astrologers do not burn their books in front of the bishop and turn to the Catholic faith with the promise of never returning to their past error, they must be expelled from the empire.

162. An interesting exception is the emperor Julian the Apostate, who in his zeal to restore the traditional religion encouraged all sorts of divination and was reported to have complete faith in his destiny on account of a personal omen (Ammianus Marcellinus 21.2.7; cf. Grodzynski 1974, 285). This illustrates the interpenetration of all types of divination: he had a night vision in which he was told that Constantius would die when Jupiter entered Aquarius and Saturn was in the twenty-fifth degree of Virgo (Ammianus Marcellinus 21.2.2).

163. Libanius, *Orations* 14.16 (362): one Aristophanes was confined, flogged, and had curial duties imposed for having introduced an astrologer to the prefect of Egypt; cf. Ammianus Marcellinus 29.2.5: Bassianus loses his property.

164. Ammianus Marcellinus 29.1.5–42, 2.9, 2.27.

165. John of Antioch, fr. 210 = *Fragmenta Historicorum Graecorum* 4.618 (Müller).

166. Chronographia 390 (Dindorf); cf. *Chronicon Paschale* 1.606 (Dindorf).

167. Marcellinus Comes, *Monumenta Germaniae Historica, Auctores Antiquissimi* 11.2 (Mömmsen).

168. Tester 1987, 95.

169. Cumont 1918.

170. *Astronomica* 1.384f. Manilius speaks of the constellations of the southern hemisphere. "cetera non cedunt: uno vincuntur in astro, / Augusto, sidus nostro qui contigit orbi, / legum nunc terris, post caelo maximus auctor" (The rest do not yield: they are conquered by one star, Augustus, the constellation who touches our world, now the author of laws on earth, later greatest in the sky).

171. *Mathesis* 2.30.5. "But indeed no astrologer could foretell anything true about the fate of the emperor; for the emperor alone does not lie under the courses of the stars and he is the only one whose fate the stars have no power to decree. Since he is the lord of the whole world, his fate is governed by the judgement of the highest god, and because the territory of the whole world lies under the powers of the emperor, he too is accounted among the number of those gods whom the supreme power has set up to create and conserve all things."

172. 1.10.13–14. He offers Constantine as an example of the workings of Fate and effectively acknowledges the power of the stars over Constantine as he prays to them "to guarantee unending rule for him and his descendants."

173. Bouché-Leclercq 1899, 250, 252. On the former he comments: "For the people of the late empire every higher class exploits a lower one and lives at its expense. Astrologers would seriously declare that the superior planet claimed a tithe from its inferior when they were in square aspect, that is to say in a hostile relation." Δορυφορία, or *comitatus,* the theorists probably likened the satellite planets to *apparitores,* or lictors, which led them to put them "in front" rather than "behind" their lord in one version. Etiquette is complicated

but seems to be influenced by court ceremonial. For astrological references, see Liddell, Scott, and Jones 1968, s.vv.

174. The philosophical attitude attributed to Trajan (*successorem suum nullus occidit:* "no one kills his successor") does not appear to have caught on, though Marcus Aurelius is supposed to have quoted it to L. Verus on Avidius Cassius: *SHA, Avidius Cassius* 2.

175. See also Riedinger 1956.

176. Magi: *Mt.* 2.1–12. Eclipse at the death of Christ: *Mt.* 27.45, *Mk.* 25.33, *Lk.* 23.44; celestial signs to announce his return: *Mt.* 24.29, *Mk.* 13.24–25, *Lk.* 21.25.

177. *Letter* 8.11.10; letter before *Ode* 22.

178. Tatian (A.D.136/40–?202), *Oration to the Greeks* 8–12; Clement (c.150–211/5), *Miscellanies* 6.148.1–3; Tertullian, *Against Marcion* 1.18; *On Idolatry* 9.3. (He may have discussed astrologers in greater detail in his missing *On Fate.*)

179. Hippolytus, *Against Heresies* 4.1–27; Sextus Empiricus, *Adversus Mathematicos* 5.50–105.

180. The Peratics were a Gnostic sect.

181. *Against Heresies* 4.2., trans. J. MacMahon. Epiphanius of Salamis in his *Remedy against Eighty Heresies,* written in 375–77, attacks eighty "heretical sects" including "Stoicism," under whose name he discusses the fate (εἱμαρμένη) associated with the planets.

182. On the details of the Gnostics' use of astrology, see appendix B.

183. *Philocalia* 23.1–21. The commentary is intercut with an extract from *Against Celsus* (2.20, secs. 12–13) and followed by an extract from the *Travels of Peter,* also used in the pseudo-Clementine *Recognitions* (23.22ff.)

184. He does add the argument from the precession of the equinoxes to the stock arguments (*Philocalia* 23.18).

185. Eusebius of Caesarea (265–339/40) is an exception; he follows Origen in respecting a nonfatalist astrology (*A Preparation for the Gospel* 6).

186. We know of the existence of previous discussions in Latin: an *On Fate, or against Astrologers* of Minucius Felix (2d/3d c.) as well as Tertullian's *On Fate.*

187. See Riedinger 1956; Gundel and Gundel n1966, 101; and Amand 1941.

188. Boll 1894, 181–238.

189. These figures were not described as kings until the sixth century, when there was a move to present the prophecies of Isaiah, Psalms, and Habukkuk as fulfilled. On the subject of Christian discussions about the star, Riedinger 1956, 130–46, is most detailed.

190. See nn. 170–72.

191. Ignatius, *Letter to the Ephesians* 19; Tertullian, *On Idolatry* 9.

192. *Excerpts from Theodotus* 74.2: "We are born again, becoming higher than all the other powers . . . [76.4] . . . from baptism he is called a servant of God even by the unclean spirits and they now tremble at him whom shortly before they obsessed . . . [78.1] . . . Until baptism Fate is real, but after it the astrologists are no longer right" (trans. P. Brown). Cf. Marius Victorinus, *Commentary on Epistle to the Galatians* 2.3, *Patrologia Latina* (*PL*) 8.1175–76 (4th c.). For other examples, see Riedinger 1956.

193. Basil, *Sermons* 25, esp. chapter 6 (*Patrologia Graeca* (*PG*) 31.1469A–1475A); John Chrysostom, *Sermon on Matthew* 6 (*PG* 57.64, 12–65, 46); Diodorus of Tarsus (*PG* 103.829–77) cf. Gregory of Nazianzus: *On Foreknowledge* 37.424A–429A) followed by the Antioch school): δύναμιν τινά θειοτέραν, εἰς ἄστρον μὲν σχηματιζομένην, τὴν δε τοῦ κοινοῦ Δεσπότου κηρύττουσαν γένεσιν. ([the star was] a divine power with the form of a star, announcing the birth of the lord of the universe).

194. There always remained room for prodigious celestial phenomena in astrology.

195. See n. 193.

196. Epiphanius, *Remedy against Eighty Heresies* 66.13; *PG* 42.48.

197. Gundel and Gundel 1966, 329.

198. See e.g., Epiphanius, *Remedy against Eighty Heresies.*

199. It is also most severely forbidden for Christians to pray to the sun, moon, and stars or to swear by them (*Constitutions of the Apostles* 5.12.1, 2, and 5). Epiphanius reports a story of one Aquila, supposedly dating from ca. A.D. 120, who, having been converted in Jerusalem, refused to give up his astrology and was excommunicated (*PG* 43.262). In 449 we hear of a similar case: Sophronius, bishop of Emesa, accused of astrology, phialomancy, and other divination, was brought to trial in the presence of the "Robber Council" of Ephesus. The accusations, interestingly in view of the connections with heresy noted, were clearly made because he was suspected of being a Nestorian (Honigmann 1944). Doubtless, there were many such cases.

200. See Barlow 1950, 108, IX, X; and Chadwick 1976.

201. *Canons of the Apostles* 1.55.61; Procopius, *Secret History* 11.76.13 (Haury). Cf., for this period, Cassiodorus' condemnation (*PL* 70.148).

202. See Fontaine 1953; *Canons of the Apostles* 1.232.29.

203. Sozomen, *History of the Church* 3.6. He later returned and was attacked for embracing Sabellianist doctrines. Socrates (*History of the Church* 2.9) says that the people rioted when he was appointed so that he fled.

204. *Life of Saint Symeon* 157, p. 138–39 (Van den Ven).

205. Letter to Leontius, preceding *Ode* 22; *Letters* 8.119–13.

206. Bonnaud 1931.

207. Cumont 1903, 436.

208. He follows Nilsson 1933, 245ff.

209. Nock 1972, 489; Livy 39.16.6–7.

210. Brown 1978, 76: "The influence of the stars was not ineluctable but baffling. Astrological beliefs condensed an image of man and of his relationship with society that assumed he lay open to conflicting choices and was subject to a full range of paradoxical triumphs and disasters. Astrology brought down into men's views of their lives and personalities the complexities and conflicts which they saw in the planets as these moved like backgammon counters across the fixity of the heavens" (see Tatian, *Oration to the Greeks* 9).

211. Cf. Riedinger 1956, 14: "But not only the period of Empire groaned under the 'yoke of Fate.'" Cramer (1956, 146) refers to a "small minority which in Rome opposed the unquestioning fatalism of the Stoics and their allies the astrologers."

212. E.g., most recently Fowden 1986, 91–94. He never really questions the nature of the experts' "belief" in strict determinism.

213. Manilius 2.13; Firmicus, *Mathesis* 1.10.

214. Long and Sedley (1987, 33 ff.) give the texts and discuss the refinements within the Stoic conceptions of Fate, focusing particularly on different types of causes.

215. Vettius Valens (2d c., see Neugebauer 1954) 5.9, p. 210, 6–9.

216. Tertullian, *On Idolatry* 9: We know that there is an alliance between magic and astrology. Cf. *Apologeticum* 35. Cf. also Tacitus, *Annals* 2.27, 2.32, 12.22. See n. 160 for the Theodosian Code.

217. Proclus, *In Rempublicam* 2.344–45 = Riess. Fr.1: "We have . . . the theurgical art, which gave us an invocation to see face to face the very powerful goddess ('Ανάγκη) and

taught us how one should approach her when one has seen her. It is, in fact, in a manner more extraordinary than when one approaches the other gods, if it is true that Petosiris, who indicates it in his writing, is a sure testifier, he who has had dealings with all sorts of gods and angels." On Petosiris, supposed author of the "astrological bible" with Nechepso, see Kroll 1935 and now Pingree 1974. On the revelations obtained by Petosiris, cf. Vettius Valens 6.1 (231, 10f.). Firmicus (1.6.2) is similarly not content with complete passivity, though he would not go so far as to practice theurgy: "Let the human race regard the power of the stars with the constant veneration of a suppliant. Let us call upon the gods in supplication and piously fulfil our vows to them so that we may be reassured of the divine nature of our own minds and may resist in some part the hostile decrees of the stars."

218. *Life of Plotinus* 10. The active use of the verb ἀστροβολέω is a hapax, but associated words are linked with the withering affect of the Dog Star (see *Thesaurus Graecae Linguae* 1[2] (1831–56 s.v.). MacKenna (rev. B. S. Page 1957) translates: "he even ventured sorcery, seeking to crush Plotinus with star-spells," while Armstrong (Loeb 1966) renders it as "trying to bring a star-stroke on him by magic."

219. 1968, 72ff.

220. Antigonus, whose retrospective horoscope I use, is second century.

221. Rhys Bram 1975, 2. All following translations are hers.

222. Pingree's ed. xiv–xvi. Dorotheus, 3.2.19–44; 3.1.27–65; 4.1.15; 5.5.15; 5.5.26.

223. Augustus' edict of A.D. 11 mentioned above remained in force. Inquiries about the death of a slave's master or about the emperor continued to be punished with great severity in the succeeding centuries (Paulus, *Opinions* 5.21.3–4; Ulpian, *Comparison of the Laws of Moses and the Romans* 15.2.3). Manetho, in his *Apotelesmatica* 6.735–37, expresses his fear of dealing with royal star configurations, because of the likelihood of arousing official wrath; cf. Cramer 1956, 186.

224. Neugebauer and Van Hoesen 1959, 91.

225. Firmicus 2 pr., Dorotheus 1 pr. E.g., Rhys Bram 1975, vii; Gleason 1989; Laistner 1941 (*manuals*); Gundel and Gundel 1966, 337 (*Lehrbuch*). Hopkins (1978, 233) refers to Firmicus' *Mathesis* as a "textbook." As for scholars' irritation, consider Housman on Manilius: "Liars need not have long memories if they address themselves to fools, who have short ones. An astrological poet writing his third book may safely forget his second, because an astrological reader will never remember it" (3:vi). Neugebauer and Van Hoesen (1959) are also understandably irritated when they cannot understand how an astrologer reaches a conclusion or uses a term "wrongly": see, e.g., 19, 28, 36. They explain a "departure from the orthodox" by chronology (36). Since I first wrote this I have been delighted to find that Tester (1987) realizes that these so-called handbooks are no use for casting a horoscope without the mathematical apparatus and frequently laments their "confusion" as adding to the difficulties.

226. The following explanation draws on that of S. J. Tester (1987, 4–9).

227. This relative position varies with the precession of the equinoxes.

228. Ancient horoscopes were actually depicted by square rather than circular diagrams. This diagram is for clarity only.

229. In *Codex phil. gr. Vindob.* (*Vienna Codex: CCAG* 6, pp. 67–71). Variant in *Codex Parisinus gr.* 2501 (*Paris Codex: CCAG* 8.2): 22°.

230. This is a common problem. As Tester (1987) observes, considerations of the problems of the obliquity of the ecliptic are ignored in the *Tetrabiblos;* the astrologer would need the *Almagest* (2.7–9) to solve them. Manilius makes reference to the inadequacy of "the vulgar method of calculation" (assuming that each sign takes two hours to rise: 3.225)

and then ends up using it (483–509). Dorotheus does make reference to the variation of rising times, when he refers to "crooked" signs (1.1.7), but he is far from clear.

231. E.g., Firmicus 8.18 uses degrees, but this is not always so in the rest of the book.

232. Astronomically, aspects are certain angular distances, made at the center of the earth, between a line from one planet and a line from another. They are measured in degrees along the ecliptic.

233. The texts are found in *CCAG* 6, pp. 67–71; and 8.2, pp. 82–84. The translations of this passage and the one below are adapted from Neugebauer and Van Hoesen 1959 (who translate only part of the full text of the horoscope). The variant for the Sun's position is given in *Paris Codex* 2501 (*CCAG* 8.2). In the text and diagram of the *Vienna Codex* the figure for Saturn is given as 16, so I have followed this for my diagram. (A further variant, in *Paris* 2417, is 10.) Neugebauer and Van Hoesen take 5, as the closest to the positions they have calculated for that hour. As far as my calculations go, however, it makes no real difference, as Mercury and Saturn are still in conjunction.

234. Neugebauer and Van Hoesen (1959, 90) observe that Saturn would come into conjunction rather than quartile with the Ascendant and the Moon.

235. *CCAG* 6, p. 68, 4–9, omitted in the *Vienna Codex;* and *CCAG* 8.2 (parenthetical observations mine).

236. Bouché-Leclercq 1899, 404.

237. Abridged: *CCAG* 8.2, p. 84. 63d year: ibid. 6, p. 68, 15.

238. See in what house, sign, and degrees the Giver of Life is located; the ruler of that sign, in what house, sign, and degrees; the Life giver, as above; and to what extent the Giver of Life and the benefic planets are aspected to the Sun and Moon.

239. Vettius Valens 3.10–12, pp. 138–44; Ptolemy, *Tetrabiblos* 3.10, pp. 129, 1–142, 15; Paul of Alexandria 35, pp. 90–94 (Boer); Heliodorus' *Commentary* on Paul 38–40, pp. 126–44 (Boer). Vettius Valens and Ptolemy are second century; Paul, the author of the Ἐισάγωγη (introd.), not to be confused with his fifth-century namesake, is fourth century; and the commentary attributed to Heliodorus is sixth century. On procedures for determining death, see Bouché-Leclercq 1899, 404–28. Manilius is perhaps the simplest, but in the second half of his book 3 there are two mutually incompatible systems: the first begins from the Sun's sign, the second from the Ascendant's sign. In both the influence over months and years, etc., is attributed to the signs. Ptolemy and others ascribe the influence to the planets. Two centuries later Paul is halfway between the two types of system. He describes a system of chronocrators (time lords), like the second system of Manilius but goes on to ascribe influence to planets in the signs (cf. Tester 1987, 41–42; 84–85).

240. In chapter 7 Gellius notes that the dangers of the climacteric have been noted for a long time and tells us that the night before last he came across a reference to it in one of Augustus' letters to Gaius and quotes as follows: "Greetings, my dear Gaius, my dearest little donkey . . . especially on days like today my eyes are eager for my Gaius, and wherever you have been today, I hope you have celebrated my 64th birthday in health and happiness. For you see, I have passed the climacteric common to all old men, the 63rd year."

241. 1.16, 17; 2.9–12, 24.

242. *SHA, Hadrian* 2.4.

243. Cramer 1956, 169.

244. See n. 233.

245. *CCAG* 6, pp. 67, 16–69, 1; προσκύνησις: pp. 69, 29–70, 5.

246. Bouché-Leclercq 1899, 576 n. 1.

247. *Excerpts from Theodotus,* a Gnostic (69–71); Brown 1978, 76.

248. 3.4.6: Mars in the second house by night. 5.2.17: Jupiter in the terms of the Ascendant by night. 3.6.5: Venus is in the second house in a nocturnal chart. 4.21.2: Mars in trine with the MC in a nocturnal chart, not well located. 4.19.5: Saturn the ruler of the chart. 5.2.20: The Moon in the terms of Mercury with the Ascendant in a nocturnal chart: they are always moving, often merchants. 3.9.6: Mercury and Saturn together by night in the twelfth house.

249. The House of Necessity in the House of the Moon, Mars, or Saturn; the House on an angle, when one of the above planets is on the anafora or catafora of any angle.

250. According to Firmicus' definition (2.9), Mars would not be in an evening rising, but Antigonus describes the planet in these terms.

251. 2.33.6: Moon in Saturn's house. 2.32.1: Mercury in Saturn's house. 2.33.13: Moon in Mercury's terms. 2.32.2: Mercury in Jupiter's terms. 2.31: Venus in Jupiter's terms. 2.1.3: The lords of the triplicity of Venus are badly located.

252. 1.10.29. This seems to be the implication of the passage, since the lords of both the triplicities of the conjunction of the Moon and Jupiter are badly located, unless the condition that the Moon be full is added.

253. *SHA, Hadrian* 14.8.

254. Particularly striking is the Hermetic passage, where even after rebirth the initiate son is portrayed as being as ignorant as before: *Corpus Hermeticum* 13: *A Secret Discourse of Hermes Trismegistus to His Son Tat Concerning Rebirth.*

255. Goody 1968, 49–55.

256. 341C–D. This letter is the only one at all likely to be by the author of the dialogues.

257. 8 pr.; 5 pr. 2.

258. See Gordon 1976.

259. Lloyd 1983, 2. He rightly rejects it as a definition of magic. Here I only want to draw on popular associations of the word.

260. Firmicus was, as it happens, a retired lawyer (4.1). Justinian's preface to the *Digest* shows a clear intention of removing contradictions in his new code, to be made up of the jurisprudential writings of the past but also of including every expert on law. It may be that the contradictions evident are simply the result of haste, but perhaps the lawyers were more concerned to make sure nothing important was left out. John Crook (unpub.) has observed that most legal writings were simply expansions of the basic propositions of the civil law; whole branches of law are derived from the elaboration of a few laconic words. Like astrologers, jurists worked within the frame of a tradition and set great store by genealogy (see, e.g., *Digest* 1.2.2.). Also there was an agonistic context, though the public disputes seem to have vanished with the juristic schools in the second century (Honoré 1962).

261. This, among other references, suggests that Ptolemy himself was not a professional astrologer but was simply summarizing the other part of his art. This would explain the relative simplicity of much of his scheme and the vagueness of interpretation. For the sentiment of this quotation, cf. *Tetrabiblos* 3.1.6, p. 109, 21–110, 3.

262. A revealing remark on the importance of keeping things esoteric comes from Villani, the biographer of the thirteenth-century Guido Bonatti, who remarks that in his book Bonatti treats the subject of astrology so clearly that he seems desirous of teaching it to women (Tester 1987, 189).

263. Vettius Valens 7.1, p. 251, 4–6. Valens makes use of the model of the mysteries quite frequently: see also, e.g., 4.11 (p. 164, 12–21), 5.2 (p. 201, 18–23), 5.12. (p. 228, 24–

28), 8.5 (p. 288, 28–30), 9.8 (p. 332, 11–14), 9.10 (pp. 337, 28–338, 2), 9.16 (p. 344, 24–29 [oath again]). Cf. Firmicus 2.14. At the preface to book 7 Firmicus demands an oath "as Orpheus, Plato and the Pythagoreans demanded of their disciples."

264. Vettius Valens 4.11; p. 163, 25. There is also a similar initiatory style: at 2.15 he introduces one list of twelve "places," only to introduce a more complex one at 4.12. He refers to his wish to make books an easy way into the art for his new pupils and others not yet trained at 3.15, pp. 149, 23ff.

265. He introduces the "Egyptian decans" in the same vein as fearful secrets that the ancients left in obscurity, though they are but a drop in an ocean of variables.

266. The ἀγών formed part of Greek education from an early stage (Beck 1975, 38–43).

267. Eunapius, *Lives of the Sophists* 497–98. See the remarks above (intro.; chap. 2), on the importance of such stories.

268. On the medical ἀγών, see chapter 3.

269. *Commentary on Hippocrates' "On Regimen in Acute Diseases"* (*Vict. Acut.*) pp. 129, 12–130, 32 = K.15.440–46.

270. The papyrus itself refers to the use of both tables of rising times and of a water clock in determining the Ascendant. On tables, see also Neugebauer and Van Hoesen 1959, no. 8, col. 1, 12–13, and commentary, p. 24. As they point out, *Tetrabiblos* 3.3; pp. 110, 1–111, 2, compares use of instruments and tables of rising times for the determination of the Ascendant but clarifies little, since Ptolemy assumes knowledge on the part of his readers.

271. For examples in "Rhetorius," see Neugebauer and Van Hoesen 1959, nos. L401, 440, 488, and 516. Pingree 1977 casts doubt on the dating and identity of this figure.

272. I am grateful to John Ray and Sarah Clackson for help with the linguistic difficulties here.

273. Hébert 1961 (cited in Bloch 1968, 295).

274. Hephaestion of Thebes 1.1.9; 4, 23–25, 4 (Pingree). Bouché-Leclercq 1899, 207f.

275. *Bricolage* was Lévi-Strauss's term for the creative construction of "mythical thought" on the model of a professional do-it-yourself expert, who builds with a limited but versatile set of tools (Lévi-Strauss 1974 [1962], 16–36). Iatromathematics was one such creative extension of the basic elements of astrology (see app. A). For another example, see *CCAG* 8.2, p. 196ff., ed. Wuilleumier, which shows how an astrologer used the characters of the planets to predict the outcome of chariot races. The colors of the teams were given to different planets; Jupiter represented victory and Saturn defeat; the Sun would assist the Reds, being fiery; the Moon's influence would depend on its state, etc. The infallible method of Theodorus mentioned is a neat example of the agonistic style of addition of variables: οὐδὲ ταύτην μὲν παραδραμών, ἀλλὰ ἀποβλέπων καὶ πρὸς ταῦτα λεπτοτέραν ἐποιήσατο τὴν κατακόπησιν (not missing that out, but paying attention to it, and in addition he made the distinction drawing more subtle). Wuilleumier (1927) argues that this Byzantine document preserved earlier sources.

276. On the meanings of the Moon, see Préaux 1973.

277. Hahm 1977.

278. *SHA, Severus Alexander* 44.4.

279. See, e.g., 1899, 428: "of this chaos of nonsensical systems, the bulk of which is like the lather of fermenting brains" cf. 254, 422, etc.

280. In physiognomics involution operates on a much simpler basic scheme. In medicine we find progressive hairsplitting on the model of διαίρεσις (*diairesis,* division), whose origin was Platonic, but which became the hallmark of the τέχνη (*technē*). While with astrology we have a constant addition of variables to consider, in the subdivision of types of

pulse, we have the addition of extra variables at different levels in the hierarchy of classification, whose basic structure is easier to perceive.

281. E.g., *Tetrabiblos* 2.9.19, p. 90, 1–13.

282. R. R. Newton (1977) concluded that the probability that Ptolemy actually observed the stars himself was around 10^{-200}! Newton's argument, however, has been much contested. See Gingerich 1980.

283. Wright 1984.

284. See Juvenal, *Satire* 6.565–81. Not every literary astrologer thought it appropriate to discuss catarchic astrology: neither Ptolemy nor Paul of Alexandria, nor his commentator Heliodorus, mentions it, nor does Firmicus deal with it.

285. Καταρχαί from the fifth century in Neugebauer and Van Hoesen: nos. L475, L478 are about journeys. L486 is on the arrival of a prefect in Alexandria and L487 on distressing letters contrary to expectation. L479 is a typical inquiry about a ship not arrived in Smyrna from Alexandria. L483 less typically asks "concerning a small lion, whether he will be tamed."

286. See *CCAG* 6, pp. 64, 26–65, 21, for a complex example: it is about the lost linen of a slave girl and examines all the positions of the planets. *CCAG* 7, pp. 90–95 affords a simplified one. The passage, translated in part by P. G. Maxwell-Stuart (1975), displays a schema to be used for finding thieves, composed by a Christian astrologer, of unknown date and name.

Chapter 2

1. *Physiognomonics* would be the more correct etymological derivation, but *physiognomics* is a more familiar term.

2. Johann Caspar Lavater (1741–1801), born in Zurich.

3. E.g., Tytler 1982; Cowling 1988. E. C. Evans, who has written most on ancient physiognomics in English, has confined her original contributions to examinations of the relations between the discipline's tenets and literary works. Evans 1935, 1941, 1945, 1969; cf. Couissin 1953.

4. English astrologer, prominent in the civil war on the Parliamentary side (1602–81).

5. Kerby-Miller 1950, 208, cited in Tytler 1982, 47.

6. See, e.g., Macmullen 1966, 95–162.

7. Suetonius, *Titus* 2. On metoposcopes predicting death, cf. Pliny, *HN* 35.88.

8. See, e.g., Gilman 1976; Cowling 1988; Didi-Huberman 1982; Balferretti 1975. Cesare Lombroso (1836–1909) offers the best-known primary material. See Lombroso 1864, 1876, 1893.

9. The Foucauldian concept of "biopower" certainly offers opportunities: one could chronicle, following the work of Aline Rousselle, the direct impact of physiognomical ideals on elite bodies, from the nurse's molding and swaddling at birth on through the strictures on decorum at all stages of education. See "Le corps opprimé: l'enfant" in Rousselle 1983. Maud Gleason (1990) follows this line of inquiry.

10. Foerster: *Scriptores Physiognomici* 1:lxxv. Henceforth all the texts in Foerster will be referenced according to the same convention as Galenic texts in Kühn's edition. Thus, this reference would read F.1.lxxv.

11. Polemo actually does curse one of the people he uses as an example: F.1.130, 5–6.

12. Gorgias, *Helen* 10; Plato, *Euthydemus* 288B–C; *Protagoras* 315A; *Menexenus* 235A; *Phaedrus* 271C 10; cf. De Romilly 1974.

13. Plutarch, *Pericles* 8. The Second Sophistic was the label attached by Philostratus, the chronicler of these Sophists operating under the Roman empire, in order to imply that

there was a second wave that was in some way akin to the Sophists in the fifth century B.C. Though misleading, it is a useful label for the Sophists of the period centering on the second century A.D. For Sophists and sorcery, see Bowersock 1969, 116–17.

14. The term, originally referring to the conjuring up of souls, is most famously used of rhetoric in Plato's *Phaedrus* (261a, 7–8).

15. Arist. *Rhet.* 1.2.1356a2; 4–13; cf. 1.15.1376a23–29: advice to show the opponent's worthlessness. Quint. *Inst.* 6.2.8–19.

16. On oneiromancy, see Pack 1941. On common learning: see Foerster's selection of quotations, F.2.241ff., especially Cicero, *De Fato* 4.7; *De Divinatione* 1.36.79, 2.46.96, 42.89; *De Natura Deorum* 2.6.17, 16.42. Vitruvius 6.1.3, 9–11. Sextus Empiricus *Outlines of Pyrrhonism* 1.85; *Adversus mathematicos* 5.95–101. Tertullian, *De Anima* 20, 25. Clement of Alexandria, *Paedagogus* 3.5.29–33. Hippolytus, *Refutatio omnium haeresium* 4.15–27; Firmicus, *Mathesis* 1.1, 3–4. Lactantius, *De Opificio dei:* 8.11, 12.12. Alexander of Tralles: *De Oculis* 2; Puschmann 1896, 174, 11–25 (F.2.241, 20–249, 8).

17. On Rufus and Galen's commentaries, see Wasserstein 1982. See also Galen's remarks in *On the Temperaments* 2.5 (p. 67, 27–29) K.1.611.5; on hair types of the races and their κράσεις, pp. 74.16–75.2, etc.) and below.

18. Hippocratic foundation: Galen, *Quod animi mores,* 57, 10–13 = K.4.798. Similarities: see, e.g., Galen's advice on studying the eyes even of the healthy for the character of the soul as well as of the sick for prognosis (*Therapeutics to Glaucon* [*Glauc.*] K.11.11).

19. Galen, *On Prognosis* pp. 100, 7–102, 27; 102, 27–104, 8 = K.14.633–34. Polemo, F.1.268f. The first Galen passage is an example of a *topos* in medical writing: Galen refers to the story of Erasistratus' discovering "the young man's love for his father's concubine," a story told with variants by various writers; there is a similar story told of Hippocrates: see Nutton 1979, 195–96. Valerius Maximus, in his account of the same anecdote, offers an astrologer called Leptines as an alternative to Erasistratus (5.7), illustrating the closeness of all three disciplines.

20. For the blood, see the remarks taken from Loxus Medicus at Anon. sec. 2 = F.2.4.

21. Polemo: madness F.110, 25–112, 1; 156, 17–20 (epilepsy?); 164, 19–21; cf. Anon. sec. 41 = F.2.59; Celsus *On Medicine,* 3.18; Caelius Aurelianus, *On Acute Diseases* 1.4ff., 42ff, 3.107; *On Chronic Diseases* 1.144ff. Epilepsy (Anon. sec. 29 = F.2.45–46), Caelius Aurelianus, *On Chronic Diseases* 1.60); apoplexy (Anon. sec. 39 = F.2.56, F.1.114, 21–116, 1 (conjectured); deafness Anon. sec. 82 = F.2.110.

22. K.19.530, 3–10. On the *Prognostica de decubitu ex mathematica scientia,* see chapter 1, n. 133.

23. Loxus: Anon. sec. 1 = F.2.3. Adamantius' use of Oribasius: see n. 55. Timocrates: Philostratus, *VS* 1.25 (536); Clement, *Miscellanies* 1.21.135.

24. See E. C. Evans 1945, 287–96, especially 291f. For examples of relevant passages, see F.2.283, 25–299, 22.

25. Evans 1945, 25. Galen is, in fact, in this treatise mainly concerned with arguments about moral philosophy with Platonists and Stoics.

26. *Temp.* 2.6, pp. 71.12–73.5. K.1.622–25.

27. *PHP* pp. 320, 29–322, 8 = K.5.463–4.

28. K.1.332, 2–334, 11. Kollesch (1988) has questioned the authenticity of this treatise, most famous of all in the Galenic canon in medieval times.

29. *Outlines of Pyrrhonism* 1.85.

30. Years of life: *HN* 11.273–74. Endorsements: *HN* 11.138: face and eyebrows reveal

emotion; 134: blinking cowardly; 70.185, hairy heart: brave and resolute (backed up by the dissection of Aristomenes the Messenian); 79.200: belly as indication of greed and stupidity with reference to animals.

31. *Oneirocritica* 2.69. Pack (1941) argues that this is because of Artemidorus' association with Ephesus and consequent enmity with Smyrna and its physiognomists.

32. See the evidence collected in Anderson 1989.

33. Aristotle, *Rhet.* 1.9.1367b7–11: "We must also take into account the nature of our particular audience when making a speech of praise, for as Socrates used to say, it is not difficult to praise Athenians with an Athenian audience. If the audience esteems a given quality, we must say that our hero has that quality, no matter whether we are addressing Scythians or Spartans or philosophers. Everything, in fact, that is esteemed we are able to represent as noble"; 1.2.1356b 32–35: "rhetoric will not consider what seems probable in each particular case . . . but that which seems probable to a class of persons" (both trans. W. Rhys Roberts). Adaptation to audience mood in forensic oratory: 2.1.1377b 28–1378a 3.

34. Bottéro 1974, 70f.

35. Cited in Bottéro, 82, 108–9.

36. Naturally, divining the character is, in a sense, divining the future in foretelling how a person will behave.

37. Rare exceptions are the metoposcopes, both the one who examined Britannicus and the one cited by the first-century grammarian Apion, who divined the ages and length of life of subjects of portraits by Apelles (Pliny, *HN* 35.88). The learned treatises seem to minimize the predictive function. Polemo does discuss ways in which he used physiognomics to tell the future and concludes with praise of this use of the art (F.1.282, 6–292, 27). These examples, however, end a sequence of character types, and three at least involve divination of intention (by pathognomical analysis): the unmasking of a liar and hypocrite (F.1.290, 20–292, 22) and two prophecies that the bride at a wedding would be (consentingly) abducted before the ceremony by her true lover (F.1.286, 1–290, 12). Only the prediction of the bereavement of the woman whose clothes leave only her nose and eyes visible and of the man threatened by death not from external disease seem pure prediction (F.1.282, 11ff.). The theme of attempted disguise on the part of the subject also recurs (cf. n. 2).

38. Cf. Joly 1962, 10, who points out that Bouché-Leclercq only devotes one page of his great work on astrology to "les qualités de l'âme" (Bouché-Leclercq 1899, 433).

39. Diogenes Laertius, 2.45; Cicero, *De Fato* 5.10; cf. *Tusculan Disputations* 4.37.80.

40. Socrates: Apuleius, *De Dogmate Platonis* 1.1; cf. Xenophon, *Memorabilia* 3.10.5. Pythagoras: Aulus Gellius, 1.9; Porphyry, *Vita Pythagorae* 13.

41. *Anthologia Palatina* 7.661 (Theocritus 10.1, p. 196 [Gow-Page]).

42. As Gleason (1989) points out, attempts to deceive observers about one's true nature form a common theme in discussions of physiognomics: see Polemo F.1.256, 7–258, 21. Anon. sec. 11 = F.2.19–20, sec. 39, sec. 52, sec. 72, sec. 132. Cf. Caelius Aurelianus, *On Chronic Diseases* 4.9.131–32.

43. Diogenes Laertius 7.173 (3d c. A.D.); Dio Chrysostom (c. A.D. 40–113 [?]); *Orations* 33.53–54 does not name Cleanthes. Cf. Anon. sec. 11 = F.2.20. Clement of Alexandria refers to κιναίδοι (effeminates) and adulterers "shamelessly making through their noses sounds of lewdness and fornication to provoke lust . . . sometimes they make a sound in their nose like a frog" (*Paedagogus* 3.5.29).

44. Petronius, *Satyricon* 126.3. The context is humorous; she can tell that the hero demands money for his favors. Whether this can be taken as evidence for any penetration of

physiognomical learning into the lower ranks of society is doubtful. Philostratus mentions a *grammaticus* who is also a physiognomist (Megistias of Smyrna) at *VS* 2.27 (618), but he is unlikely to be a humble schoolteacher.

45. *Epidemics* 2.6.1. Cf. 2.5.1; 2.5.16; 2.5.23; 2.6.14, 19; 6.4.19; *On Regimen* 1.36.

46. 6.15: Περὶ τῶν σοφιστῶν φυσιογνωμονικός (Physiognomical Work on the Sophists). Cf. Athenaeus 14.656.

47. Aristotle, *Generation of Animals* 4.3.769b. Pseudo-Aristotle, *Physiognomonica* (*Phgn.*) 805a19f.

48. Pliny *HN* 11.273–74. Diogenes Laertius 5.25 (based on Ariston of Ceos, late 3d c. B.C.). Cf. Aristotle, *Fragments* 14 (Rose).

49. See F.1.xviii f. For an attempt to subject it to a logical analysis: *Analytica Priora* 2.27.70b6–39. For related interests, see especially *Historia Animalium* 1.9.491b12–492b, 3 (metoposcopy and the signification of eyes, eyebrows, eyelids, and ears); 1.1.488b, 25 (animals' characters); *De Anima* 2.9.421a23–27 (hardness of flesh and natural endowment); *De Partibus Animalium* 2.2.647b1–651a4 (cf. Anon. sec. 2: blood's influence on soul), 3.4.667a9f. (heart's influence on soul; cf. Polemo F.1.110, 17–39), 4.5.774b1–3 (hairier: more lustful), 5.7.786b35–787a, 2 (deep voices are superior). *Politics* 7.6.1327b19–36 (effect of climate on mores). Of disputed works: *Problemata* 10.48.896a38–39 (chiromancy); 34.1.963b18–19 (porous teeth: short-lived). See also F.2.256, 12–271, 24 and Evans 1969, 7–10, 22–4.

50. Von Premerstein 1908, 46ff. He depends, however, on the identification of "the enemy of the emperor" with the conspirator Lusius Quietus (on which see chap. 3). Cf. Christ, Schmid, and Stählin 1961 (1924) 2.2, 693.

51. *Codex Bodleianus Clarkianus* 11 fd. 77, in *Anecdota Oxoniensium* 4.255.

52. *Codex Leidensis* 1206. Date: Hoffmann: F.1.96 (757 years after the Hegira). At F.1.lxxx Foerster gives the date as 1356, having calculated using the wrong date for the Hegira, though he uses the correct date of 622 when calculating the date of the Constantinople epitome (lxxxvii).

53. The problems of the Arabic are discussed in Gleason 1989, 412; cf. Hoffmann's preface (F.1.95–96).

54. Apart from Adamantius these are the MS *Matritensis* N. 73, fols. 219–23 (F.1.cxxiv-v, 320–47, 351–59, 386–424), a slightly different, less reliable fragment of an epitome that can sometimes be used to establish the correct reading in difficult passages; "Pseudo-Polemo" (F.1.cxxv-cxxx and 298–431); and the seventeenth-century Arabic Constantinople epitome (F.1.lxxxvii). Adamantius' epitome is the basis of this work by an unknown Byzantine transmitted by several MSS that attribute it to Polemo himself. It is completed by some late editions (F.1.427–31). The Anonymous Latin author also sometimes preserves a fuller version of Polemo.

55. F.1.ci-ciii. Rose (*Anecdota Graeca* 1, 25) connects him with the author of a medical work, the Περὶ ἀνέμων (On Winds) (ed. ibid. 29–48), and with the author cited by Oribasius (*Synopsis* 3.24, 25, etc.), and by Paul of Aegina (7.26), for medical recipes, who would have lived in the first half of the fourth century.

56. On Loxus, see Misener 1923.

57. No author's name is given in the oldest MSS. See Kelter 1890, 48; Evans 1969, 76; and Sabbah 1978, 423, 563.

58. Jüttner 1967. It is not certain when he died, but Fronto heard him declaim in Italy in 143 (*Epistles* 2.5.3).

59. Reardon 1971, 107–9.

60. Boulanger 1923, 93. Donald Russell (1983, 4), on the other hand, considers it lacks the ῥοῖζος (rushing style) for which Polemo was famous.

61. *VS* 1.22 (525).

62. Thus, Millar 1977, 385ff., who cites several instances in which the success of the hearing was materially affected by the reactions of the emperors to the orators. It was "an unquestioned assumption" that rhetoric was crucial (433–34 on *Inscriptiones Latinae Selectae* 6680). Cf. Marrou 1956, 294, who points to the "efficacité politique" resulting from the universally recognized prestige of the oratorical art. Bowie himself, while suggesting that the epideictic style was unsuitable for political life, admits that there are three passages suggesting that Sophistic rhetoric was regarded as politically useful (Plutarch, *Precepts of Statecraft* 814a–c; Dio Chrysostom, *Orations* 18.2–3, 47.1). For Philostratus' evidence, see especially *Lives of the Sophists* (*VS*) 2.5 (570), 2.9 (582), 2.30 (622–23), and 2.30 (626).

63. Philostratus, *VS* 1.25 (531–44). Notable events include: embassy to Hadrian brings gifts to Smyrna: 531; free travel / entourage: 532; imperial letter to Smyrna defending his use of Hadrian's money / dedication of the Olympieion: 533; accredited in Hadrian's will / insult to Antoninus: 534; forgiven: 540; and cf. embassy to Trajan: 1.21 (520–21). Further testimonials to his legendary abilities occur at 1.22 (524–25), 1.24 (529), 2.1 (564), 2.10 (589), 2.15 (595), 2.16 (597), and 2.25 (609).

64. *VS* 1.25 (531). The quarrel is referred to as one of the feuds over an ass's shadow by Dio Chrysostom (*Orations* 34.48). For other feuds in Asia Minor over rights to imperial cult centers, see Tacitus, *Annals* 4.55; and Dio Cassius 59.28.1. For the subsequent history of the quarrel (over honorific titles): *Sylloge Inscriptionum Graecarum*[3] 849d, no. 2. (On the particular incident, see section 8a.)

65. καὶ ὅσα ἐπετύχομεν παρὰ τοῦ κυρίου Καίσαρος Ἁδριανοῦ . . . (and how much we got from Lord Caesar Hadrian [through Polemo] . . .), *Inscriptionnes Graecae ad res Romanas pertinentes* 1431.1.33.

66. Delivery (ὑπόκρισις) in Aristotle was one-third of the training. While he compared it to acting, he speaks of the voice only: *Rhet.* 3.1.1403bff. Theophrastus probably added bodily movements: Diogenes Laertius 5.48. In the Roman orators it was one-fifth of the training: Cicero, *De Inventione* 1.7.9; *De Oratore* 1.131, 142; *Rhet. ad Her.* 1.2.3; Quint. *Inst.* 3.3.1ff. In general, see: *Rhet. ad Her.* 3.11.19–15.27; Quint., *Inst.* 11.3.1–184 (*actio*).

67. *VS* 1.25 (537). This was a tactic normal in *contiones* (popular addresses: *Rhet. ad Her.* 3.15.27), though Quintilian had reservations about excessive use of *inambulatio* (walking around: *Inst.* 11.3.126; cf. Cicero, *De Oratore* 3.59.220).

68. Maximus of Tyre, *Philosophoumena* 25.3; Dio Chrysostom, *Orations* 31.162–63. On the gait, cf. Clement of Alexandria, *Paedagogus* 3.11.73.

69. For near-contemporary rhetorical handbooks, see "Hermogenes," "Menander Rhetor," and Theon. E.g., Hermogenes, *Progymnasmata,* main divisions: race and city, family, events at birth, upbringing, education, bodily and mental qualities, accomplishments, actions, external blessings, length of life, manner of death, number of children (15, 18–17, 2). Aphthonius under the biggest heading—actions—considers divisions by soul, body, and fortune (22, 6). Theon under ἀγαθά (good things) considers things to do with the soul and character, the body and externals. "Menander" justifies describing physical beauty, concentrating on glance, beard, eyes, hair, and so on but advises: "to avoid scandal, work up his personality and considerable dignity" (398, 14f.). Ψόγος (invective) was taken to use the same topics to opposite effect (Aristotle, *Rhet.* 1.9.1368a33–37; Aphth. 27, 17–18 (Rabe); Theon (Spengel) 2.112, 17–18; *Rhet. ad Her.* 3.6.10 and 14.): e.g., the dubious

parentage, the ominous omens at birth, poverty, evils of appearance, the terrible institutions founded. (Quint. *Inst.* 3.7.19ff., on *vituperatio.*) Less attention is devoted to it in the rhetorical treatises; only Theon and Aphthonius discuss it under a separate heading, perhaps because it was less dignified and thus less suitable for discussion in a rhetorical treatise: Quintilian (*Inst.* 12.9.8ff.) advises sparing use of invective for the ideal orator, as too much is unworthy. For the figures used to describe the person: Cicero, *De Oratore* 3.204; *Orator* 138; *Topics* 83, Quint. *Inst.* 6.2.17. Ἔκφρασις: (*ekphrasis*) Hermog. 22, 7–10; Aphth. 36, 21–37, 3; Theon 2.118, 6–120, 11 may be used of anything, εἰκονισμός (*eikonismos*) of people only. εἰκονισμός: Polybios (Spengel 3.108). χαρακτηρισμός/*effictio: Rhet. ad Her.* 4.49.63 (of bodily form). Tryphon (Spengel 3.201, 27ff.), Cocondrios (ibid., 241), Polybios (ibid., 108, 32). ἠθολογία: Quint. *Inst.* 6.2.17. *Descriptio: Rhet. ad Her.* 4.39.51; Cic. *De Oratore* 3.204; *Orator* 138; *Topics* 83. *Notatio,* review of character: *Rhet. ad Her.* 4.50.63.

70. This comes from *Phgn.* (808b2–4); cf. Aristotle, *De Partibus Animalium,* 675b26ff.; and Pliny, *HN* 79.200.

71. 2.27.70b, 6f. Citations from Burnyeat (unpub.), 22. I am much indebted to his paper in what follows.

72. Mode of reasoning translates συλλογισμός (*syllogismos*). *Rhet.* 2.22.1395b21–26. Cf. 1.11.1355a, 8–14.

73. "Dispositions follow bodily characteristics and are not in themselves unaffected by bodily impulses. Conversely that the body suffers sympathetically with affections of the soul is evident in love, fear, grief and pleasure" (805a1–2, 5–8; trans. W. S. Hett).

74. τὸ γὰρ δύνασθαί τινων ὄντων ἀναγκαῖον θεῖναι ἴδιον ὑπολαμβάνομεν φιλοσοφίας. (We take the ability to reason what is necessary, given certain conditions, to be the especial property of philosophers.)

75. Burnyeat (unpub.) has recently argued that the equation of an enthymeme with a truncated syllogism is mistaken.

76. *Rhet.* 1.2.13.1357a16ff.; 2.23.2–3.1295b22–26, 3.18.4.1419a18–19. Cf. Burnyeat (unpub.), 20.

77. Demetrius on the enthymeme: 30–33; the characterization of it as an incomplete syllogism: 32. Alexander Numenius' observation is reported by the Byzantine scholar Planudes: *Rhetores Graeci* 5, 403 (Walz).

78. Quint. *Inst.* 5.14.1, 24: "It has a major premiss and a minor premiss, but no conclusion: So it is an imperfect syllogism." Cf. 5.10.3: "Some call it a rhetorical syllogism, others an imperfect syllogism, because its parts are not so clearly defined or of the same number as the normal syllogism, since such precision is not specially needed by the orator." It should be stressed that this is not the only understanding of the enthymeme in the orators of the period; another influential view was that the enthymeme was a conclusion from incompatibles. What is important is that the enthymeme was commonly associated with an abbreviation of the syllogism.

79. Here the translator has probably read κητῶν (of sea monsters) for κυνῶν (of dogs). The former appears in Adamantius in the previous observation in which the sea monster's characteristics are savage-mindedness, foolishness, and impiety (see F.1.373, 9–74, 4). Anon. (sec. 48) also translates *maris beluae* (sea monster).

80. Dagron (1987, 71–72) thinks this facility is peculiar to animals. For him the use of other kinds of humans (women, foreigners), or of characteristic expressions for particular emotions, must be tautological. Burnyeat (1982) suggests that, in any case, for the Stoics the concept of knowledgeable seeing overrides the distinction between direct observation and inference.

81. Sassi (1988, 74), who presents physiognomical reasoning as being an enthymeme, or rhetorical syllogism in the second figure, in which the middle term *B* is predicated both in the major premise (the rule) and in the minor premise (the result), recasts the process of reasoning along the lines of Peirce's depiction of abduction (see chap. 3): *Rule:* All animals with psychic characteristic 'A' have the physical characteristic 'B.' *Result:* The animal 'C' has the physical characteristic 'B.' *Case:* The animal has the psychic characteristic 'A.'

82. Examples in rhetorical theory: Aristotle makes them the rhetorical equivalent of induction, as enthymemes are the equivalent of deduction. *Rhet.* 1.2.1356b, 2.25.1402b. If no enthymemes can be used, examples are to work for proof. If enthymemes can be used, examples may be used as witnesses, supplementary to the former: *Rhet.* 2.20.1394a. On examples generally, cf. Isocrates, *To Demonicus* 34; *Rhetoric to Alexander* 8.1429a-1430a. Invalidation of examples: Arist. *Rhet.* 2.25.1403a6–10; *Rhet. ad Her.* 2.29.46; Quint. *Inst.* 5.13.24; Cicero, *De Inventione* 1.30.49; Apsines (Spengel 1.375–76). On παράδειγμα (example) as a form of ὁμοίωσις (comparison), see below.

83. Reardon 1971, 109.

84. F.1.114, 6–116, 14. This comes after a promise to be brief, a promise often associated with the most detailed subdivision (see chap. 3 on Galen).

85. F.1.120, 9. Galen, too, often refers to a further stage of knowledge, which may be achieved by reading another of his books, or by long practice. See chap. 3.

86. F.1.158, 22–160, 2. The MS has "you will be able to know the situation of yourself and others."

87. See, e.g., F.1.112, 23–24; 136, 17–19; 148, 2–6; 156, 20–22; 166, 19–22; 192, 8–18; 208, 9–11.

88. Blinking: Pliny, *HN* 11.134; squint: 122, 24ff.; paleness: 244, 9–10.

89. Cf. André 1982, 19. See Sassi 1984a; 1988, 62–66, on the connections between drama from early Greece to New Comedy, the masks described by Pollux and modeled in Lipari, and physiognomical types.

90. Reading μιαρία (brutality) for the original, in which the Latin rendering *irrisionem* (a mocking character) follows the Arab translator's mistake (see F.1.lxxxii).

91. Sexes: F.1.192, 8ff.; animals: 170, 24ff.; races: 236, 9ff.; animals and sexes: 170, 6–9.

92. The eyes are accorded first place according to common opinion, as Foerster's quotations indicate (Cicero, *De Legibus* 1.27; Pliny, *HN* 11.145; Quint. *Inst.* 11.3.75–76; Lactantius, *De Opificio Dei* 8.11, 8.92). It is also the emphasis of rhetorical training (Cicero, *De Oratore* 3.59.221). In what Geneva Misener (1934) has termed "iconistic descriptions" (the accounts of personal appearance common to Egyptian tax collectors, advertisers of runaway slaves and retrospective biographers), however, the eyes are not singled out for special emphasis.

93. Sec. 10. On animal signs, cf. sec. 132.

94. The coding of character in Suetonius, who had certainly read physiognomical texts, is ambiguous enough for Couissin (1953, 244) to interpret Augustus as the incarnation of the eagle type and Evans (1969, 53) to understand him as an obvious lion type.

95. Cf., for such lists, Lucian, *De Saltatione* 29; Alciphron 4.19.6; Quint. *Inst.* 11.3.74, 178.

96. Bompaire 1923, 109. *Rhet.* 2.2–17.1378a–1391b. Cf. *Nicomachean Ethics* 4.7.1127a21–27, which discusses ἀλαζών (the braggart), αὐθέκαστος (the self-willed man), εἴρων (the dissembler). Furley (1953), however, argues that Theophrastus' *Characters* has nothing to do with the ethical works; it is purely for rhetorical purposes. What is clear, at any rate, is that lists of character portraits were made for rhetorical use.

97. Quint. *Inst.* 9.3.99. On the influence of Theophrastus: ibid. 6.2.17.

98. Polemo lists the bold/strong type, the timid/cowardly, the literature lover, the apathetic, the impudent, the lover of elegance, the prudent/clever, the sad man, the androgyne or effeminate, the placid, the mocking, the avaricious, the malevolent or foolish, and the bitter, before proceeding to those whose destinies he foretold (F.1.268, 20ff.).

99. Despite the circumstantial sound of these accusations, fabrication of these types of accusation is sanctioned in rhetorical treatises. See Barton 1994.

100. Caster (1938, 79–93) has examined the tradition in order to explain how Lucian's treatment of Alexander of Abonoteichos uses it: "the most revolting accusations arise from pure and simple commonplaces of invective—the ancient audience would have been astonished had (the enemies of the polemicist) not been prostituted or assassinated someone." These themes of διαβολή: murder, attempted murder, theft, depraved morals, and lack of culture were all taught in the schools.

101. Head: F.1.236, 2–6. Mouth: 226, 21–28, 3. Nose: 228, 16–18. Cf. 214, 12f.: when the throat is rather hollow, do not praise it; attack instead.

102. The tense is not clear from the Arabic. F.1.148, 6–9; Anon. sec. 34.

103. See, e.g., Quint. *Inst.* 6.2.18: "Denique ἦθος omne bonum et comem virum poscit. Quas virtutes cum etiam in litigatore debeat orator, si fieri potest, approbare, utique ipse aut habeat aut habere credatur." (In sum, ēthos in all its forms demands that the speaker is a man of good character and courtesy. He needs to possess or be believed to possess those virtues for the possession of which it is his duty, if possible, to commend his client as well.) At 2.4.20 Quintilian remarks, in the context of praise and blame, that the character is molded by contemplation of vice and virtue.

104. F.1.138, 1–142, 3: A.D. 123; see Bowersock 1969, appendix 2.

105. Von Premerstein 1908, 46–71. See n. 49.

106. *In Pisonem* 1.1. Cf. *Pro Caecina* 10.27; *Post Reditum in Senatu* 6.13; *In Vatinium* 2.4; *In Verrem* 2.2.44. 108; *De Oratore,* 2.46.266.

107. *Tractatus Coislinianus* 8 (argued by Janko 1984, 42–90, to be Aristotle's lost *On Comedy*). Cic. *De Oratore* 2.236; cf. 238, 239, 248, 264, 266. See Plass 1988.

108. Pack (1941), following Mesk 1932, noted this, though he preferred to see it as a defensive use on Polemo's part. He compares the defensive tone of Adamantius F.1.298, 7ff., probably taken from Polemo's *prooemium.* The focus on contemporary examples in physiognomics, at least, goes back to its origins: note the title of Antisthenes' work of the fifth century: "Περὶ τῶν σοφιστῶν φυσιογνωμονικός" (Physiognomical Treatise about the Sophists). See n. 46.

109. Signs are *testes* (witnesses) or *indices* (informers); verbs like *denuntio* (denounce) and *prodo* (betray) are used regularly for their role. It is possible that the Arabic has intensified the judicial metaphor; in the variants in the manuscripts of Anon., however, the verb *indicare* (inform, give evidence about) is most common, and other verbs with judicial associations are prominent (see André 1981, 46).

110. The term τόπος has had different meanings for different authors; for many rhetoricians, following Aristotle, it is a kind of reasoning procedure. Here my use of italics with the transliterated form (topos/topoi) indicates the common meaning of *commonplace.*

111. Diogenes Laertius 1.33: some ascribe the observation to Socrates, some to Thales; a similar comment is attributed to Plato by Plutarch (*Marius* 46.1).

112. Much effort was devoted by the authors of rhetorical τέχναι (*technai*) toward subdividing the generic term of comparison. E.g., the Augustan Tryphon (Spengel 3.191, 23–192, 19; 200, 3f.) divides the generic term ὁμοίωσις (*homoiosis*) into three types; cf.

Polybios (ibid. 106). Cocondrios (ibid. 239) divides into six, while Herodian puts one of the six on a level with ὁμοίωσις Up to nine categories of one subdivision were possible: Polybios, ibid. 108. Quintilian refuses to subdivide too minutely: 5.11.30. Clearly, the general concept verged on example and was seen to bridge the gap between proof and ornament: *Rhet. ad Her.* 4.45.59; Cicero, *De Inventione* 1.30.49; Quint. *Inst.* 5.11.125, 14.34, 8.3.72.

113. Fraenkel 1950, 2:101ff.; 3:773.

114. *Rhet.* 3.2.10.1405a, 1.9.1368a.

115. In the Greek tradition, at least, the slave would make a fourth here (cf. Vegetti 1979; Sassi 1988), yet the slave is interestingly absent in Polemo, though it is a theme in the Peripatetic treatise (e.g., 811a1–4, 812b36–813a1). Perhaps there is a lack of consensus that would allow natural correlates to his servile condition in the Greek context, after the third century B.C. Polemo does once refer to an indication of servile character at F.1.204, 16–17 (thick legs and heels / stupidity). In Rome the looks of the slave of New Comedy may have been influential, in cases like the accusation of servile coloring leveled at Piso (see above), as Sassi (1988) suggests. Quintilian records an orator suggesting that his opponent had the face of a slave, though this was in the particular context of a case concerning his status: *Inst.* 6.3.32.

116. Examples of *descriptio* also use animals: *Rhet. ad Her.* 4.39.51.

117. Anon. sec. 10. On the attribution to Loxus, see Misener 1923.

118. F.1.194, 4–14, with contributions from Adamantius in square brackets (350, 12–351, 3). He offers γονύκροτος (knock-kneed) as the alternative to "beautiful" knees. The Arabic text is obscure in the last sentence: "a short stride, a dawdling walk, soft limbs; she is slow in her movements, but quick to fall over (?)."

119. Adamantius (F.1.350, 10–12) describes the female as ἀγεννές, πικρόν, δολερόν, κουφόνουν, ἄδικον, φιλόνεικον, θρασύδειλον (mean-spirited, bitter, cunning, frivolous, unfair, fond of quarrels, and brazen).

120. Tragedy: Hall 1989. Old Comedy: Henderson 1975, sec. 472. Roman Comedy: Lilja 1965, 68–70. Greek oratory: Süss 1910, 250. Roman oratory: Nisbet 1961; and Richlin 1983. The signs remained the same in the Christian context, as Clement of Alexandria makes clear: *Paedagogus* 2.7, 3.3ff.

121. On paradigms of effeminacy, see Gleason 1990, 394–99; and Edwards 1993, chapter 2.

122. The two accusations are not infreqently paired. Clement of Alexandria, *Paedagogus* 3.3.15–19 (F.2.304, 11–17), referring to a metoposcope. Philostratus tells us that Polemo actually spoke on the theme of "the adulterer unmasked" (VS 1.25 [532]). Favorinus was accused of adultery (by a man of consular rank), despite his eunuchism, according to Philostratus: it was presented as one of his paradoxical features (*VS* 1.8 [489]).

123. *Phgn.* 808a13–16; Polemo: F.1.276, 14–19; Adamantius F.1.415.4–6; *Matrit.* F.1.415, 9–11–416, 6–9. Pseudo-Polemo: 415, 15–17–416, 11–14, Anon. sec. 115 (F.2.134–135): κιναίδοι *(kinaidoi) /molles* sec. 98 = F.2.123–24: *androgyni.*

124. The Arabic text breaks off halfway through, so the following quotation is reconstructed with the help of Adamantius. The square brackets indicate Adamantius' version, the round Polemo's (F.1.276, 15–19; 415, 4–6, 416, 1–4).

125. Philostratus, *VS* 1.25 (536).

126. For the details of his life, see Philostratus, *VS* 1.8 (490).

127. Philostratus, *VS* 1.8 (490); 1.25 (537); (536).

128. Philiscus: *VS* 2.30 (623); Alexander: *VS* 2.5 (570–71).

129. Inferred from his disquisition on exile: Φαβωρίνου Περὶ φυγῆς (Favorinus' *On Exile*): Barigazzi 1966. On the reasons for using this as evidence, see appendix C.

130. Lucian (*Demonax* 12.13. F.), learning that Demonax was ridiculing his oratory as effeminate, went to ask him who he was to mock his lectures. "A man whose ears are not easy to deceive," replied D. and, when F. asked him what was his technical preparation for beginning philosophy, came up with the punchline "My virility." Another time F. asked D., "What is the doctrine to which you hold most in philosophy?" "Who told you I was a philosopher?" said D. and laughed as F. was going away. F. asked why he was laughing. "Because it seems nice that you, who don't have one, should want to judge a philosopher by his beard!" Polemo indulged in this milder wit himself occasionally: Philostratus, *VS* 1.25 (541).

131. Anon. translates Polemo here by *tensam frontem* (furrowed brow).

132. Drowning *androgyni:* MacBain 1982. *Androgyni* in the Monstrous Races: Friedman 1981; Wittkower 1951. *Monster* as a term of insult: Nisbet 1961.

133. Reverdin 1961; Dover 1974; Momigliano 1975; Whitehead 1977; Van der Vliet 1984; Hall 1989. See, e.g., of rough contemporaries, "Apollonius of Tyana," *Epistles* 21; Plutarch, *De Malignitate Herodoti* (*Mor.* 854E–874E); Scopelian at *VS* 1.21 (520); Lucian (a Syrian!): see Bompaire 1958, 228.

134. The concept of latitude is secondary to characterizing localities by the longest hours of daylight. See n. 142.

135. Vitruvius, *On Architecture* 6.1.6: Greece; 6.1.10: Rome. The earlier Greek version: Aristotle, *Politics* 7.6, 1327b29ff. For the Greeks it remained in Greece: Anon., *Life of Pythagoras,* in Photius, *Biblioteca* Cod. 249. See below on Ptolemy.

136. Trans. F. Granger. Cf. Pliny, *HN* 3.39.42; Seneca, *On Anger* 2.15.5.

137. Galen, *QAM* p. 64, 10–19. K.4.805.

138. Philosophical works: *De Natura Deorum* 2.6.17, 2.16.42. *De Fato* 4.7; *De Legibus* 1.9.26–27; 1.36.79. Speeches: *Pro Flacco* 7.17, 8.19, 11.24, 24.57 (Greek *levitas* [fickleness] and barbarian cruelty), 15.36 (Greek inconstancy: testimony worthless), 25.61, 2.62 (contrasts between Western and Asiatic Greeks: Asiatics fickle and cruel, testimony worthless), 27.65 (proverbs denigrating particular Asiatic groups), 28.71 (extravagance and fickleness); *In Verrem* 2.2.7 (Sicilians not fickle and lazy, as other Greeks); *De Lege Agraria* 2.95 (Sicilians liars). On the Northern barbarians: *In Pisonem* 53 (implies Piso is a Gaul); *Pro Fonteio* 21–33 (Celts godless; their garb, speech and gait are outlandish; they should not be believed). See Wardman 1976 and Sherwin-White 1967.

139. Dover 1974, 84f.; Whitehead 1977; Levin 1950.

140. See, e.g., Horace, *Odes* 3.24 (simple lives of Scythians, etc.); Tacitus, *Germania;* Dio Chrysostom, *Orations* 36 (the Borysthenic oration); Clement of Alexandria, *Paedagogus* 3.3.24–25; Pseudo-Quintilian, *Declamations* 3.16; Diogenes Laertius 1.101–2 (Anacharsis); Apsines: Spengel 1.339, 342, 351, 355 (theme: the Scythians stopped being nomadic and became ill). In general, cf. Bompaire 1958, 229ff.

141. Bompaire 1958, 222.

142. For the geographical/astronomical divisions of the earth, see Bouché-Leclercq (1899, 327–47). Cf. Dagron 1987, 78 n. 7.

143. Manilius 4.742–805; Dorotheus Sidonius 427–28; Paul of Alexandria 1.2.1. See Bouché-Leclercq 1899, 332.

144. In the Constantinople epitome of Polemo's treatise they are lacking in courage and look terrified.

145. 2.4.1 (76, 5). Boll (1894) notes some departures from the details of Ptolemy's

Geography and argues that the whole is derived from Posidonius. Bouché-Leclercq (1899) is skeptical: the triplicities must be Ptolemy's, even if the scheme according to parallels is Posidonius'.

146. Pure Greek type (F.1.242, 11–244, 2): "the build is half-way between tall and short, fat and thin; he is upright, with an attractive face and expression, his complexion is white with a tinge of red, he is fairly fleshy, with medium-sized hands and forearms. . . . He has a head neither big nor small, with a thick, strong neck, soft, red hair, both curly and combed straight[?], a square face, thin lips, a straight, moderate nose, and eyes which are moist, amber[?]-coloured and very mobile." Ideal male, opposite of the female, see above (F.1.194, 14–15); i.e., at least, presumably, a large head and mouth, coarse, light[?]-coloured hair, a wide face, a thick neck, a strong chest, strong, sinewy legs with little flesh on them and a clear[?] voice. Lion: F.1.196, 7–15: "A large head, wide brow, prominent eyebrows, deepset amber[?]-coloured eyes, a thick nose, thick jaw and mouth, a broad throat, strong neck and curly hair which reddens with age; huge shoulders[?], strong flanks, thighs and hips with little flesh on them, a broad chest, very sinewy fore- and hind legs, and similar knee joints, a clear voice, a walk with separated steps, deliberate, very modest[?]" Clement of Alexandria, too, links the male with the lion by his hairiness; a sign of strength and rule (*Paedagogus* 3.3.18).

147. See F.1.xcvii–xcix for comparisons of the *Codex Leidensis* with the Constantinople epitome. This list in Polemo mentions only Egyptians, Macedonians, Phoenicians, Cilicians, and Scythians, though other races are mentioned elsewhere.

148. Sherwin-White 1967, 3–4. Strabo on the Celtiberi in the past (θηριώδης, beastliness, 3.2.15), Lusitanians (δυσήμεροι, ἀγριώδης [untamed, wild], 3.3.6–8). Caesar on *feri barbari,* "wild barbarians" (some Gauls are, some are not: see *De Bello Gallico* 1.31.5 and bk.1 generally). Tacitus: Germans and Britons are no longer new and strange but beyond Suebia *mira feritas* (amazing beastliness, 46.1). Pliny, *HN* 6.50–55; 194–95. See Wiedemann 1986.

149. Dio Chrysostom (*Orations* 5) and Apuleius (*Florida* 6) evidence the interest of audiences in fabulous beasts from these regions.

150. Pliny, *HN* 7.2.23–32. See Reardon 1971 on Phlegon of Tralles and other paradoxographers of the Second Sophistic. The paradoxographers in general are collected in Westermann 1963 (1839) and Giannini 1965. Erudite delight: Lucian's sketch of the range of monstrous races living within a whale (!) (*Verae Historiae* 1.34ff.).

151. For Aristotle, in the context of reproduction, the birth of monsters is the triumph of the animal substrate, in that the influence that makes the embryo develop into a human is lacking. It is in this connection that he mentions the physiognomist who συνέπειθε πολλάκις λέγων (often persuaded [people] in saying) that every person can be classified as belonging to one of three animal types (*Generation of Animals* 769b20–22).

152. *Odyssey* 21.295, 304; *Iliad* 1.262f.; Plutarch *Theseus* 30; Diodorus Siculus 4.70; Hyginus *Fabulae* 31, 33; Pausanias 7.18.1; Aelian, *De Natura Animalium* 12.1.

153. In the Περὶ βλασφημιῶν (Taillardat) one finds κένταυρος (centaur, 414) and κέρκωψ (man-monkey, 417). Cf. F.2.278, 26–29, 5.

154. The "golden mean" is clearly related to the valuation of proportion and, thus, symmetry. Sambursky (1961, 30) observes that symmetry and proportion are at the roots of Greek science, art, and ethics. The Polycleitan canon delimits the good body; only the temperate soul is good; great importance is attached to geometrical equality (Plato, *Gorgias* 508A). These related notions are the basis of humoral theory: symmetry is an equal distance between extremes: Galen, *On Temperaments* p. 33, 5–6.

155. See Tytler 1982; and Baltrusaitis 1957.

156. For Dagron 1987 (see n. 79) the reference to animals was the foundation stone of physiognomics, because the other two methods (topoi) only function tautologously.

157. Zoological method, F.1.170, 24ff. List of ninety-four animal species (including *gallina* and *gallus,* [hen and cock], 172, 5–190, 3).

158. Ptolemy, *Tetrabiblos* 3.12.10, pp. 145–47.

159. Physiognomics lay too close to astrology to be popular with the church: see Hippolytus, *Refutatio Omnium Haeresium* 4.15.

160. Dagron 1987, 75–76. F.1.304, 5–11.

161. See, e.g., Midgely 1979 (philosophy); John Berger 1971, 1977 (art criticism); Thomas 1983 (modern history); Willis 1974 (anthropology).

162. Berger 1971, 1977. I do not count the ubiquitous "pets" of the industrialized world, since they are treated more as people than animals by their owners. Any sign of animal nature in a pet is an embarrassment.

163. Loraux points out that even this praise is put into question (1978, 63–65).

164. Loraux 1978, 60. She rejects the idea that it is a totemic relation, because there is no totemic system in the Lévi-Straussian sense.

165. Cf. Tapper 1989; and Aristotle *Rhet.* 1.9.35.1367b: closeness of counsel and praise. Clearly, the fables of Aesopian type are the best example of this.

166. Cf. Vegetti 1979.

167. So in Attic orators θηρίον (wild beast) is a normal derogatory term (see Dover, 1974, 74), and in Ciceronian invective *belua* or *bestia* (beast) is a primary insult (*In Pisonem* 1.1 and 8; Nisbet *ad loc.* Cf. *Philippic* 2.30). See also Lilja 1965; and Suetonius, Περὶ Βλασφημιῶν (On Insults).

168. Alternative to rough: *deficiens* (weak), to coarseness (*asperitatis*), *strenuitatis* (vigor), *malignitatis* (MS *aviditatis,* greed). F.1.156, 7–10, 252, 3–4.

169. F.1.196, 1–7. Anon. sec. 8 = F.2.13.

170. Toynbee 1973. See especially the Late Antique mosaic from Antioch-on-Orontes.

171. Quint. *Inst.* 11.3.160; cf. *VS* 1.25 (536). See Gleason 1989, 404 n. 59.

172. Zagianaris 1977.

173. L'Orange 1947, 12f., 22f., 110f. Evans 1935, 1969. Dagron 1987, 75.

174. Gordon 1980, 26f. (Seneca *De Benevolentia* 2.9.1; Aulus Gellius 5.9; Aelian, *De Natura Animalium* 7.23, 5.39).

175. Pliny feels he should refute these stories: 8.17.19.

176. Anon. sec. 122 = F.2.138–39; see Misener 1923.

177. *Comica Adespota* Fr. 478. *Lysistrata* 1014–15.

178. *Ox:* huge orbs of eyes—foolish, gentle, naive (F.1.108, 10–12); hollow eyes—noisy, tumultuous (192, 4–8); eyes turned up—foolish, lazy, evil-minded, greedy, lustful, drunken, licentious (122, 4–7). *Ass:* foolish, etc. (122, 4–7), noisy, etc. (192, 4–8). *Ram/goat:* lazy, reckless (266, 5–8). *Pig:* "If eyebrow hair so long it reaches sides of forehead and temples—much lust and pig-like nature" (254, 18–256, 1). *Goat:* glittering eyes, of marble color, or a lot of thigh hair—debauched (248, 1–4; 252, 7–9). *Cock:* shining, lively eyes—womanizer (248, 8–10). If the neck is like a cock's crest—no knowledge or intelligence (220, 16–18). But though the *dog* is vile and quarrelsome (226, 10–13), immodest (248, 4–6), irritable (268, 11–14), and flattering (262, 23–264, 2), as a well-bred hound it compares with lions (228, 7–9), and the *horse,* though noisy, violent, and rash (262, 13–17), has a great mind (254, 12–13). Thus, it basks in the glory of man's exalted pursuit, the hunt.

179. See Henderson 1975, 131–33: female: see under χοῖρος (piglet), δέλφαξ (pig), ὗς (pig), ταῦρος (bull), κύων, etc.; and see horse (84), ram (87), bull (89), dog (88). Male: pig (110f.), sow (113f.), dog (117f.), bull (120), horse (?) (84). Adams (1982, 28–34) is a little more skeptical. This suggestion comes from Leach's analysis of English animal names (1964).

180. *Seasnake:* lips as big as mouth in the example of a tyrannical, insidious poisoner (148, 23–150, 23). *Crab:* man with small, red eyes and thus called "Crab," from Lydia (144, 4–16). Not prudent or intelligent, with a very cutting tongue, a greedy rascal. *Tortoise:* the description of this example has unfortunately been lost (190, 19–20).

181. Crocker 1977, 42, following Fernandez 1971.

182. Dio Cassius, 55 (56) 9; Cumont 1918.

183. *VS* 2.30 (622).

184. *On Prognosis* p. 68, 18–21 = K.14.600. For Attalus and Maximus, see Nutton ad loc. For the potential political power of doctors, see also the entire diatribe in the *prœmium* to *On Prognosis* and especially the attack on those ("the Methodists") "who announce they can teach the arts in a very short time and so assemble a host of pupils through whom they themselves acquire influence in their cities."

185. Millar 1977, 435.

186. Anderson (1989) sets out the evidence for the audience of the Sophists and their political role.

187. *Rhet.* 3.14.1415b.

Chapter 3

1. See the remarks in my introduction. Though earlier writers than Galen are credited with the "discovery" of the diagnostic value of the pulse, he was involved in the process of bringing about this consensus on its value, which must be the process examined in a socializing understanding of science (Brannigan 1981). I consider his predecessors in this regard below.

2. Ginzburg (1983 [1980], 81). It corresponds to the concept of μῆτις discussed by Detienne and Vernant 1978 (1974). They blame Plato for being the first to condemn this craftsman's knowledge as inferior, not qualifying as real ἐπιστήμη.

3. He follows up the remarks of the art critic Edgar Wind (1964), who speaks of the artist's "giv[ing] himself away, as a criminal might be spotted by a fingerprint" and of the interest of "modern psychology" in our "inadvertent little gestures" in his appreciation of the "Morelli method."

4. He draws on the work of Bottéro (1974) cited in chapter 2.

5. Ginzburg 1983, 113. *Coniector,* as in Cicero, *On Divination* 1.58.132.

6. Morelli and Freud were trained as doctors, as was Conan Doyle, who makes Holmes pursue some aspects of medical studies, though in a somewhat unorthodox fashion: Watson is horrified to learn before meeting his prospective fellow lodger that such is his zeal for exact knowledge that he beats the corpses in the dissecting rooms in order to establish the potential for bruising after death. Ginzburg also points out the early involvement of medical symptomatology in the Mesopotamian treatises on divination and pauses to glance at Hippocratic medicine, which, he argues, "clarified its methods by analyzing the central concept of the symptom [σημεῖον]" in its attempt to establish histories of each disease.

7. Galen, *On Plethora* (*Plenit.*) K.7.580, 18–581, 6; *On Curing through Blood-Letting* (*Ven. Sec.*) K.11.285, 10–12; *Therapeutic Method* (*Meth. Med.*) K.10.205, 15–206, 6; *On*

Regimen in Acute Diseases (*Dict. Acut.*) p. 197, 1–12 = K.15.585; *Hygiene* (*San. Tu.*) p. 57, 28–34 = K.6.129. On the precise meaning of στοχαστικὴ τέχνη, see the remarks of Allen (forthcoming).

8. Truzzi 1983. Sebeok and Umiker-Sebeok 1983; Carettini 1983; and Eco 1983. Sebeok and Umiker-Sebeok point out that Peirce also had medical connections and, indeed, makes reference to Galen (1983, 29). For a thorough exegesis of "abduction" in Peirce's work, see Fann 1970.

9. On *firasa*, see Mourad 1939. On the Stoics, see chapter 2.

10. Baring-Gould 1968, 1:159.

11. See *Protreptic* (*Protr.*) 5, p. 107, 4–6 = Kaibel, p. 4, 16–19 = K.1.7; *On His Own Books* (*Lib. Prop.*) 11, p. 116, 20–26 = K.19.40; *On the Method of Healing* (*Meth. Med.*) 1.4, K.10.32, 5ff.; *Ven. Sec.* K.11.256, 2–18; *On Prognosis* (*Praecog.*) p. 120, 12 = K.14.55. In *The Best Doctor Is a Philosopher* (*Opt. Med.*) 1, p. 1, 1–9 = K.1.53, Galen attempts to attribute a geometrical model to his ideal Hippocrates. Cf. Vegetti 1981 and Deichgräber 1970, 100, 103.

12. The complex relationship between the need for reason and experience in medicine is discussed in Frede 1981.

13. The autodidact is idealized especially in *On Examining the Best Physicians* (*Med. Cogn.*), while the impression that he offers the key to fame and fortune is left particularly in *On Prognosis*.

14. The term appears most frequently in the work of Galen, most obviously infused with religious discourse (*On the Usefulness of the Parts* [*UP*]. At 7.14, 1, pp. 418, 19–419, 8 = K.3.576–77, he claims that the "mystery" he offers is not inferior to those at Eleusis, or Samothrace, in showing the wisdom, providence, and power of the creator of animals and implicitly compares himself to a hierophant. Interestingly, it is in this context that he claims originality in relation to other anatomists. At 12.6, 2, p. 196, 5–15 = K.4.21, he equates knowledge of the demonstrative method with initiation into the mysteries. In *Temperament and Force of Simple Drugs* (*Simp. Med.*) 7.1, K.12.2, 2–8, in the second prooemium, he refers to the fact that books of the mysteries are not meant to be read by the profane; though some laymen may read them, his books are not for the untrained.

15. Sebeok and Umiker-Sebeok remark on Holmes's self-presentation as thaumaturge, in Eco and Sebeok 1983, 44–46.

16. See chapter 1 n. 127. "Whereas some of his contemporaries, like Pamphilus and Xenocrates, were less scrupulous about what they accepted, Galen's reliance upon astronomy and dreams is conditioned by the logical demonstration by which they are tested." (Nutton 1979, 172). Nutton (1985) offers a useful illustration of the great variety of healers.

17. Strong attacks on Sophists and orators, e.g., *Praecog.* p. 74, 3–8 = K.14.605, *Commentary on Hippocrates's Prognostics* (*In Hipp. Progn.*) 1.4, p. 205, 3–8 = K.18B.15–16; cf. *PHP* p. 651, 14–16 = K.5.651, 1–3; p. 179, 6–12 = K.5.221, 6–8. On Galen's ambivalent attitude to rhetoric generally, see Pearcy 1983.

18. Bowersock (1969) devotes chapter 5 ("The Prestige of Galen") to Galen.

19. *Meth. Med.* 8.3, K.10.560, 4–561, 7. See Kollesch 1981.

20. Scarborough (1981) inserts a proper note of skepticism about Galen's account of his achievements with his investigation of contemporary evidence, which does little to bear out the picture in the corpus. Nutton (1984) does something, however, to rescue Galen's high reputation with his contemporaries. *On Prognosis* narrates his rise to fame, emphasizing the effects of his amazing prognoses and cures. For this rhetoric to work, as he makes clear, influential friends had to play brokering roles.

21. Edelstein (1967, 65) notes that ever since the work of Ermerins (1832) modern scholars have interpreted prognosis as the objectively significant knowledge of what the outcome of the sickness will be and that Littré and Daremberg, the editors of the Hippocratic corpus, formulated the "still accepted judgement" that prognosis constitutes the scientific achievement of ancient medicine (Littré [1839–61] 1.451ff., 413–14; Daremberg 1855, 121–22. Lloyd (1968) puts forward the view that Edelstein overstressed the propaganda angle and neglected the parallels with modern medicine: ancient doctors "recognized that knowledge of the outcome of the disease would enable the doctor to heal his patients better."

22. "The lay public who watched in amazement the doctor's prognoses come true was not always going to accept that reasoning and observation lay behind these astonishing successes or to be prepared to learn the theory of prognosis" (Nutton 1979, 233).

23. Peirce's mature formulation, according to Fann (1970), was that the three processes were to be seen as successive in scientific practice. Abduction invents or proposes the hypothesis; it is the only logical operation that introduces any new ideas. This is followed by deduction, which explicates the hypothesis, deducing from them the necessary consequences that may be tested, and finally by induction, as the experimental consequences are actually tested.

24. Hankinson (1988) points out the history of explicit effort to base divination on a rational foundation, accessible to everyone, not just those with a talent for prophecy, and the denials of difference in method between scientific and inductive inference from Plato onward (*Phaedrus* 244C) and most subtly argued by the Stoics. See, e.g., Diogenes Laertius 7.149; and Cicero, *On Divination* bk. 1.

25. The ἦθος was the first of Aristotle's canonical elements of rhetoric, and it refers to all the factors that lead to the audience's putting their trust in the speaker. See introduction, chapter 2.

26. As Scarborough (1981, 8) notes, Marcus Aurelius himself comments disparagingly on doctors, among other βάναυσοι τεχνίται (vulgar craftsmen), who honor their own specific skill more than the reason they share with the gods: *Meditations* 6.35.

27. *Opt. Med.* p. 6, 23–27, 24, esp. 6–8 = K.1.60–61. Cf. *Meth. Med.* 7.1, K.10.457, 4–8, 9.4; K.10.608, 15–609, 16, 2.5; K.10.114, 15–115, 4.

28. *Logical method* (*Inst. Log.*) 11.1, p. 24, 15–16; *On the Construction of the Medical Art* (*Const. Art.*) p. 225, 16ff. = K.1.226; *Praecog.* p. 74, 2–6 = K.14.605; *On the Errors Particular to Each Soul* (*Pecc.*), p. 47, 13–48, 7 = K.5.60–62; *Thrasybulus* (*Thras.*) p. 35, 25–36, 7 = K.5.810. Galen devoted a compendious treatise in fifteen books to the canons of scientific proof (*On Demonstration* [*Dem.*]), famous under the empire and in the Islamic world, of which fragments have been collected by Müller (1897). He also wrote commentaries on Aristotle's *Analytics* (cf. K.8.764, 19–765, 4; 705, 18–706, 3), on Theophrastus, Chrysippus, on Plato's logic, in all nineteen titles and fifty-eight books in *Lib.Prop.* pp. 115–24 = K.19.39–43, along with another forty or so shorter works on matters philosophical. For the stress on this philosophical program, see also remarks in *Praecog.*, p. 74, 2–6 = K.14.605; *Med. Cogn.* 5.3–5, p. 69; *On the Parts of Medicine* (*Part. Med.*) 6.6, p. 42, 2–3; *PHP* 2.3.12–13, p. 112, 7–12 = K.5.222, 2.5.67; p. 140, 21–22 = K.5.254; 9.8.1, p. 590, 12–13 = K.5.782. Most of the first two books of *Meth. Med.* are also devoted to arguing for the importance of demonstrative method to the doctor. It is striking that the ethical is inextricably involved with philosophical method; those who fail to adopt the correct (philosophical) method are presented as failing morally (e.g., *Meth. Med.* K.10.114, 15–115, 4; see below). Barnes (1991, 56–60) discusses the link between lack of logic and moral

failings: such doctors become tyrants (*Meth. Med.* 1.9, K.10.76, 8–10; 2.5, 105, 8–106, 1; 2.5, 109, 3–6; 9.4, 609, 3–16) rather than persuading or teaching; on the other hand, they become slaves to their patients' whims. In the end, in their ignorance, they kill their patients (ibid. K.10.390, 1ff.; 815, 1–10, 909, 10–16, 2; cf. Barnes 1991, 59).

29. *On the Formation of the Foetus* (*Foet. form.*) K.4.695, 3–696, 3.

30. *Lib. Prop.* p. 117, 4–7 = K.19.40. Interestingly enough, from the point of view of a rare coincidence with modern justifications of the truth of science, he mentions technological successes such as clocks and engineering works as proofs of this truth in this context. Here his father's occupation as an architect seems to have been influential.

31. Diaeresis: *PHP* pp. 566, 10–572, 15 = K.5.753–60; *Ven. Sect.*, K.11.258, 14–259, 2; *Opt. Med.*, p. 1, 17–2, 3; p. 6, 10–22 = K.1.59; *On Abnormal Breathing* (*Diff. Resp.*), K.7.894, 18–895, 13. On the pulses: *On the Varieties of Pulses* (*Diff. Puls.*) K.8.600, 16–602, 3.; K.8.608, 1–609, 17; K.8.735, 14–736, 5.

32. On accusations of relying on μαντική and premonitions for his cures, see Nutton 1979, 169; and *On the Varieties of Fevers* (*Diff. febr.*) 2.7, K.7.354, 4–6. In *On Precipitating Causes* (*Caus. procat.*) 3.18, p. 5, 17–23, he ascribes these attacks to their ignorance. He does, however, make use of premonitions (*On Diagnosis through Dreams* [*Somn. Dig.*] K.6.835, 11–14): καὶ δή τινα μαντικῶς ὑπ' αὐτῆς [sc. τῆς ψυχῆς] προδηλοῦνται. καὶ γὰρ τοῦτο τῇ πείρᾳ μαρτυρεῖται. (Sometimes [the soul] reveals something of a prophetic nature, as is witnessed by experience). Cf. *Praecog.* p. 134, 26f = K.14.666–67. In this he stands in opposition to the Methodists (*In Hipp. Progn.* 1.1, p. 197, 8–12 = K.18B.1). See *Nat. Fac.* 1.12, pp. 121, 24–122, 3 = K.2.29, the passage in which he mentions astrology quoted above (see chap. 1).

33. Divination suffers from a double image, differing according to the moral use. The malicious mode (γοητεία) is what Galen is really worried about. He claims at one point that his opponents only use geometry and arithmetic to calculate their expenses, the stars and prediction only to find out how much money they will inherit (p. 72, 30–74, 2 = K.14.604–5).

34. διέβαλλε (he slandered): p. 84, 8 = K.14.615.

35. See Nutton 1979, 166; and Birley 1972: he was *Consul ordinarius* in 173, a scion of one of Asia Minor's greatest dynasties and a friend of Fronto (see *PIR*²C 1024).

36. Trans. Nutton, p. 124, 14–20 = K.14.655–56. Cf. *Protr.* p. 103, 17–104, 4 = Kaibel, p. 1, 15–20 = K.1.2. Galen, in his *Commentary on the Hippocratic Oath,* observed that it was appropriate that Asclepius, the god of healing, should have been the son of Apollo, since doctors need prophecy to tell the future for their patients. (Rosenthal, the editor [1956], expressed doubts about its authenticity, but Nutton [1990, 254] dismisses them.) Kudlien (1981) has examined Galen's attitude to religious matters and his reverence for Asclepius in particular.

37. διαλεκτικῶς, ἔφη, συνελογίσω τὴν εὕρησιν τοῦ γενησομένου. (p. 86, 29–30 = K.14.618).

38. *In Hipp. Epid.* 6, 4.10, p. 204, 6–7 = K.17B.146.

39. *Loc. Aff.* 5.8, K.8.361, 12–366, 5.

40. Cf. Galen, *On Medical Names* (*Nom. Med.*), p. 21, 14f. Here he argues that his own predictions were attained by rational calculation, not by acting as a prophet, augur, or astrologer, whose predictions did not allow for changing circumstances. Cf. *Const. Art.* 17, K.1.292, 2–4.

41. Sebeok and Umiker-Sebeok, in Eco and Sebeok 1983, 44–46.

42. At *Praecog.* 7, pp. 104, 24–110, 12 = K.14.635–41, there is a case that offers some

parallels: Galen and his client both refer jovially to his extraordinary powers of divination, when he works out that Boethus' young son has been secretly eating and where he has hidden the food. Here he reveals, however, how he worked it out, and Boethus thinks that anybody should be able to use his or her common sense in this way. For other cases of detection by nonmedical means, see the case of Justus' wife, for which Galen works out that she is in love with the dancer Pylades; the case of the steward, whose illness Galen traces to his worry about being found to have lost his master's money (*Praecog.* pp. 100, 7–104, 8 = K.14.630–35); and the case of the wealthy drug addict, whose self-ministrations, despite his staunch denials, are discovered by Galen, when his suspicions are aroused by the coloring of his tongue by the drug; *On Prognosis through the Pulse* (*Praesag. puls.*) 1.1, K.9.218, 8–220, 3.

43. A typical comment of Watson's comes at Baring-Gould 1968, 432: "I trust that I am not more dense than my neighbours, but I was always oppressed with a sense of my own stupidity by my dealings with Sherlock Holmes. Here I had heard what he had heard, I had seen what he had seen, and yet from his words it was evident that he saw clearly not only what had happened, but what was about to happen, while to me the business was still confused and grotesque." Holmes certainly is not very helpful: at one point in "The Sign of Four," when Watson inquires what his theory is with regard to some footmarks, he relies with typical brusqueness: "My dear Watson, try a little analysis yourself. . . . You know my methods. Apply them, and it will be instructive to compare results." The unfortunate Watson complains that he cannot conceive of anything that will cover the facts.

44. Cf. Nutton 1972, 54.

45. See Nutton 1972, 62.

46. Amazing prognoses and dialogues: *Diff. Puls.* 3.3, K.8.656, 1–17. Dispute over the heavy pulse with a nonagenarian follower of Archigenes: ibid., 653, 15–655, 17. Full pulse dispute: Ibid. 2.3, K.8.569–74.

47. See especially *Opt. Med.* This is not an attitude confined to Galen: in the *Digest* we find that in the choice of doctors to be salaried by the city *probitas morum* (moral probity) is as important as *peritia artis* (expertise in the art): 50.9.1. and 4, cited in Nutton 1979, 58. The importance of moral character for the civic physician is confirmed in inscriptions (*Insciptiones Graecae* 12.5.719; *IGR* 3.534; 4.1087; cf. Nutton 1985, 35). Nutton (1985, 28–29) compares the claims of Vitruvius for architecture (1.1f.), Onasander's for the general (*Strat.* 1–2), and Lucian, whose satirical defense of solo dancing (*De Saltatione*), shows how well worn a *topos* these moral themes were. Astrologers, too, made such claims (see chap. 1).

48. *Med. Cogn.* 8.9–9.3, 99–103; cf. *Meth. Med.* 9.4, K.10.608, 15–609, 16; and see chapter 3.

49. Probably the Sextus Quintilius Condianus, who was consul in 180 (Nutton 1979, *ad loc.*), though Birley (1972) argues that he was the young Commodus, nicknamed Sextus as the sixth child of Marcus and Faustina.

50. *Diff. Puls.* 1.1. K.8.493, 1–497, 12. *On Discernment of the Pulse* (*Dign. Puls.*) K.8.773, 8–12.

51. Cf. *Meth. Med.* K.10.76, 15–18, and 608, 15–9, 16, in which Galen draws the contrast between himself and the others. This theme of moral decline is elaborated, in particular in the prooemia, briefly in technical treatises (e.g., *On the Faculties of Purgatives* [*Purg. Fac.*]): a rise in crime and in sophistry since ancient times, K.11.323.1ff.), at length in less-technical treatises (*Med. Cogn., Opt. Med., Meth. Med., Protr.*). E.g., "In ancient times, when men were not obsessed, as they are (now), with the pursuit of luxury, students

of this art: the virtuous kings and the sons of divine kings and their kinsmen, were worthy of this (art) on account of their superior innate virtues. Those kings educated their sons in this (art), and at that time, none of them had ever thought that it was shameful to take up this art of Apollo and Asclepius. At present, its status has declined; it is suitable (only) for slaves and despicable men . . . [practitioners] only aim is to gain money, power and position" (*Med. Cogn.* 1.1–13, pp. 41–47). On the Galenic *topos* that love of fame and money leads doctors off the straight and narrow, see Nutton 1979, 220.

52. Deichgräber 1970. Cf. *Med. Cogn.* 1.1–1.13, pp. 41–47). For the moral ideal of a doctor untainted in the midst of luxury and seductive pressure, cf. Hippocrates, *Epidemics* 6.4.7.

53. *Praecog.* p. 128, 25–30 = K.14.660.

54. Cf. Hippocrates, *Decorum* p. 25, 17–19; 21f. (of around 200 B.C.)

55. *In Hipp. Epid. 6* pp. 205, 11–207, 21 = K.17B.148–52; cf. Deichgräber 1970, 40f.

56. *Lib. Prop.* 12, p. 121, 12–13 = K.19.45. It is clear from *Lib. Prop.* that Galen specifically imagines and caters for different audiences in his works and considers the problem of their falling into the hands of the wrong recipient; cf. *Commentary on Hippocrates's On Fractures* 1.1, K.18B.321, 1–322, 2.

57. *Diff. Puls.* 2.2–4. K.8.578, 15–590, 3, especially 586, 19–587, 11. *Opt. Med.* p. 2, 15–20 = K.1.55, 5–9.

58. Cf. Athenaeus in Oribasius, *Medical Collection* 39.21, p. 141, 5–9.

59. For lay interest in medicine, see also Bowersock 1969, 59–75.

60. On the φιλόκαλοι as audience, see Manuli 1983. On the use of the word by Galen and in the Second Sophistic generally, see Nutton 1979, 193.

61. That is not to say that he claims that they read his work, only that he put on display lectures for them (in this period we must imagine sufficient knowledge of Greek on the part of the cultivated elite for this to be plausible).

62. *Praecog.* 11, pp. 126, 16–130, 10 = K.14.657–611.

63. *Praecog.* p. 82, 15–16 = K.14.613.

64. *Praecog.* p. 80, 15–18 = K.14.612.

65. *Praecog.* pp. 90, 6–92, 33 = K.14.620–24.

66. Galen is obviously a foreign doctor at Rome himself, and at *Praecog.* p. 116, 16–19 = K.14.647, he is proud to recount how much money he got from Boethus.

67. See Juvenal, *Satire* 3; Dio Chrysostom, *Orations* 7; and Nutton 1979 *ad loc.*

68. He asserts that other doctors who only praise Hippocrates without practicing his precepts are like athletes who approve of training but fail to prepare for competition: *Opt. Med.* 1, p. 53, 1ff. = K.1.53.

69. Galen tells us that he wrote one of his works (*On the Movement of the Thorax and Lungs*) as an epideictic speech for a fellow student to deliver on his return to his hometown from Rome, a typical occasion for a Sophistic display (*On Anatomical Procedures* [*Anat. Admin.*] K.2.217, 6–11).

70. He devoted several works to the refutation of Favorinus' views: the only extant treatise deemed to be authentic is the fragment of *On the Best Doctrine* (*Opt. Doct.*) / Favorinus fr. 28, p. 179–94 Barigazzi. He also wrote against his *Against Socrates* (*Lib. Prop.* 12, p. 121,1 = K.19.45) and on Epictetus (ibid. 11, 120, 6 = K.19.44, 8).

71. *Anat. Admin.* 7.16, K.2.619, 16–621, 1 (Galen and his pupils dissect an elephant in front of many physicians unwilling to accept his predictions about the anatomy of the heart); *On Phlebotomy against the Erasistrateans in Rome* (*Ven. Eras. Rom.*) K.11.194, 6–7 (refers to his custom of speaking in public each day on any questions put forward); cf.

193, in which Teuthras tries to provoke Galen to debate and then retreats; *Praecog.* (ἀγών) pp. 94, 19–100, 6 = K.14.626–30.

72. *Med. Cogn.* 9.6, p. 105 (Galen performs many dissections [including one of an ape] in front of spectators at a medical competition in Pergamum, challenging his opponents to replace its intestines).

73. On Ephesus, see Keil 1905. Here there were formal contests with lists of victors publicly displayed. There were four sections in which candidates could compete at the Great Asclepeia, συντάγματος (free choice of medical theme on which to orate?), προβλήματος (theme chosen by the judges), χειρουργίας (surgical demonstrations), and οργάνων (medical instruments). The order in which these four appear, with words before deeds, is notable. Despite the archaeologists' ideas, these are unlikely to have been official examinations of civic physicians, of whose existence we may remain in doubt, but were, rather, the usual challenge matches, in the context of a civic festival. See also *Die Inschriften von Ephesos,* 1160–70, 4101; and Knibbe 1982, 136, no. 146, which dates the contests securely back to at least the A.D. 130s. For Smyrna, see Lebas and Waddington 1870. Nutton (1979, 187) believes that the practice of holding these public competitions originated in the Hellenistic custom of public lectures for the education of the citizens and only became competitive in Roman times. We know that, at least later, these competitions were often held in theaters or specially built auditoria as well as outside, which throws some light on the importance of the spectacular. John Chrysostom, *PG* 63, p. 655, cited in Nutton 1979, 188.

74. *Ven. Eras. Rom.,* K.11.194, 6–7, *Lib. Prop.,* p. 95, 2–5 = K.19.13; cf. 189, 1, for the date of 163 (see Nutton 1979, 186).

75. Lycus: *Lib. Prop.* p. 100, 15ff. = K.19.20, Sophist: K.8.571, 5–572, 8, old man: K.8.572, 8–573, 16.

76. *Thras.* pp. 97, 8–98, 4 = K.5.894–96.

77. Alexander: *Praecog.* pp. 97, 5–98, 8, K.14.627–8; imaginary dispute: *Diff. Puls.* 1.1. K.8.494, 10–495, 9.

78. E.g., *Diff. Puls.* 656, 1–2; *Praecog.* pp. 134, 14–138, 4 = K.14.666–69; *Med. Cogn.* 8.5, pp. 95–97. See also Nutton 1979, 160.

79. *Ven. Eras., Ven. Eras. Rom.,* see Brain 1986.

80. *Lib. Prop.* p. 95, 19–21, K.19.14; cf. *Ven. Eras. Rom.* K.11.191, 13–17.

81. *Praecog.* p. 96, 11–15 = K.14.627: "those with loud voices are much better at producing a convincing demonstration"; cf. *Anat. Admin.* 8.4, K.2.663, 14–16.

82. Furley and Wilkie 1984, 36. The experiment Galen describes involves ligating the artery in two places and cutting between the two. On Erasistratus' account, however, the blood could still have been diverted from the veins nearby to fill the vacuum. Wilkie makes some useful observations on the differences between the experimental norms of antiquity and those of the present day (ibid., 47–57).

83. Dio Chrysostom, *Orations* 33.6. Here the doctor is pictured surrounded by bones, which he arranges and rearranges as he describes pores and secretions. Dio comments that the audience is agape, fooled like children at this θεωρία . . . καὶ πομπή (spectacle and parade).

84. *Lib. Prop.* 13, pp. 96, 7–9 = K.19.14–15.

85. *Dign. Puls.* K.8.768, 13ff; cf. *Meth. Med.* 9.4, K.10.608, 15–609, 3; *PHP* p. 198, 23–27 = K.5.319; p. 378, 38–380, 7 = K.5.528.

86. *Loc. Aff.* K.8.158, 6–11.

87. Singer unpub., chap. 1. Cf. *Meth. Med.* 9.4, K.10.609, 13–16.

88. *Elem. Sec. Hipp.* p. 33, 7–11 = K.1.457–58.

89. Hippocrates: K.11.166, 16–167, 4; 167, 8–10; 168, 9–12; 340, 8–10; *San. Tu.* p. 50, 11–17 = K.6.111; Coans: *PHP,* pp. 510, 5–8 = K.5.685. See Lloyd 1991, 400 n. 8.

90. See Von Staden 1982.

91. Lloyd 1991, 399ff., suggests that they may not have been atypical, but there is little evidence to support this.

92. Nutton (1972, 53) comments that a certain archaism is characteristic of the "Second Sophistic" and refers to this as a "refuge against doubt." This is not to say that it was a persuasive weapon used equally by everybody. The Methodists choose not to venerate Hippocratic tradition in this way (though Asclepiades does not entirely escape the role of "father of the tradition," along with Thessalus and Themison.) But even the Empirics claim "the ancients" for their side (Celsus, *On Medicine,* preface).

93. Smith 1979, 61ff. See especially *On the Order of His Own Books* (*Ord. Lib.*) p. 86, 13–87, 23 = K.19.56–58.

94. *Med. Cogn.* 6.7–8, p. 85. For an ingenious interpretation of Hippocrates, in which Galen reads him so eccentrically that he can claim others need his help to understand him, see *San. Tu.* 2.4, pp. 48, 19–53, 26 = K.6.105–19.

95. *Praecog.,* p. 70, 15–17 = K.14.602; *Med. Cogn.* 2.1, p. 47. cf. *Const. Art.* 17, K.1.294: here doctors are presented as having no doubts about the validity of prognosis, and Hippocrates is not mentioned.

96. *Praecog.,* p. 136, 18–19 = K.14.668; cf. cupping glass: ibid. p. 132, 26–31 = K.14.664, and p. 134, 1–6 = K.14.665. Cf. *Therapeutics to Glaucon* 1.16, K.11.68, 15–18; *On Crises* (*Cris.*) 3.11, p. 210, 17–20 = K.9.766.

97. The divisions between sects now look more fluid and context relative than they did in Wellmann's time.

98. *Praecog.,* pp. 128, 32–130, 1 = K.14.660–61.

99. *Diff. Puls.* K.8.497, 13–17.

100. Marcellinus similarly gives Hippocrates credit, frequently mentioning him as a major authority (*On Pulses,* 32ff., 45ff., 56ff., 70ff., 275ff., 355ff., 506ff.).

101. See the evidence collected in Daremberg and Ruelle 1879, 616. Cf. *Praecog.* p. 130, 3–6 = K.14.660–61, in which he claims that he only added the theory of pulses to the Hippocratic art of prognosis, "which was all that he had not worked out, just as all his successors down to our time have made various additions, one after another." Galen makes similar excuses for the lack of Hippocratic writings on anatomy: Hippocrates did not need to write about it, as anatomical instruction was oral and kept within the family (*Anat. Admin.* 2.1, K.2.280, 1–83, 1).

102. See Edelstein 1967, 184.

103. *San. Tu.* 2, 2–6, pp. 39, 7–61, 9 = K.6.84–133, on massages, seems like a miniature version of the pulse polemic, as I shall summarize it below. At p. 43, 14ff. = K.6.94ff., Galen attacks trainers who make many distinctions in types of massage; they have failed to follow the simple precepts of Hippocrates. As with Archigenes, we are led to expect that Galen will simplify and rationalize the varieties. But his real quarrel is over the logical failures of these untrained trainers. The divisions these people make are not to count as differentiae of massages, when they say they differ according to accidental, not essential, features. But he thinks their mistakes will easily be detected: his real polemic is against the trainer Theon. Galen is ingenious in excusing Hippocrates for leaving out varieties while accusing Theon of this very crime. And here the elaboration begins: at p. 51, 1–10 = K.6.113, Galen produces a table, like those in the pulses, to show that Theon has only mentioned six qualities and quantities of massages, when he should have had nine. Galen

proceeds to mention even more variables according to climate, temperature, place, season, hour of the day, individual constitution, and so on (pp. 55–7 = K.6.120–33). In discussion of massages for particular needs (3.2, pp. 75, 15–80, 7 = K.6.169–80 [apotherapy for athletes], 3.6, pp. 86, 20–88, 19 [massages for fatigues], and 3.13, pp. 101, 6–102, 20 = K.6.228–32 [morning and evening massages]) he mentions differences according to whether a napkin, powder, or bare hands, with their degrees of softness, are used, the numerous different types of oils and their different quantities (pp. 86, 31–87, 13 = K.6.195–97), the kinds of movements, circles, strokes, and directions: not only moving from top to bottom or bottom to top, but also subvertically, obliquely, transversely, and subtransversely, terms he has to explain (p. 42, 24–31 = K.6.92). Despite the usual protestation about not engaging in useless disputes about names, he cannot resist discussing nomenclature. Here, certainly, there is more careful attention to cause and effect, and it is possible that a few of his opponents' distinctions are jettisoned, though most seem to reappear in discussion of massages for particular occasions. Overall, though, the pressures of the ἀγών seem to have led to extra variables needing to be considered. Shortly afterward, in the third book, he takes Theon to task again for not distinguishing kinds of fatigue, after alluding to the failures of others' distinctions (3.5, pp. 83, 1–96, 17 = K.6.189–218). Logically, there should be fifteen. If one adds the different forms of constriction and the different states of the body associated with indigestion, sexual activity, sun, sleeplessness, and grief, the permutations become difficult to number (p. 96, 1–4 = K.6.217). Galen leaves plethora, dyspepsia, constipation, vomiting, headaches, and so on to discuss later.

104. E.g., Ptolemy, *Tetrabiblos* 1.20.45; 1.21.49; Firmicus Maternus, *Mathesis* 4.22.8–19; Vettius Valens, *Anthologies* 5.6, p. 222, 1–13.

105. Marcellinus, *On Pulses* 260–67. Cf. Deichgraber 1956.

106. Breasted 1930. See 1:104.

107. There are some problems with the text here, however: see Magazis et al. 1978, 88.

108. On whom see now von Staden 1989.

109. *Praesag. Puls.* 2.2, K.9.272, 12ff.

110. He discusses, in addition to Herophilus and his fellow Alexandrian Erasistratus, figures such as Bacchius of Tanagra, Zeno of Laodicea, Chrysermus, Alexander Philalethes, Demosthenes Philalethes, Heraclides of Eretrea, Aristoxenus, Heraclides of Tarentum, Asclepiades of Bithynia, Athenaeus, Agathinus of Sparta, Archigenes of Apamea, Cassius Iatrosophistes, and Magnus of Ephesus. See also the definitions in *Def. Med.,* listed below (n. 131).

111. *Def. Med.:* K.19.375, 16–378, 3; 402, 18–412, 15, on which see Kollesch 1973. *Puls. Ant.* K.19.346–462; 629–42. These treatises, like those of Marcellinus, Rufus (?), and Pseudo-Soranus, never mention Galen and seem to reflect the influence of Archigenes, or earlier pulse theorists. Hence, in the absence of other decisive indications, they are usually assumed to predate Galen (see, e.g., Harris 1973, 237, 251, 267, 271).

112. *Def. Med.* K.19.376, 8–11: σφυγμός ἐστιν ἄγγελος ἀψευδὴς τῶν ἐν βάθει κεκρυμμένων καὶ τῶν ἀφανῶν προφήτης καὶ τῶν ἀδήλων ἔλεγχος ἐν ἁρμονικῇ κινήσει καὶ μαντικῇ πληγῇ διάθεσιν ἀόρατον προαγορεύων.

113. Rufus: Daremberg-Ruelle 1879, 219–32; Pseudo-Soranus: Rose, *Anecdota Graeca* 2.263, 19–266, 14, and 275, 1–280, 13.

114. Importance: *Praesag. puls.* 1.1, K.9.208, 10ff. Sign of vital force: ibid. 1.11, K.9.420, 16–421, 6. *Meth. Med.* 1.2, K.8.770; *Praecog.* p. 128, 3ff. = K.14.658; 138, 13ff. = K.14.670; *Const. Art.* 17, K.1.294, 2–4.

115. This, he claimed, no earlier doctors had taught, though Herophilus had begun (*Diff. Puls.* K.8.274, 16–275, 4).

116. *Dign. Puls.* K.8.773, 2–6; cf. K.9.274, 12ff.

117. *Dign. Puls.* 1.1, K.8.773, 14–774, 2; 1.8, 808, 14–15; 2.1, 826, 17–827, 3; 2.2. 859, 16–860, 3.

118. *Dign. Puls.* 1.8, K.8.806, 12–808, 1. Cf. Harris 1973, 406.

119. *Praecog.* 138, 23–140, 14 = K.14.670–71.

120. Cited in Temkin 1973, 182 n. 120.

121. *Lib. Prop.* 5, p. 110, 25–27 = K.19.33; cf. *Simp. Med.* 6.1, K.11, 796, 16–797, 2; *San. Tu.* p. 51, 25–32 = K.6.114. For the need for a teacher, cf. *On the Composition of Drugs by Type* (*Comp. Gen.*) K.13.560, 7–561, 6, in which he talks of books falling into the wrong hands, those not learning medicine from a teacher, altogether ανεισάκτους and ἀγυμνάστους (uninitiated and untrained).

122. *Puls. Tir.* K.8.477, 15–18; cf. F.1.192.

123. K.8.619, 11–620, 1; cf. 637, 9ff.

124. For variant classifications, see, e.g., *Def. Med.*'s categories, listed below (n. 131); or Ps-Soranus' similar list (Rose, *Anecdota Graeca* 275–80).

125. K.8.753, 12–15; 698, 2; cf. *Lib. Prop.* 5, p. 111, 5 = K.19.33.

126. Cf. Harris 1973, 255. E.g., Galen says that Archigenes differentiates unevenness (ἀνωμαλία) from irregularity rather obscurely. The chief objection is that he does not stick to the notion of "differentia" as denoting a class of pulse, i.e., the specific qualities of a single beat, because of the introduction of notions of rhythm and order, etc.

127. 608, 3–613, 4. His scorn for Archigenes' failures is unrelenting: ἐπειδὴ σύνθετον ἀδιάρθρωτόν τε καὶ ἀδιώριστον ἔχει τὴν διδασκαλίαν, καὶ παντάπασιν ἰδιωτικήν τε καὶ ἀδιώριστον τε καὶ ἀτέχνον ("since he keeps instruction all of a piece, without distinction or division, and in every way unprofessional, lacking in order, and lacking [the foundations of] *technē*" 609, 3–4).

128. "Archigenes, as it were, badly butchered it."

129. 577, 18–578, 3. Rufus (231, 14–232, 1), however, attributes a different, tenfold division, adding βάρος—ποσόν πληγῆς (weight, size of beat) and σκληρότης—σύστασις (hardness, solidity), of which the first at least follows the threefold division into the extremes and the mean (8.591, 602). Wellmann thinks that this was Archigenes' real scheme.

130. Thus, if Wellmann's reconstruction (1895, 175–76) is right, Galen only excludes the category of strength under the rubric τὸ ποσὸν τῆς πληγῆς (the size of the beat), though he does have a τὸ τῆς πληγῆς ποιόν (the type of beat) category corresponding to Archigenes' σφοδρότης—τὸ παρὰ τὸν τόνον τῆς δυνάμεως (strength, intensity of force). Otherwise, his initial scheme is basically the same as Archigenes'.

131. *Puls. Tir.* 460, 17–461, 5. The author of *Def. Med.* offers the following simple categories, using a threefold division: size, fullness, hardness, wetness, dryness, heat, strength, speed, frequency, order, equality, rhythm (divided only into eurhythmic, arhythmic, cacorhythmic, and pararhythmic), and adds the quivering, oblique, worming, mouse-tailed, double-hammer, spiderlike, intermittent, fading, deficient, gazelling, recurrent, and anting. Ps-Soranus' *On Pulses* (Rose: 275–80) has a similar list, in which there is even less hierarchical ordering of the different types.

132. I.e., the big, ([?]subdivided into long, broad, and high), the small ([?] subdivided into short, narrow, and low, and the medium, together with the six pairs mentioned above

(short/low, short/narrow, long/wide, long/high, wide/high, narrow/low: see Wellmann 1895, 1., 177–78 and K.8.606, 615).

133. K.8.595, 1–596, 11. How exactly this works as a sixfold differentiation is unclear to me, but the text seems corrupt here; here there seem to be six differences between the biggest and the moderate, as in and 620, 6–8. Thus, presumably, there are six more between the smallest and the moderate. In 618, 6–16, however, there seem to be four only.

134. See, e.g., chapters 25–26 (549, 18–556, 16).

135. Marcellinus (*On Pulses* 129–32), however, while mentioning this, says that he has come across it himself often in cases of delirium and heart disease. Some of these special types of pulse appear in all the writers from Herophilus onward, and they are prominent in the book Galen writes for beginners: *On Pulses for Beginners* (K.8.460, 1–17).

136. See Harris 1973. At *Diff. Puls.* K.8.537, 4–542, 13, it is simply classified as the third type of pulse unequal in one part, at *On the Causes of Pulses* (*Caus. Puls.*) K.9.75, 17–80, 6, it seems to be an exclusively arterial phenomenon, while at *Praesag. Puls.* K.9.303, 12–309, 19, it is the single-beat version of the "interrupted" pulse, whose "systematic" version is the intermittent or "beat-dropping" pulse, i.e., caused by a defect in the heart as well.

137. *Praecog.* pp. 138, 24–142, 14 = K.14.670–73.

138. See Nutton 1979, 227.

139. *In Hipp. Progn.* p. 369, 19–25 = K.18B.301.

140. *Praecog.* p. 140, 12–14 = K.14.671; *Diff. Puls.* K.8.768, 15–19; 859, 16–860, 3; *Praesag. Puls.* K.9.274, 12–16; K.9.420, 7–10; *Cris.* p. 100, 2–16 = K.9.599; p. 90, 22–24 = K.9.584.

141. E.g., Harris 1973, 429.

142. Ideler, *Phys. med. gr.* 1, p. 261, 1–262, 2. Unfortunately, we have little trace of writers on the urines apart from Galen and the Hippocratics to set against Theophilus' picture; texts such as the early imperial Athenaeus' *On Urines* remain in unedited MSS.

143. Ideler, *Phys. med. gr.* 1, pp. 262–83.

144. *Part. Med.,* in which he takes on board the criticism that different subdivisions are possible (49). He says that this is unimportant so long as there are no omissions.

145. See above.

146. Temkin 1973, 68.

Conclusion

1. I mention some cases in point in the concluding section of chapter 2.
2. Chapter 1.
3. See appendix A.
4. Adamantius F.1.298, 14–299, 2. Cf. chapter 3.
5. Galen, see chapter 3. Ptolemy, *Tetrabiblos* 1.2.13, p. 7, 20ff..
6. Galen, see chapter 3. Adamantius F.1.297, 15–16.
7. Hesse 1980, 22.

References

Adams, J. N. *The Latin Sexual Vocabulary.* London, 1982.

Africa, T. W. *Science and the State in Greece and Rome.* New York, London, and Sydney, 1968.

Alföldi, A. "Commandants de la flotte romaine à Cyrène," In *Mélanges d'archéologie, d'epigraphie et de l'histoire offerts à J. Carcopino,* ed. J. Heurgin, G. Picard, and W. Seaton. Paris, 1966: 25–34.

Allbutt, C. *Greek Medicine in Rome.* New York, 1921.

Allen, J. "Failure and Expertise in the Ancient Conception of an Art." In *Scientific Failure,* T. Horowitz and A. I. Janis. Forthcoming.

Amand, D. *Fatalisme et liberté dans l'antiquité grecque.* Louvain, 1940.

Anderson, G. "The Pepaideumenos in Action: Sophists and Their Outlook in the Early Empire." *Aufstieg und Niedergang der römischen Welt. Geschichte und Kultur Roms im Spiegel der neueren Forschung. Teil 2. Principat.* 33.1 (1989): 79–208.

André, J. "Introduction" to *"Traité de physiognomie" (Anonyme Latin).* Paris, 1981.

Ashmore, M. *A Question of Reflexivity: Wrighting Sociology of Scientific Knowledge.* D.Ph. diss., York, 1985.

———. *The Reflexive Thesis: Wrighting Sociology of Scientific Knowledge.* Chicago, 1989.

Bachelard, G. *L'Actualité de l'histoire des sciences.* Paris, 1951.

Baldwin, B. "Executions under Claudius." *Phoenix* 18 (1964): 119–28.

Balferetti, L. *Cesare Lombroso.* Turin, 1975.

Baltrusaitis, J. *Abérrations: quatre essais sur la légende des formes.* Paris, 1957.

Barigazzi, A. "Introduzione" to *Favorino di Arelate: opere.* Florence, 1966.

Baring-Gould, W. S. *The Complete Sherlock Holmes.* 2 vols. London, 1968.

Barlow, C. W. *Martini Episcopi Bracarensis opera omnia.* New Haven, Conn., 1950.

Barnes, B. "Paradigms: Scientific and Social." *Man* n.s. 4 (1969): 94–102.

———. *Scientific Knowledge and Sociological Theory.* London, 1974.

———. *Interests and the Growth of Knowledge.* London, 1977.

Barnes, B., and Mackenzie, D. "On the Role of Interests in Scientific Change." In *On the Margins of Science: The Social Construction of Rejected Knowledge,* ed. R. Wallis, 49–66. Keele, 1979.

Barnes, B., and Shapin, S., eds. *Natural Order: Historical Studies of Scientific Culture.* London, 1979.

Barnes, B., and Bloor, D. "Relativism, Rationalism and the Sociology of Knowledge." In *Rationality and Relativism,* ed. M. Hollis and S. Lukes, 21–47. London, 1982.

Barnes, J. "Galen on Logic and Therapy." In *Galen's Method of Healing,* ed. K. Kudlien and R. Durling, 50–102. Leiden, 1991.

Barnes, J., Brunschwig, J., Burnyeat, M., and Schofield, M., eds. *Science and Speculation: Studies in Hellenistic Theory and Practice.* Cambridge, 1982.

Barton, T. S. "The *Inventio* of Nero: Suetonius." In *Reflections of Nero: Culture, History and Representation,* ed. J. Masters and J. Elsner, 48–63. London and Chapel Hill, 1994.

———. "Augustus and Capricorn Again." Forthcoming in *Journal of Roman Studies* 85, 1995.

Bayet, J. "L'Immortalité astrale d'Auguste ou Manilius commentateur de Virgile." *Revue des Etudes Latines* 17 (1939): 141–71.

Beard, M., and North, J. A., eds. *Pagan Priests: Religion and Power in the Ancient World.* London, 1990.

Beck, F. A. G. *Album of Greek Education: The Greeks at School and at Play.* Sydney, 1975.

Berger, J. "Animal World." *New Society,* November 25, 1971, 1042–43.

———. "Animals as Metaphor," "Vanishing Animals," and "Why Zoos Disappoint." *New Society,* March 10, 1977, 504–5, March 31, 1977, 664–65, April 24, 1977, 122–23.

Birley, A. R. "A New Nickname for Commodus and a Date for Fronto's Death." *Chiron* 2 (1972): 463–73.

Bloch, M. "Astrology and Writing in Madagascar." In *Literacy in Traditional Societies,* ed. J. Goody, 277–97. Cambridge, 1968.

Bloch, R. *Les Prodiges dans l'antiquité classique.* Paris, 1963.

Bloor, D. "Wittgenstein and Mannheim on the Sociology of Mathematics." *Studies in the History and Philosophy of Science* 4 (1973): 173–91.

———. *Knowledge and Social Imagery.* London, 1976.

———. "Polyhedra and the Abominations of Leviticus." *British Journal for the History of Science* 11 (1978): 245–71.

———. "Durkheim and Mauss Revisited: Classification and the Sociology of Knowledge." *Studies in the History and Philosophy of Science* 13 (1982): 267–97.

———. *Wittgenstein: A Social Theory of Knowledge.* London, 1983.

Blum, C. *Studies in the Dream-Book of Artemidorus.* Uppsala, 1936.

Bodei, R. "Hermann Usener nella filosofia moderna: tra Dilthey e Cassirer." In *Alien Wisdom: The Limits of Hellenization,* ed. A. Momigliano, 23–42. Cambridge, 1975.

Boeffle, A. *Le Ciel des romains.* Paris, 1989.

Boll, F. *Studien über Claudius Ptolemaeus.* Jahrbücher für classische Philologie, Supplementband 21, 1894.

———. *Sphaera: Neue griechische Texte und Untersuchungen zur Geschichte der Sternbilder.* Leipzig, 1903.

Boll, F., and Bezold, C. *Sternglaube und Sterndeutung: Die Geschichte und das Wesen der Astrologie.* 3d ed., revised by W. Gundel. Leipzig, 1926.

Bompaire, J. *Lucien écrivain: imitation et création.* Paris, 1958.

Bonnaud, R. "Notes sur l'astrologie latine au VIe siècle." *Revue Belge de Philologie et Histoire* 10 (1931): 557–77.

Borsarello, J. *Les Pouls en médicine chinoise.* Paris, 1981.

Bottéro, J. "Symptômes, signes, écritures." In *Divination et rationalité,* ed. J.-P. Vernant, 70–199. Paris, 1974.

Bouché-Leclercq, A. "*Haruspices.*" In *Dictionnaire des antiquités,* ed. C. Daremberg and D. Saglio, 2.2: 17–33. Paris, 1896.

———. *L'Astrologie grecque.* Paris, 1899.

Boulanger, A. *Aelius Aristide et la sophistique dans la province d'Asie au IIe siècle de nôtre ère.* Paris, 1923.

Bowersock, G. *Greek Sophists in the Roman Empire.* Oxford, 1969.

———. "The Pontificate of Augustus." In *Between Republic and Empire: Interpretations of Augustus and His Principate,* ed. K. A. Raaflaub and M. Toher, 380–94. Berkeley, 1990.

Bowie, E. L. "The Importance of the Sophists." *Yale Classical Studies* 27 (1982): 29–59.

Brain, P. *Galen on Bloodletting: A Study of the Origins, Development and Validity of His Opinions.* Cambridge, 1986.

Brannigan, A. *The Social Basis of Scientific Discoveries.* Cambridge, 1981.

Brea, L. B. *Menandro e il teatro greco nelle terracotte liparesi.* Genoa, 1981.

Breasted, J. H. *The Edwin Smith Surgical Papyrus.* 2 vols. Chicago, 1930.

Brind'Amour, P. "Problèmes astrologiques et astronomiques soulevés par le récit de la mort de Domitien chez Suétone." *Phoenix* 35 (1981): 338–44.

Broughton, T. R. S. *The Magistrates of the Roman Republic.* New York, 1951.

Brown, P. *The World of Antiquity from Marcus Aurelius to Muhammad.* London, 1971.

———. *The Making of Late Antiquity.* Harvard, 1978.

Buchner, E. "*Horologium Solarium Augusti.*" In *Kaiser Augustus und die verlorene Republik,* ed. W.-D. Heilmeyer et al. Berlin, 1988.

Burgess, T. C. *Epideictic Literature.* 1902. Reprint. New York and London, 1987.

Burke, K. D. *A Grammar of Motives.* 1945. Reprint. Berkeley, 1969.

———. *A Rhetoric of Motives.* 1955. Reprint. Berkeley, 1958.

———. *The Philosophy of Literary Form: Studies in Symbolic Action,* rev. and abridged,1957. Reprint. Berkeley, 1973.

Burnyeat, M. F. "The Origins of Non-Deductive Inference." In *Science and Speculation: Studies in Hellenistic Theory and Practice,* ed. J. Barnes et al., 193–238. Cambridge, 1982.

———. "The Enthymeme." Unpub. MS.

Cambiano, G. "Scienza organnizzata e scienza 'selvaggia' in Hermann Usener." In *Alien Wisdom: The Limits of Hellenization,* ed. A. Momigliano, 43–64. Cambridge, 1975.

Carettini, G. P. "Peirce, Holmes, Popper." In *The Sign of Three,* ed. U. Eco and T. Seboek, 135–53. Bloomington, Ind., 1983.

Caster, M. *Etudes sur Alexandre le faux prophète de Lucien.* Paris, 1938.

Černý, J., Parker, R. A., and Kahle, P. "The Old Coptic Horoscope." *Journal of Egyptian Archaeology* 43 (1957): 86–100.

Chadwick, H. *Priscillian of Avila: The Occult and the Charismatic in the Early Church.* Oxford, 1976.

Christ, W. von, Schmid, W., and Stählin, O. *Geschichte der griechischen Literatur.* Vol. 2 i.ii, *Handbuch d. Altertumswissenschaft,* 7.ii, Munich 1920–61.

Coarelli, F. *Roma Sepolta.* Rome, 1984.

Colin, J. "Encolpio e il piatto d'argento con lo zodiaco." *Rivista di Filologia Classica* N.F. 29 (1951): 97–144.

Collins, H. "An Empirical Relativist Programme in the Sociology of Scientific Knowledge." In *Science Observed: Perspectives on the Social Study of Science,* ed. K. Knorr-Cetina and M. Mulkay, 85–113. London and Beverly Hills, Calif., 1983.

———. "Stages in the Empirical Programme of Relativism." *Social Studies of Science* 11 (1981): 3–10.

———. "The Sociology of Scientific Knowledge: Studies of Contemporary Science." *Annual Review of Sociology* 9 (1983): 265–85.

Cooter, R. "Deploying Pseudo-Science: Then and Now." In *Science, Pseudo-Science and*

Society, ed. M. P. Hanen et al., 17–28. Waterloo, Ont., 1980.

Couissin, J. "Suétone physiognomiste dans les 'Vies des XII Césars.'" *Revue des Etudes Latines* (1953): 234–256.

Cowling, M. *The Artist as Anthropologist.* London, 1988.

Cramer, F. H. "The Caesars and the Stars." *Seminar* 9 (1951): 1–35.

———. *Astrology in Roman Law and Politics.* Philadelphia, 1956.

Crawford, M. H. *Coinage and Money under the Roman Republic: Italy and the Mediterranean Economy.* London, 1985.

Crocker, J. C. "The Social Functions of Rhetorical Forms." In *The Social Uses of Metaphor: Essays in the Anthropology of Rhetoric,* ed. J. C. Crocker and J. D. Sapir, 33–66. Philadelphia, 1977.

Cumont, F. "L'Eternité des empereurs romains." *Revue d'Histoire et de Littérature Religieuses* 1 (1896): 435–52.

———. "La Polémique d'Ambrosiaster contre les paiens." *Revue d'Histoire et de Littérature Religieuses* 8 (1903): 417–40.

———. *Astrology among the Greeks and Romans.* 1912. Reprint. New York, 1960.

———. "Astrologica." *Révue Archéologique* 3 (1916): 1–22.

———. "Astrologues romains et byzantins." *Mélanges d'Archéologie et de l'histoire* 37 (1918).

———. "Les *Prognostica de decubitu* attribués à Galien," *Bulletin de l'Institute de l'Histoire Belge* 15 (1935): 119–32.

———. *L'Egypte des Astrologues.* Brussels, 1937.

Curry, P. "Revisions of Science and Magic." *History of Science* 23 (1985): 279–34.

———, ed. *Astrology, Science and Society: Historical Essays.* Woodbridge, Eng., 1987.

Dagron, G. "Le Saint, le savant, l'astrologue: étude de thèmes hagiographiques à travers quelques recueils de questions et réponses des Ve-VIIe siècles," *La Romanité chrétienne en orient: héritages et mutations,* 142–56. London, 1984.

———. "Image de bête ou image de dieu: le physiognomie animale dans la tradition grecque et ses avatars byzantins." In *Poikilia,* 69–80. Festschrift for J.-P. Vernant, Paris, 1987.

Daremberg, C. V. *Oeuvres choisies d'Hippocrate.* Paris, 1855.

———. *Histoire des sciences médicales.* 2 vols. Paris, 1870.

Daremberg, C. V., and Ruelle, C. E. *Oeuvres de Rufus d'Ephèse.* Paris, 1879.

Dauge, Y. A. "Le Troisième livre de l'Enéide: astrologie et energétique de la metamorphose." *Pallas: Revue des Etudes Antiques* 30 (1983): 25–48.

Deichgräber, K. "*Professio Medici.* Zum Vorwort des Scribonius Largus." *Akademie der Wissenschaften und der Literatur. Abhandlungen der geistes-und sozialwissenschaftlichen Klasse,* Jahrgang 1950.9. Mainz: 853–79.

———. "Galen als Erforscher des menschlichen Pulses: ein Beitrag des Wissenschaftlers. *De Dignotione Pulsuum* 1. 1." *Sitzungsberichte der Deutschen Akademie der Wissenschaften zu Berlin. Klasse für Sprachen, Literatur und Kunst,* Jahrgang 1956.3. 3–41.

———. *Medicus Gratiosus: Untersuchungen zu einem griechischen Arztbild.* Wiesbaden, 1970.

Delattre, A. L. "Musée Lavigerie de St. Louis de Carthage." *Musées de L'Algérie et de Tunisie* 8, no. 2 (1899–1900).

Descoeudres, J. -P. "The Australian Expedition to Pompeii: Contributions to the Chronology of the Fourth Pompeiian Style." *Cahiers d'Archéologie Romande* 43 (1987): 135–48.

Detienne, M. *Dionysus Slain.* Trans. M. and L. Muellner, of *Dionysos mis à mort.* Paris, 1977. Baltimore, 1979.

Detienne, M., and Vernant, J.-P. *Cunning Intelligence in Greek Culture and Society.* Hassocks, Eng., 1978. Trans. J. Lloyd, of *Les Ruses de l'intelligence: la métis des grecs.* Paris, 1974.

Devitt, M. *Realism and Truth.* Oxford, 1984.

Dicks, D. R. "Astronomy and Astrology in Horace." *Hermes* 91 (1963): 60–73.

Didi-Huberman, G. *L'Invention de l'hysterie: Charcot et l'iconographie de la Salpêtrière.* Paris, 1982.

Domaszewski, A. von. "Die Thierbilder der Signa." *Archäologisch-Epigraphische Mitteilungen* 15 (1892): 182–93.

Douglas, M. *Purity and Danger.* London, 1966.

———. "Preface" to *Implicit Meanings,* ix–xxi. London, 1975.

Dover, K. J. *Popular Morality in the Time of Plato and Aristotle.* Oxford, 1974.

Dreyfus, H. L., and Rabinow, P. *Michel Foucault: Beyond Structuralism and Hermeneutics.* Brighton, Eng., 1982.

Duhem, P. *L'évolution de la mécanique.* Paris, 1903.

———. *Les Origines de la statique.* 2 vols. Paris, 1905–6.

———. ΣΩΖΕΙΝ ΤΑ ΦΑΙΝΟΜΕΝΑ. *Essai sur la notion physique de Platon a Galilée.* Paris, 1908.

———. *The Aim and Structure of Physical Theory.* Trans. P. P. Wiener, of 2d ed. of *La Théorie physique: son objet, sa structure.* Paris, 1914. Princeton, 1954a.

———. *Le Système du monde: histoire des doctrines cosmologiques de Platon à Copernic.* 2 vols. 2d ed. Paris, 1954b.

Dumont, M. "Le Succès mondain d'un fausse science, la physiognomie de Johann Caspar Lavater." *Actes de la Recherche en Sciences Sociales* 54 (1984): 2–30.

Durkheim, E. *The Elementary Forms of the Religious Life.* Trans. J. W. Swain. London, 1915.

Dwyer, E. J. "Augustus and the Capricorn." *Mitteilungen des Deutschen Archäologischen Instituts, Römische Abteilung* 80 (1973): 59–67.

Eco, U. "Horns, Hooves, Insteps: Some Hypotheses on Three Types of Abduction." In *The Sign of Three,* ed. U. Eco and T. Sebeok, 198–220. Bloomington, Ind., 1983.

Eco, U., and Sebeok, T., eds. *The Sign of Three.* Bloomington, Ind., 1983.

Edelstein, L. *Ancient Medicine: Selected Papers of Ludwig Edelstein,* ed. O. and C. L. Temkin. Baltimore, 1967.

Edmondson, R. *Rhetoric in Sociology.* London, 1984.

Edwards, C. *The Politics of Immorality in Ancient Rome.* Cambridge, 1993.

Eichler, F., and Kris, E. *Die Kameen im Kunsthistorisches Museum.* Vienna, 1927.

Elia, O. *Pitture di Stabia.* Naples, 1957.

Espérandieu, E. *Recueil général des bas-reliefs, statues et bustes de la Gaule romaine.* 15 vols. Paris, 1908–.

Evans, E. C. "Roman Descriptions of Personal Appearance in Roman History and Biography." *Harvard Studies in Classical Philology* 46 (1935): 43–84.

———. "The Study of Physiognomy in the Second Century A.D." *Transactions of the American Philological Association* 72 (1941): 287–98.

———. "Galen the Physician as Physiognomist." *Transactions of the American Philological Association* 76 (1945): 96–108.
———. "Physiognomics in the Roman Empire." *Classical Journal* 45 (1950): 277–82.
———. "Physiognomics in the Ancient World." *Memoirs of the American Philosophical Society* 59, no. 5 (1969).
Fahnestock, J. "The Heroine of Irregular Features: Physiognomy and the Conventions of Heroine Description." *Victorian Studies* 24 (1981): 325–50.
Fann, K. T. *Peirce's Theory of Abduction.* The Hague, 1970.
Fardon, R. *Power and Knowledge: Anthropological and Sociological Approaches.* Edinburgh, 1985.
Farrington, B. *Science and Politics in the Ancient World.* London, 1939.
———. *Greek Science.* 2 vols. London, 1944–49.
Fernandez, J. W. "Persuasions and Performances: On the Beast in Every Body . . . and the Metaphor in Every Man." In *Myth, Symbol, and Culture,* ed. C. Geertz. New York, 1971.
Feyerabend, P. *Against Method: Outline of an Anarchistic Theory of Knowledge.* London, 1975.
Fichtner, G. *Corpus Galenicum: Verzeichnis der Galenischen und pseudoGalenischen Schriften.* Tübingen, 1985.
Fleck, L. *Genesis and Development of a Scientific Fact.* Chicago and London, 1979. Trans. of *Entstehung und Entwicklung einer wissenschaftslichen Tatsache.* Basel, 1935.
Fontaine, J. "Isidore de Séville et l'astrologie." *Revue des Etudes Latines* (1953): 271–300.
Foucault, M. *Discipline and Punish: The Birth of the Prison.* Trans. A. Sheridan. New York, 1979.
———. *The History of Sexuality.* Vol. 1: *An Introduction.* Trans. R. Hurley. New York, 1980.
Fowden, G. *The Egyptian Hermes: A Historical Approach to the Late Pagan Mind.* Cambridge, 1986.
Fraenkel, E. *Commentary on the "Agamemnon" of Aeschylus.* Oxford, 1950.
Frede, M. "On Galen's Epistemology." In *Galen: Problems and Prospects,* ed. V. Nutton, 65–86. London, 1981.
Friedman, J. B. *The Monstrous Races in Mediaeval Life and Thought.* Cambridge, 1981.
Fuhrmann, H. "Archäologische Grabungen und Funde in Italien, Albanien und Libyen, Oktober 1939–Oktober 1941." *Archäologischer Anzeiger* 56 (1941): 329–733 (bound with *Jahrbuch des Deutschen Archäologischen Instituts).*
Fuhrmann, M. *Das systematische Lehrbuch. Ein Beitrag zur Geschichte der Wissenschaften der Antike.* Göttingen, 1960.
Furley, D. J. "The Purpose of Theophrastus' Characters." *Symbolae Osloenses* (1953): 56–60.
Furley, D. J., and Wilkie, J. S. *Galen on Respiration and the Arteries.* Princeton, 1984.
Furtwängler, A. *Die Antiken Gemmen.* 3 vols. Leipzig, 1900.
———. *Beschreibung der Geschnittenen Steine im Antiquarium.* Berlin, 1896.
Gellner, E. "Is Belief Really Necessary." In *The Devil in Modern Philosophy,* ed. I. C. Jarvie and J. Agassi, 52–61. London, 1974.
Geneva, A. "The Study of Astrology." *London Review of Books,* November 27, 1987.
Getty, R. J. "*Liber et Alma Ceres* in Vergil 'Georgics' 1.7." *Phoenix* 5 (1951): 96–107.
Giannini, A. *Paradoxographorum Graecorum Reliquiae.* Milan, 1965.

Gilbert, G. N., and Mulkay, M. *Opening Pandora's Box: A Sociological Analysis of Scientists' Discourse.* Cambridge, 1984.

Gilman, S. L., ed. *The Face of Madness: Hugh Diamond and the Invention of Psychiatric Photography.* Cornell, 1976.

Gingerich, O. "Was Ptolemy a Fraud?" *Quarterly Journal of the Royal Astronomical Society* 21 (1980): 388–99.

Ginzburg, C. "Spie: radici di un paradigma indizionario." In *Crisi della ragione,* ed. A. Gargani, 57–106. Turin, 1979. Trans. in *The Sign of Three,* ed. U. Eco and T. Sebeok, 95–136, Bloomington, Ind., 1983.

Gleason, M. "The Semiotics of Gender: Physiognomy and Self-Fashioning in the Second Century C.E." In *Before Sexuality: The Construction of Erotic Experience in the Ancient Greek World,* ed. D. M. Halperin, J. J. Winkler, and F. I. Zeitlin, 389–416. Princeton, 1989.

Goldenweiser, A. "Loose Ends of Theory on the Individual Pattern and Involution in Primitive Society." In *Essays in Anthropology Presented to A. L. Kroeber,* ed. R. Lowie, 99–104. Berkeley, 1936.

Goody, J., and Watt, I. P. "The Consequences of Literacy." In *Literacy in Traditional Societies,* ed. J. Goody, 27–68. Cambridge, 1968.

Gordon, R. L. "The Sacred Geography of a Mithraeum: The Example of Sette Sfere." *Journal of Mithraic Studies* 1 (1976): 119–265.

———. "Reality, Evocation and Boundary in the Mysteries of Mithras." *Journal of Mithraic Studies* 4 (1980): 19–99.

———. "From Republic to Principate: Priesthood, Religion and Ideology." In *Pagan Priests: Religion and Power in the Ancient World,* ed. M. Beard and J. A. North, 177–98. London, 1990.

Griffith, F. L. "The Old Coptic Horoscope of the Stobart Collection." *Zeitschrift für Ägyptische Sprache* (1900): 71–85.

Grodzynski, D. "Par la bouche de l'empéreur." In *Divination et rationalité,* ed. J.-P. Vernant, 267–94. Paris, 1974.

Gross, A. G. *The Rhetoric of Science.* Cambridge, Mass., 1990.

Gundel, H. G. "Weltbild und astrologie in den griechischen Zauberpapyri." *Münchener Beitrage zur Papyrusforschung und Antiken Rechtsgeschichte* 53, Munich, 1968.

Gundel, W. "Kometen." *Pauly Wissowa: Real-Encyclopädie* (1922), 11:1143–93.

———. "Textkritische und exegetische Bemerkungen zu Manilius." *Philologus* n.s. 35 (1926): 309–38.

———. "Libra." *Pauly Wissowa: Real-Encyclopädie* (1926), 13.1:116–37.

———. "Skorpios." *Pauly Wissowa: Real-Encyclopädie* (1927), 3A:588–609.

Gundel, W., and Gundel, H. G. *Astrologumena: die astrologische Literatur in der Antike und ihre Geschichte.* Sudhoffs Archiv, Beiheft 6. Wiesbaden, 1966.

Hacking, I. "Language, Truth and Reason." In *Rationality and Relativism,* ed. M. Hollis and S. Lukes, 48–66. London, 1982.

Hahm, D. E. *The Origins of Stoic Cosmology.* Athens, Ohio, 1977.

Hall, A. R. "Microscopic Analyses and the General Picture." *Times Literary Supplement,* April 26, 1974, 437–38.

Hall, E. *The Invention of the Barbarian: Greek Self-Definition through Tragedy.* Oxford, 1989.

Hanen, M. P., Osler, M. J., and Weyant, R. G., eds. *Science, Pseudo-Science and Society.* Waterloo, Ont., 1980.

Hankinson, R. J. "Stoicism, Science and Divination." In *Method, Medicine and Metaphysics,* ed. R. J. Hankinson, 123–60. Edmonton, 1988.

Hannestad, N. *Roman Art and Imperial Policy.* Aarhus, 1986.

Harding, S. G., ed. *Can Theories Be Refuted? Essays on the Duhem-Quine Thesis.* Dordrecht and Boston, 1976.

Harris, C. R. S. *The Heart and the Vascular System in Greek Medicine from Alcmaeon to Galen.* Oxford, 1973.

Heath, T. L. *Aristarchus of Samos.* Oxford, 1913.

———. *A History of Greek Mathematics.* Oxford, 1921.

Hébert, J.-C. "Analyse structurale des géomancies comoriennes, malgaches et africaines," *Journal de la Société des Africanistes* 31 (1961): 115–208.

Heeg, J. "Uber ein angebliches Diokleszitat." *Sitzungberichte der Königlich-Preussischen Akademie der Wissenschaften* (Jahrgang 1911): 911–1007.

Heidel, W. A. *The Heroic Age of Science.* Baltimore, 1933.

Heilmeyer, W. D., Martin, H. G., and E. La Rocca, eds. *Kaiser Augustus und die verlorene Republik. Eine Ausstellung im Martin Gropius-Bau, Berlin, 7 Juni–14 August 1988.* Berlin, 1988.

Heinemann, F. "Eine Vorplatonische Theorie der τέχνη." *Museum Helveticum* 18 (1961): 105–30.

Henderson, J. *The Maculate Muse: Obscene Language in Attic Comedy.* Yale, 1975.

Hesse, M. "The Explanatory Function of Metaphor." In *Logic, Methodology and Philosophy of Science,* ed. Y. Bar-Hillel, 249–59. Amsterdam, 1965.

———. "Is There an Independent Observation-Language?" In *The Nature of Scientific Theory,* ed. R. G. Colodny, 35–77. Pittsburgh, 1970.

———. "Reasons and Evaluation in the History of Science." In *Changing Perspectives in the History of Science,* ed. M. Teich and R. Young, 127–47. London, 1973.

———. "The Strong Thesis in the Sociology of Science." Part 1 in "Models of Method in the Natural and Social Sciences." *Methodology of Science* 8 (1975): 163–78.

(All Hesse articles in *Revolutions and Reconstructions in the Philosophy of Science.* Brighton, Eng., 1980.)

Hirst, P. Q. "Is It Rational to Reject Relativism?" In *Reason and Morality,* ed. J. Overing, 85–103. London, 1985.

Hölscher, T. "Ein römischer Sternziegel mit Victoria und Capricorni." *Jahrbuch des Zentralmuseums Mainz* 12 (1965): 59–73.

———. "Historische Reliefs." In *Kaiser Augustus und die verlorene Republik,* ed. W.-D. Heilmeyer et al., 351–400. Berlin, 1988.

Hommel, P. *Studien zu den römischen Figurengiebeln der Kaiserzeit.* Berlin, 1954.

Honigmann, E. "A Trial for Sorcery on August 22, 449." *Isis* 35 (1984): 281–84.

Honoré, A. M. *Gaius.* Oxford, 1962.

Hopkins, K. *Conquerors and Slaves.* Cambridge, 1978.

Horine, E. M. "An Epitome of Ancient Pulse-Lore." *Bulletin of the History of Medicine* 10 (1941): 209–49.

Housman, A. E. "Manilius, Augustus, Tiberius, Capricornus and Libra." *Classical Quarterly* 7 (1913): 109–14.

Janko, R. *Aristotle on Comedy: Towards a Reconstruction of Poetics II.* London, 1984.

Joly, R. "La Caracterologie antique jusqu'à Aristote." *Revue Belge de philologie et d'histoire* 40, no. 1 (1962): 5–28.
Jones, W. H. S. *The Medical Writings of Anonymous Londiniensis.* Cambridge, 1947.
Jüttner, H. *De Polemonis Rhetoris Vita Operibus Arte.* Hildesheim, 1967 (Ph.D. diss. Breslau, 1897, repub. in *Breslauer Philologische Untersuchungen* 8, no. 1 [1898]).
Keil, J. "Ärzteinschriften aus Ephesos." *Jahreshefte des österreichischen archäologischen Instituts in Wien* 8 (1905): 128–38.
Kelter, E. *Apulei quae fertur physiognomia quando composita sit.* Ph.D. diss. Kiel, 1890.
Kerby-Miller, C., ed. *Memoirs of the Extraordinary Life, Works and Discoveries of Martin Scriblerus.* By J. Arbuthnot, A. Pope, and J. Swift. New Haven, 1950.
Klingender, F. *Animals in Life and Thought to the End of the Middle Ages.* London, 1971.
Knibbe, D. "Neue Inschriften aus Ephesos." *Jahreshefte des österreichischen archäologischen Instituts in Wien* (Hauptblatt) 53 (1981–82): 87–150.
Knorr-Cetina, K., and Mulkay, M., eds. *Science Observed: Perspectives on the Social Study of Science.* London and Beverly Hills, Calif., 1983.
Kollesch, J. *Untersuchungen zu den pseudogalenischen Definitiones Medicae.* Berlin, 1973.
———. "Galen und die Zweite Sophistik." In *Galen: Problems and Prospects,* ed. V. Nutton, 1–12, London, 1981.
———. "Anschauungen von den ἀρχαί in der Ars medica und die Seelenlehre Galens." In *Le opere psicologiche di Galeno,* ed. P. Manuli and M. Vegetti, 215–30. Naples, 1988.
Koyré, A. *From the Closed World to the Infinite Universe.* Baltimore, 1957.
———. *Metaphysics and Measurement.* London, 1968.
Kraft, K. "Zum Capricorn auf den Münzen des Augustus." *Jahrbuch für Numismatik und Geldgeschichte* 17 (1967): 17–27.
Kragh, H. *An Introduction to the Historiography of Science.* Cambridge, 1987.
Kroll, W. "Nechepso." *Pauly Wissowa: Real-Encyclopädie* 16, no. 2 (1935): 2160–67.
Kudlien, F. "Galen's Religious Belief." In *Galen: Problems and Prospects,* ed. V. Nutton, 117–27, London, 1981.
Kuhn, T. S. *The Structure of Scientific Revolutions.* 1962. Reprint. Chicago, 1970.
Kuriyama, S. *Varieties of Haptic Experience: Chinese and Ancient Greek Pulse-Lore Compared.* Ph.D. diss., Harvard, 1987.
Laistner, M. L. W. "The Western Church and Astrology in the Early Middle Ages." *Harvard Theological Review* 34 (1941): 251–75.
Lambrechts, P. "La Politique 'apollinienne' d'Auguste et le culte impériale." *Nouvelle Clio* 5 (1953): 65–82.
Lasswitz, K. *Geschichte der Atomistik im Mittelalter bis Newton.* 2 vols. Hamburg, 1890.
Laudan, L. *Progress and Its Problems: Towards a Theory of Scientific Growth.* London, 1977.
Lavater, J. K. *Physiognomy; or the Corresponding Analogy between the Conformation of the Features and the Ruling Passions of the Mind.* Trans. S. Shaw, of *Physiognomische Fragmente.* London (?), 1800.
Leach, E. "Anthropological Aspects of Language: Animal Categories of Verbal Abuse." In *New Directions in the Study of Language,* ed. E. H. Lenneberg, 23–63. Cambridge, Mass., 1964.
———. *Social Anthropology.* Cambridge, 1983.
Lebas, P., and Waddington, W. H. *Voyage archéologique.* Paris, 1870.

Lecouteux, C. "Les Panotéens: sources, diffusion, emploi." *Etudes Germaniques* 35 (1980): 253–66.

Lehmann-Hartleben, K. "Ein Altar in Bologna." *Mitteilungen des Deutschen Archäologischen Instituts, Römische Abteilung* 42 (1927): 163–76.

Lemay, R. "The True Place of Astrology in Mediaeval Science and Philosophy: Towards a Definition." In *Astrology, Science and Society,* ed. P. Curry, 57–73. Woodbridge, Eng., 1987.

Levin, S. "The Significance of Ethnic Classes in Greek and English." *Transactions of the American Philological Association* 40 (1950): 130–52.

Lévi-Strauss, C. *Totemism.* R. Needham, rev. trans. of *Le Totémisme aujourd'hui* (1962). London, 1969.

———. *The Savage Mind.* Trans. of *La Pensée sauvage* (1962). 2d ed. London, 1974.

Liddell, H. G., Scott, R., and Jones, H. S. *A Greek-English Lexicon.* Oxford, 1968.

Liebeschuetz, W. *Continuity and Change in Roman Religion.* Oxford, 1979.

Lilja, S. "Terms of Abuse in Roman Comedy." *Annales Academiae Scientiarum Fennicae,* ser. B 141.3 (1965).

Littré, E. *Oeuvres complètes d'Hippocrate.* 10 vols. Paris, 1839–61.

Lloyd, G. E. R. "Ancient Medicine and Modern Controversies." *History of Science* 6 (1968): 125–29.

———. *Magic, Reason and Experience.* Cambridge, 1979.

———. *Science, Folklore and Ideology.* Cambridge, 1983.

———. *The Revolutions of Wisdom.* Berkeley, 1987.

———. *Demystifying Mentalities.* Cambridge, 1990.

———. "Galen on Hellenistics and Hippocrateans: Contemporary Battles and Past Authorities." *Methods and Problems in Ancient Science,* 398–416. Cambridge, 1991.

Lombroso, C. *Genio e follia.* Milan, 1864.

———. *L'uomo delinquente.* Turin, 1876.

———. *La donna delinquente, la prostituta e la donna normale.* Turin, 1893.

Lones, T. E. *Aristotle's Researches in Natural Science.* London, 1913.

Long, A. A. "Astrology: arguments pro and contra." In *Science and Speculation: Studies in Hellenistic Theory and Practice,* ed. J. Barnes et al., 165–92. Cambridge, 1982.

Long, A. A., and Sedley, D. N. *The Hellenistic Philosphers.* Vol. 1: *Translation of Principal Sources and Philosophical Commentary.* Cambridge, 1987.

Loraux, N. "La Race des femmes et quelques-unes de ses tribus." *Arethusa* 11 (1978): 43–87.

Mabilleau, L. *Histoire de la philosophie atomistique.* Paris, 1895.

MacBain, B. *Prodigy and Expiation: A Study in Religion and Politics in the Late Republic.* Brussels, 1982.

Mach, E. *The Science of Mechanics.* Trans. T. J. McCormack. 4th ed. Chicago, 1919.

McKay, S. *A History of Ancient Gynaecology.* Sydney, 1901.

MacMullen, R. *Enemies of the Roman Order.* Cambridge, 1966.

———. "Social History in Astrology." *Ancient Society* 2 (1971): 105–16.

Maderna Lauter, C. "Glyptik." In *Kaiser Augustus und die verlorene Republik,* ed. W.-D. Heilmeyer et al., Berlin, 1988.

Magazis, G., Hoff, H. E., and Christ, J. "Perspectives on Physiological Monitoring: Markellinos on the Pulse." *Cardiovascular Research Bulletin* 16 (1978): 83–109.

Maiuri, A. *Pompeii: I nuovi scavi e la Villa dei Misteri.* Rome, 1931.

Mannheim, K. *Ideology and Utopia: An Introduction to the Sociology of Knowledge.* London, 1936.

Manuli, P. "Lo stile del commento: Galeno e la tradizione ippocratica." In *Formes de pensée dans la collection hippocratique,* ed. F. Lasserre and P. Mudry, 471–82. Lausanne, 1983.

Marrou, H.-I. *A History of Education in Antiquity.* Trans. G. Lamb, of *Histoire de l'education dans l'antiquité.* Paris, 1948. London, 1956.

Masterman, M. "The Nature of a Paradigm." In *Criticism and the Growth of Knowledge,* ed. I. Lakatos and A. Musgrave, 59–89. Cambridge, 1970.

Mattingly, H. *Roman Coins: From the Earliest Times to the Fall of the Western Empire.* London, 1960.

———. *Coins of the Roman Empire in the British Museum.* 6 vols. London, 1923–62.

Maxwell-Stuart, P. G. "A Guide to Thieves." *Rivista di Studi Classici* 23 (1975): 333–36.

———. *Studies in Greek Colour-Terminology.* Vol. 1: γλαυκός Vol. 2: χαροπός. Leiden, 1981.

Mensching, E. *Favorin von Arelate: der erste Teil der Fragmente Memorabilien und Omnigena Historia.* Berlin, 1963.

Mercklin, E. von. *Antike Figuralkapitelle.* Berlin, 1962.

Mesk, J. "Die Beispiele in Polemons Physiognomik." *Wiener Studien* 50 (1933): 51–67.

Meyer, E. von. *Geschichte der Chemie von dem ältesten Zeiten bis zur Gegenwart.* Leipzig, 1914.

Meyer-Steineg, T. *Ein Tag im Leben des Galen.* Jena, 1913.

Midgeley, M. *Beast and Man: The Roots of Human Nature.* Brighton, Eng., 1979.

Millar, F. *The Emperor in the Roman World.* London, 1977.

Misener, G. "Loxus, Physician and Physiognomist." *Classical Philology* 18 (1923): 1–22.

———. "Iconistic Portraits." *Classical Philology* 19 (1924): 97–123.

Momigliano, A. *Alien Wisdom: The limits of Hellenization.* Cambridge, 1975.

———, ed. *Aspetti di Hermann Usener filologo della religione.* Pisa, 1982.

Montanari Caldini, R. "L'astrologia nei *Prognostica* di Germanico." *Studi Italiani di Filologia Classica* n.s. 45 (1973): 137–204.

Morris, M., and Patton, P. *Michel Foucault: Power, Truth and Strategy.* Sidney, 1979.

Mourad, Y. *La Physiognomie arabe et le Kitab-al-Firasa de Fakhr al-Din Al-Razi.* Paris, 1939.

Mulkay, M. "Some Aspects of Cultural Growth in the Natural Sciences." *Social Research* 36 (1969): 22–52.

———. "The Scientist Talks Back: A One-Act Play, with a Moral, about Replication in Science and Reflexivity in Sociology." *Social Studies of Science* 14 (1984): 265–82.

Mulkay, M., Potter, J., and Yearley, S. "Why an Analysis of Scientific Discourse is Needed." In *Science Observed: Perspectives on the Social Study of Science,* ed. K. Knorr-Cetina and M. Mulkay, 171–203, London and Beverly Hills, Calif., 1983.

Müller, I., ed. Vol. 2 of *Galeni Pergameni Scripta Minora.* Leipzig, 1891.

———. "Über Galens Werk vom wissenschaftlichen Beweis." *Abhandlungen der philosophisch-philologischen Klasse der königlich-bayerischen Akademie der Wissenschaften* 20, no. 2 (1894–95) (1897): 403–78.

———. *Handbuch der Altertumswissenschaft.* Munich, 1923–.

Neugebauer, O. *The Exact Sciences in Antiquity.* Copenhagen, 1951.

———. "The Chronology of Vettius Valens." *Harvard Theological Review* 47 (1954): 65–67.

Neugebauer, O., and Van Hoesen, H. B. *Greek Horoscopes.* Philadelphia, 1959.

Newton, R. R. *The Crime of Claudius Ptolemy.* Baltimore, 1977.

Nietzsche, F. "On Truth and Falsity in an Extra-Moral Sense." In *The Complete Works of Friedrich Nietzsche,* ed. O. Levy, vol. 2. New York, 1964.

Nilsson, M. P. "Wesensverschiedenheiten der römischen und der griechischen Religion." *Mitteilungen des Deutschen Archäologischen Instituts, Römische Abteilung* 48 (1933): 245–60.

Nisbet, R. G. M. "The *In Pisonem* as an Invective." Appendix 6 to his ed. of Cicero's *In L. Calpurnium Pisonem Oratio,* 192–96. Oxford, 1961.

Nock, A. D. "A Feature of Roman Religion." *Essays on Religion and the Ancient World,* 1:481–92. Oxford, 1972.

Nola, R., ed. *Relativism and Realism in Science.* Dordrecht, 1988.

Norsa, M., and Vitelli, G. "Il papiro vaticano greco 11: Φαβωρίνου Περὶ φυγῆς," *Studi e Testi* 53 (1931).

North, J. A. "Religion and Politics from Republic to Principate." *Journal of Roman Studies* 76 (1986): 255–57.

———. "Diviners and Divination at Rome." In Beard and North, *Pagan Priests,* 49–72.

North, J. D. *Horoscopes and History.* London, 1986.

Nutton, V. "Galen and Medical Biography." *Proceedings of the Cambridge Philological Society* 198 (1972): 50–62.

———. "Galen in the Eyes of His Contemporaries." *Bulletin of the History of Medicine* 58 (1984): 315–24.

———. "Murders and Miracles: Lay Attitudes towards Medicine in Classical Antiquity." In *Patients and Practitioners: Lay Perceptions of Medicine in Pre-Industrial Society,* ed. R. S. Porter, 23–53. Cambridge, 1985.

———. "The Perils of Patriotism: Pliny and Roman Medicine." In *Science in the Early Roman Empire: Pliny the Elder, His Sources and Influence,* ed. R. French and F. Greenaway, 30–58. London and Sydney, 1986.

———. ed. *Claudii Galeni De Praecognitione, Corpus Medicorum Graecorum* 5.8.1. Berlin, 1979.

———. ed. *Galen: Problems and Prospects.* London, 1981.

Oehler, K. *Two Interpretations of Reflexivity in the Sociology of Science: An Examination of H. M. Collins' Radical Programme.* Virginia Polytechnic Institute and State University. Typescript.

L'Orange, H. P. *Apotheosis in Ancient Portraiture.* Oslo, 1947.

Ortner, S., and Whitehead, H. *Sexual Meanings: The Cultural Construction of Gender and Sexuality.* Cambridge, 1981.

Overing, J., ed. *Reason and Morality.* London, 1985.

Pack, R. A. "Artemidorus and the Physiognomists." *Transactions of the American Philological Association* 72 (1941): 321–34.

Pagel, W. *Paracelsus. An Introduction to Philosophical Medicine in the Renaissance.* 2d ed. Basel and New York, 1982.

Parker, R. "Sex, Women and Ambiguous Animals." *Phronesis* 29 (1984): 174–87.

Partington, J. R. "The Origin of the Atomic Theory." *Annals of Science* 4 (1939): 245–82.

Pearcy, L.T. "Galen and Stoic Rhetoric." *Greek, Roman and Byzantine Studies* 24 (1983): 259–72.

Peirce, C. S. *Collected Papers of Charles Sanders Peirce.* Ed. C. Hartshorne, P. Weiss, and A. W. Burks. 8 vols. Cambridge, Mass., 1935–66.

Perelman, C., and Olbrechts-Tyteca, L. *The New Rhetoric: A Treatise on Argumentation.* Trans. J. Wilkinson and P. Weaver. Paris, 1958. Notre Dame, 1969.

Pinch, T., and Pinch, T. "Reservations about Reflexivity and New Literary Forms: Or Why Let the Devil Have All the Good Tunes?" In *Knowledge and Reflexivity,* ed. S. Woolgar, 178–97. London and Beverly Hills, 1988.

Pingree, D. "Petosiris." *Dictionary of Scientific Biography,* 10:547–49. New York, 1974.

———. "Political Horoscopes from the Reign of Zeno." *Dumbarton Oaks Papers* 30 (1976a): 133–50.

———. *Dorothei Sidonii. Carmen Astrologicum. Interpretationem Arabicam in linguam Anglicam versam una cum Dorothei fragmentis et Graecis et Latinis.* Leipzig, 1976b.

———. "Antiochus and Rhetorius." *Classical Philology* 72 (1977): 203–23.

Plass, P. *Wit and the Writing of History: The Rhetoric of Historiography in Imperial Rome.* Madison, Wis., 1988.

Pollini, J. *Studies in Augustan Historical Reliefs.* Ph.D. diss. Berkeley, 1978.

Popper, K. R. *Conjectures and Refutations: The Growth of Scientific Knowledge.* London, 1963.

———. *The Open Society and Its Enemies.* London, 1945.

Porter, R. "Making Faces: Physiognomy and Fashion in Eighteenth-Century England." *Etudes Anglaises* 38 (1985): 385–96.

Poster, M. *Foucault, Marxism and History: Mode of Production versus Mode of Information.* Cambridge, 1984.

Préaux, C. *La Lune dans la pensée grecque.* Brussels, 1973.

Premerstein, A. von. "Das Attentat der Konsulare auf Hadrian im Jahre 118." *Klio* Beiheft 6 (1908): 46–71.

Price, S. R. F. "The future of dreams, from Freud to Artemidorus." *Past and Present* 113, no. 3 (1986): 1–37.

Puschmann, T., ed. *Alexander von Tralles.* Vienna, 1878.

———. *A History of Medical Education in Antiquity.* Trans. E. H. Hare. London, 1921.

Quine, W. V. O. "Two Dogmas of Empiricism." *From a Logical Point of View: Logico-Philosophical Essays,* 20–46. Cambridge, Mass., 1953.

Rawson, E. "The Prodigy-Lists and the *Annales Maximi.*" *Classical Quarterly* n.s. 21 (1971): 158–69.

———. "Caesar, Etruria and the *Disciplina Etrusca.*" *Journal of Roman Studies* 68 (1978): 132–52.

Reardon, B. P. *Courants littéraires dans la deuxième sophistique.* Paris, 1971.

Redfield, J. M. *Nature and Culture in the Iliad: The Tragedy of Hector.* Chicago, 1975.

Reverdin, O., ed. *Grecs et barbares.* Entretiens sur l'Antiquité Classique de la Fondation Hardt 8. Geneva, 1961.

Rhys Bram, J. *Ancient Astrology, Theory and Practice: Matheseos Libri VIII by Firmicus Maternus* (trans. and comm.). Park Ridge, N.J., 1975.

Richlin, A. *The Gardens of Priapus: Sexuality and Aggression in Roman Humor.* Yale, 1983.

Richter, G. M. A. *Catalogue of Engraved Gems of the Classical Style.* New York, 1920.

———. *Roman Portraits in the Metropolitan Museum in New York.* New York, 1948.

Riedinger, U. *Die heilige Schrift im Kampf der griechischen Kirche gegen die Astrologie von Origenes bis Johannes von Damaskos.* Innsbruck, 1956.

Riess, E. "*Nechepsonis et Petosiridis fragmenta magica.*" *Philologus* supp. 6 (1892): 325–88.

———. "The Influence of Astrology on Life and Literature at Rome." *Classical Weekly* 27 (1933): 73–78.

Ritterling, H. "*Legio*." *Pauly Wissowa: Real-Encyclopädie* 122 (1925): 1372–1829.

Romilly, J. de. *Rhetoric and Magic*. Harvard, 1974.

Rosenthal, F. "An Ancient Commentary on the Hippocratic Oath." *Bulletin of the History of Medicine* 30 (1956): 52–87.

Rousseau, J.-J. *Essai sur l'origine des langues*. Paris, 1763.

Rousselle, A. *Porneia*. Paris, 1983.

Russell, D. A. F. M. *Greek Declamation*. Cambridge, 1983.

Sabbah, G. *La Méthode d'Ammien Marcellin*. Paris, 1978.

Sambursky, S. *The Physical World of the Greeks*. London, 1963.

———. "Harmony and Wholeness in Greek Scientific Thought." *Histoire de la pensée*. Vol. 13: *Mélanges Alexandre Koyré*. Vol. 2. *Publiés à l'occasion de son soixante-dixième anniversaire. L'Aventure de l'esprit*, 442–57. Paris, 1961.

Sarton, G. *An Introduction to the History of Science*. 3 vols. Baltimore, 1927–48.

———. *The Study of the History of Science*. Cambridge, Mass., 1936.

———. *The Life of Science*. New York, 1948.

———. *Horus: A Guide to the History of Science*. Waltham, Mass., 1952.

———. *Galen of Pergamum*. Lawrence, 1954.

———. *A History of Science: Ancient Science through the Golden Age of Greece*. Cambridge, Mass., 1959.

Sassi, M. M. "Dalla scienza delle religione di Usener ad Aby Warburg." In Momigliano, *Alien Wisdom*, 65–92.

———. Review of Brea 1981. *Quaderni di Storia* 19 (1984): 275–80.

———. "I Barbari." In *Il Sapere degli antichi*, ed. M. Vegetti, 262–78. Turin, 1985.

———. *La Scienza dell'uomo nella Grecia antica*. Turin, 1988.

———. "Plutarco antifisiognomico, ovvero: del dominio della passione." Forthcoming.

Scarborough, J. "The Galenic Question." *Sudhoffs Archiv* 65 (1981): 1–31.

Scheffler, I. *Science and Subjectivity*. Indianapolis and New York, 1967.

Schilling, R. "A propos des exta: l'extispicine étrusque et la *litatio* romaine." *Rites, cultes, dieux de Rome*, 183–90. Paris, 1979.

Schnapp-Gourbeillon, A. *Lions, héros, masques: les répresentations de l'animal chez Homère*. Paris, 1981.

Schorlemmer, C. *The Rise and Development of Organic Chemistry*. Manchester, 1879.

Schuster, J., and Yeo, R. *The Politics and Rhetoric of Scientific Method: Historical Studies*. Dordrecht, 1986.

Schutz, M. "Zur Sonnenuhr des Augustus auf dem Marsfeld," *Gymnasium* 97 (1990): 432–57.

Scott, R. T. *Religion and Philosophy in the Histories of Tacitus*. Rome, 1968.

Scott Ryberg, I. *Rites of the State Religion in Roman Art*. Memoirs of the American Academy in Rome 19. Rome, 1955.

Sebeok, T. A., and Umiker-Sebeok, J. "You Know My Method: A Juxtaposition of Charles S. Peirce and Sherlock Holmes." In *The Sign of Three*, ed. U. Eco and T. Sebeok, 11–54, Bloomington, Ind., 1993.

Shapere, D. "The Structure of Scientific Revolutions." *Philosophical Review* 73 (1964): 383–94.

Shapin, S. "History of Science and Its Sociological Reconstructions." *History of Science* 20 (1982): 157–211.

Sherwin-White, A. N. *Racial Prejudice in Imperial Rome.* Cambridge, 1967.

Singer, C., ed. *Studies in the History and Method of Science.* 2 vols. Oxford, 1917–21.

———. *From Magic to Science.* London, 1928.

Singer, C., and Sigerist, H. E. *Essays on the History of Medicine Presented to Karl Sudhoff.* Oxford and Zurich, 1924.

Singer, P. N. "Preface." *Galen on the Soul: Philosophy and Medicine in the Second Century A.D.* Ph.D. diss. Cambridge, 1993.

Smith, D. *The Hundred and One Dalmatians.* London, 1956.

Smith, W. D. *The Hippocratic Tradition.* Ithaca, 1979.

Sperber, D. "Pourquoi les animaux parfaits, les hybrides et les monstres sont bons à penser symboliquement?" *L'Homme* 15 (1975): 5–34.

Staden, H. von "Haireseis and heresy." In *Jewish and Christian Self-Definition.* Vol. 3: *Self-Definition in the Roman World,* ed. B. F. Meyer and E. P. Sanders, 76–100. London, 1982.

———. *Herophilus: The Art of Medicine in Early Alexandria.* Cambridge, 1989.

Stierlin, W. *L'Astrologie et le pouvoir de Platon à Newton.* Paris, 1986.

Süss, W. *Ethos.* Leipzig and Berlin, 1910.

Syme, R. "Astrology in the Historia Augusta." *Historia Augusta Papers,* 80–97. Oxford, 1983.

Tannéry, P. *La Géometrie grecque.* Paris, 1887.

———. *Recherches sur l'histoire de l'astronomie ancienne.* Paris, 1893.

———. *Mémoires scientifiques.* 16 vols. Paris, 1912–43.

———. *Pour l'histoire de la science Hellène.* 2d ed. Paris, 1930.

Tapper, R. L. "Animality, Humanity, Morality, Society." In *What Is an Animal?* ed. T. Ingold, 47–60. London, 1988.

Tarn, W. W. "Alexander Helios and the Golden Age." *Journal of Roman Studies* 22 (1932): 135–60.

Temkin, O. *Galenism: Rise and Decline of a Medical Philosophy.* Ithaca, N.Y., and London, 1973.

Tester, S. J. *A History of Western Astrology.* Woodbridge, 1987.

Thagard, P. "Why Astrology is a Pseudo-Science." In *Proceedings of the 1978 Biennial Meeting, Philosophy of Science Association,* ed. I. Hacking and P. D. Asquith, 1:223–34. East Lansing, Mich., 1978.

———. "Resemblance, Correlation and Pseudo-Science." In *Science, Pseudo-Science and Society,* ed. M. P. Hanen et al., 237–72, Waterloo, Ont., 1980.

Thomas, K. V. *Man and the Natural World: Changing Attitudes in England 1500–1800.* London, 1983.

Thorndike, L. *A History of Magic and Experimental Science.* 8 vols. New York, 1923–58.

———. "A Roman Astrologer as a Historical Source: Julius Firmicus Maternus." *Classical Philology* 8 (1913): 415–35.

Toomer, G. J. "Galen on Astrologers and Astronomers." *Archive for the History of the Exact Sciences* 32 (1985): 193–206.

Torelli, M. *Elogia Tarquinensia.* Florence, 1975.

Toulmin, S. *Human Understanding.* Oxford, 1972.

Toynbee, J. M. C. *Animals in Roman Life and Art.* London, 1973.

Trillmich, W. "Münzpropaganda." In *Kaiser Augustus und die verlorene Republik,* ed. W.-D. Heilmeyer et al., Berlin, 1988.

Truzzi, M. "Sherlock Holmes: Applied Social Psychologist." In *The Sign of Three,* ed. U. Eco and T. Sebeok, 55–80, Bloomington, Ind., 1983.

Tytler, G. *Physiognomy in the European Novel: Faces and Fortunes.* Princeton, 1982.

Usener, H. *De Stephano Alexandrino.* Bonn, 1980.

Vallance, J. "A Second Look: Marshall Clagett's 'Greek Science in Antiquity': Thirty-Five Years Later." *Isis* 81 (1990): 713–21.

Van der Vliet, E. "L'Ethnographie de Strabon: idéologie ou tradition?" In *Strabone: contributi allo studio della personalità e dell'opera,* ed. F. Prontera, 29–86. Perugia, 1984.

Vegetti, M. *Il coltello e lo stilo: animali, schiavi, barbari e donne alle origine della razionalità scientifica.* Milan, 1979.

———. "Modelli di medicina in Galeno." In *Galen: Problems and Prospects,* ed. V. Nutton, 47–63, London, 1981.

———. "La questione dei metodi: una nota preliminare." Introduction to *Tra Edipo e Euclide: forme del sapere antico,* 11–22. Milan, 1983.

Vernant, J.-P., ed. *Divination et rationalité.* Paris, 1974.

Vernant, J.-P., and Gernet, J. "Social History and the Evolution of Ideas in China and Greece from the Sixth to the Second Centuries B.C." In *Myth and Society in Ancient Greece.* Trans. J. Lloyd, of *Mythe et société en Grèce ancienne,* 71–91. Paris, 1974. Hassocks, Eng., 1982.

Veyne, P. *Did the Greeks Believe in Their Myths?* Trans. P. Wissing, of *Les Grecs ont-ils cru à leurs mythes? Essai sur l'imagination constituante.* Paris, 1983. Chicago and London, 1988.

Vickers, B. *In Defence of Rhetoric.* Oxford, 1988.

Vidal-Naquet, P. "La Raison grecque et la cité." *Raison Présente* 2 (1967): 51–61.

Voigt, W. von. "Unter welche Gestirnen wurden Cäsar, Agrippa und Tiberius geboren?" *Philologus* 58, n.s. 12 (1899): 170–204.

Vollenweider, M.-L. *Die Steinschneidekunst und ihre Künstler in spätrepublikanischer und augusteischer Zeit.* Baden-Baden, 1966.

Waddington, W. H., Balsdon, E., and Reinach, T. *Recueil général des monnaies grecques d'Asie Mineure.* Vol. 1. Paris, 1904.

Walker, D. P. *Spiritual and Demonic Magic from Ficino to Campanella.* London, 1958.

Wallis, R., ed. *On the Margins of Science: The Social Construction of Rejected Knowledge.* Keele, 1979.

Wardman, A. *Rome's Debt to Greece.* London, 1976.

Wasserstein, A. *Galen on Airs, Waters, Places in the Hebrew Translation of Solomon Ha-Me'ati.* Jerusalem, 1982.

Wechsler, J. *A Human Comedy: Physiognomy and Caricature in Nineteenth-Century Paris.* London, 1982.

Weinstock, S. "The Author of Pseudo-Galen's *Prognostica De Decubitu.*" *Classical Quarterly* 42 (1948): 41–43.

———. "C. Fonteius Capito and the *Libri Tagetici.*" *Papers of the British School at Rome* n.s. 5 (1950): 44–49.

———. "*Libri Fulgurales.*" Papers of the British School at Rome n.s. 6 (1951): 122–53.

———. *Divus Julius.* Oxford, 1971.

Wellmann, M. *Die Pneumatische Schule bis auf Archigenes.* Berlin, 1895.

———. "Zu Diokles." *Hermes* 48 (1913): 464–68.

Westermann, A. *Scriptores rerum mirabilium Graeci.* 1839. Reprint. Amsterdam, 1963.

Whitehead, D. *The Ideology of the Athenian Metic.* Cambridge, 1977.

Whitley, R. "Black-Boxism and the Sociology of Science: A Discusion of the Major Developments in the Field." In *The Sociology of Science,* ed. P. Halmos, 61–92. Keele, 1972.

Wiedemann, T. E. J. "Between Men and Beasts: Barbarians in Ammianus Marcellinus." In *Past Perspectives: Studies in Greek and Roman Historical Writing,* ed. I. S. Moxon et al., 189–201. Cambridge, 1986.

Wind, E. *Art and Anarchy.* New York, 1964.

Wittkower, R. "Marvels of the East. A Study in the History of Monsters." *Allegory and the Migration of Symbols,* 45–74. London, 1951. Reprint from *Journal of the Warburg and Courtauld Institutes* 5 (1942): 159–97.

Woolgar, S. "Interests and Explanation in the Social Study of Science." *Social Studies of Science* 11 (1981): 365–94.

———. "Irony in the Social Study of Science." In *Science Observed: Perspectives on the Social Study of Science,* ed. K. Knorr-Cetina and M. Mulkay, 239–86, London and Beverly Hills, Calif. 1983.

———. *Science: The Very Idea.* Chichester, 1988b.

———, ed. *Knowledge and Reflexivity: New Frontiers in the Sociology of Knowledge.* London and Beverly Hills, Calif. 1988a.

Wright, P. W. G. *Astrology in Mid-Seventeenth-Century England: A Sociological Analysis.* Ph.D. diss., London, 1984.

Wuilleumier, P. "Cirque et astrologie." *Mélanges de l'Ecole Française de Rome* 44 (1927): 184–209.

Yates, F. *Giordano Bruno and the Hermetic Tradition.* London and Chicago, 1974.

Zagianaris, N. "Le Roi des animaux dans la tradition antique." *ΠΛΑΤΩΝ* 29 (1977): 26–49.

Ziman, J. *Reliable Knowledge.* Cambridge, 1978.

Index